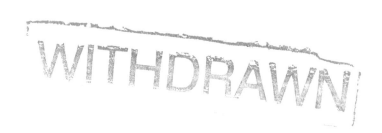

Performance Analysis of Sport IX

Sport performance analysis helps coaches, athletes and sport scientists develop a better understanding of sport performance and therefore enhances their effectiveness when devising methods for improving that performance. *Performance Analysis of Sport IX* is the latest in a series of volumes to showcase the very latest scientific research into sport performance analysis, helping to bridge the gap between theory, research and practice in sport.

Drawing on data from a wide variety of sports, the book covers every key topic and sub-discipline in performance analysis, including:

- analysis of technique
- technical effectiveness
- tactical evaluation
- patterns of play
- motor learning and feedback
- work rate and physical demands
- performance analysis technology
- analysis of elite athletes and teams
- effectiveness of performance analysis support
- observational analysis of injury risk
- analysis of officials

Effective use of performance analysis is now an essential component of the high performance strategy of any sport team or individual athlete, especially those competing at elite levels. This book is therefore essential reading for any student, researcher or practitioner working in performance analysis, and invaluable reading for any sport scientist, coach or athletic trainer looking for ways to improve their work with athletes.

Derek M. Peters is Professor of Sport, Health and Exercise Science at the University of Worcester, UK. He is a Higher Education Academy National Teaching Fellow (2008) and is accredited by the British Association of Sport & Exercise Sciences (BASES) for Interdisciplinary Research. He is the Treasury of the International Society of Performance Analysis of Sport, Professor II in the Faculty of Health & Sport Sciences at the University of Agder in Norway, Visiting Professor to the Lithuanian Sports University in Kaunas, Lithuania, and Editor-in-Chief of both *Basketball Research* and the *Graduate Journal of Sport, Exercise & Physical Education Research*.

Peter O'Donoghue is a Reader at Cardiff Metropolitan University, UK. He was Chair of the International Society of Performance Analysis of Sport and is General Editor of the International Journal of Performance Analysis in Sport. His research interests include racket sport performance and opposition effects in sports performance.

Performance Analysis of Sport IX

Edited by
Derek Peters and Peter O'Donoghue

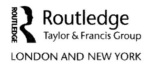

LONDON AND NEW YORK

First published 2014
by Routledge
2 Park Square, Milton Park, Abingdon, Oxon OX14 4RN

Simultaneously published in the USA and Canada
by Routledge
711 Third Avenue, New York, NY 10017

Routledge is an imprint of the Taylor & Francis Group, an informa business

British Library Cataloguing in Publication Data
A catalogue record for this book is available from the British Library

Library of Congress Cataloging in Publication Data
Performance analysis of sport IX / edited by Derek Peters and Peter O'Donoghue.
pages cm
1. Sports sciences–Research. 2. Sports–Physiological aspects.
3. Performance–Research. 4. Coaching (Athletics)–Research.
5. Athletic ability–Testing. 6. Athletes–Rating of. I. Peters, Derek M.
GV558.P35 2013
796.01'5–dc23
2013006783

ISBN: 978-0-415-64339-9 (hbk)
ISBN: 978-0-203-08044-3 (ebk)

Typeset in Times New Roman
by Cenveo Publisher Services

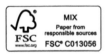

Printed and bound in Great Britain by
TJ International Ltd, Padstow, Cornwall

Contents

PART 1
Performance Analysis and Coaching   1

Figures

Tables

List of contributors

Maria Anguera, University of Barcelona, Spain.

Duarte Araújo, Faculty of Human Kinetics, Technical University of Lisbon, Lisbon, Portugal.

Sophie Arundel, Cardiff School of Sport, Cardiff Metropolitan University, UK.

Arnold Baca, Centre of Sport Science and University Sports, University of Vienna, Vienna, Austria.

Kevin Ball, Institute of Sport Exercise and Active Living (ISEAL), School of Exercise and Sport, Victoria University, Australia.

António Barbosa, UTAD, CIDESD Vila Real, Portugal.

Luís Barnabé, Faculty of Human Kinetics, Technical University of Lisbon, Portugal.

Jochen Baumeister, Institute of Sports Medicine, University of Paderborn, Germany.

Lauren Birkbeck, Nottingham Trent University, Brackenhurst Campus, Nottingham, UK.

Wes Bodden, Cardiff School of Sport, Cardiff Metropolitan University, UK.

Eleanor Boden, Duchy College, Stoke Climsland, Cornwall, UK.

Ceri Bowley, Cardiff School of Sport, Cardiff Metropolitan University, UK.

Tina Breitkreutz, Otto-von-Guericke-University Magdeburg, Germany.

Charlotte Bridgen, Myerscough College, Bilsborrow, Preston, UK.

Franck Brocherie, ISSUL, University of Lausanne, Switzerland.

James Brouner, Kingston University London, UK.

Donald Buchanan, Department of Applied Science, London South Bank University, London, UK.

Ed Burt, London Sport Institute, Middlesex University, London, UK.

Jorge Campaniço, UTAD, CIDESD Vila Real, Portugal.

Ana Isabel Carita, Faculty of Human Kinetics, Technical University of Lisbon, Portugal.

Hyongjun Choi, Dankook University, Yongin, South Korea.

David Cook, Department of Applied Science, London South Bank University, London, UK.

Jason Cook, Loughborough College, Loughborough, UK.

Jackson Cruz, Faculty of Human Kinetics, Technical University of Lisbon, Portugal.

Chris Cushion, Loughborough University, Loughborough, UK.

Dante De Rose Jr., School of Sciences, Arts and Humanities, University of Sao Paulo, Brazil.

Michael Dellnitz, Chair of Applied Mathematics, University of Paderborn, Germany.

Umberto Di Felice, Department of Biomedical Sciences and Technologies, University of L'Aquila, Italy.

Rocco Di Michele, Faculty of Exercise and Sport Science, University of Bologna, Italy.

Sandro Didier, Faculty of Human Kinetics, Technical University of Lisbon, Portugal.

Peter Dineen, London Sport Institute, Middlesex University, London, UK.

Ricardo Duarte, Faculty of Human Kinetics, Technical University of Lisbon, Lisbon, Portugal.

Abdulaziz Farooq, ASPETAR, Doha, Qatar.

António Paulo Ferreira, Faculty of Human Kinetics, Technical University of Lisbon, Portugal.

Sofia Fonseca, Faculty of Physical Education and Sports of Lusófona University, Lisbon, Portugal.

John Francis, University of Worcester, Worcester, UK.

Olivier Girard, ASPETAR, Doha, Qatar.

Fernando Gomes, Faculty of Human Kinetics, Lisbon Portugal.

Jose Guzmán, University of Valencia, Valencia, Spain.

Anita Hökelmann, Otto-von-Guericke-University Magdeburg, Germany.

Lucy Holmes, Cardiff School of Sport, Cardiff Metropolitan University, UK.

Barry Horgan, National Athlete Development Academy (NADA), Dublin, Ireland.

Sara Horne, Brunel University, UK.

Mike Hughes, London Sport Institute, Middlesex University, London, UK.

Masahiko Ishihara, Kota town office, Aichi, Japan.

Rasmus Jakobsmeyer, Institute of Sports Medicine, University of Paderborn, Germany.

Nic James, London Sport Institute, Middlesex University, London, UK.

Polly Johns, Kingston University London, UK.

Gareth Jones, University of Worcester, Worcester, UK.

Tetsu Kitamura, University of Tsukuba, Tsukuba, Japan.

Sasaki Koh, Nagoya University, Nagoya, Japan.

Leonardo Lamas, School of Physical Education and Sport, University of Sao Paulo, Brazil.

Peter Lamb, Technische Universität München, Germany.

Martin Lames, Technische Universität München, Germany.

José Leitão, UTAD, CIDESD Vila Real, Portugal.

Roland Leser, Centre of Sport Science and University Sports, University of Vienna, Vienna, Austria.

António Lopes, Faculty of Physical Education and Sports of Lusófona University, Lisbon, Portugal.

Rob Mackenzie, Loughborough University, Loughborough, UK.

Akira Maeda, National Institute of Fitness and Sports in Kanoya, Kanoya, Japan.

Ivan Malagoli Lanzoni, Department of Histology, Embryology and Applied Biology, University of Bologna, Italy.

Samuele Marcora, Center for Sport Studies, University of Kent, UK.

Franco Merni, Faculty of Exercise and Sport Science, University of Bologna, Italy.

Gregoire Millet, ISSUL, University of Lausanne, Switzerland.

Rafa Martinez-Gallego, University of Valencia, Valencia, Spain.

Takahiro Morishige, Chukyo University, Toyota, Japan.

Jun Murakami, Fukuoka University, Fukuoka, Japan.

Shunsuke Murakami, Graduate School of Physical Education, National Institute of Fitness and Sports in Kanoya.

Stafford Murray, English Institute of Sport, Manchester, UK.

Hidetsugu Nishizono, National Institute of Fitness and Sports in Kanoya, Kanoya, Japan.

Peter O'Donoghue, Cardiff School of Sport, Cardiff Metropolitan University, UK.

Nimai Parmar, London Sport Institute, Middlesex University, London, UK.

Ana Paulo, Faculty of Physical Education and Sports of Lusófona University, Lisbon, Portugal.

Antonino Pereira, IPV, Viseu, Portugal.

Derek Peters, University of Worcester, Worcester, UK.

Juan-Carlos Quintana-Duque, University of Konstanz, Germany.

Jesus Ramón-Llin, University of Valencia, Valencia, Spain.

Hayley Randle, Duchy College, Stoke Climsland, Cornwall, UK.

Clare Rhoden, University of Worcester, Worcester, UK.

Michael Richardson, Center for Cognition, Action and Perception, University of Cincinnati, Cincinnati, United States.

Catherine Roberts, Cardiff School of Sport, Cardiff Metropolitan University, UK.

Eduardo Rostaiser, School of Physical Education and Sport, University of Sao Paulo, Brazil.

Ulrich Rückert, Cognitronics and Sensor Systems Group, CITEC, Bielefeld University, Germany.

Felipe Santana, School of Physical Education and Sport, University of Sao Paulo, Brazil.

Hugo Sarmento, UTAD, CIDESD Vila Real, Portugal.

Dietmar Saupe, University of Konstanz, Germany.

Reinhard Schnittker, Institute of Sports Medicine, University of Paderborn, Germany.

John Seeley, Department of Applied Science, London South Bank University, London, UK.

Malte Siegle, Technische Universität München, Germany.

Michael Stöckl, Technische Universität München, Germany.

Hiroo Takahashi, National Institute of Fitness and Sports in Kanoya, Kanoya, Japan.

Albin Tenga, Department of Coaching and Psychology, Norwegian School of Sport Sciences, Oslo, Norway.

Robert Timmermann, Chair of Applied Mathematics, University of Paderborn, Germany.

Bruno Travassos, Department of Sport Sciences, University of Beira Interior, Covilhã, Portugal.

Valmor Tricoli, School of Physical Education and Sport, University of Sao Paulo, Brazil.

Yuichi Ueno, Ryutsu Keizai University, Ryugasaki, Japan.

Carlos Ugrinowitsch, School of Physical Education and Sport, University of Sao Paulo, Brazil.

Michele van Rooyen, Centre for Human Performance Sciences, University of Stellenbosch, South Africa.

Anna Volossovitch, Faculty of Human Kinetics, Technical University of Lisbon, Portugal.

Goran Vučković, University of Ljubljana, Ljubljana, Slovenia.

Julia West, University of Worcester, Worcester, UK.

Cassie White, Nottingham Trent University, Brackenhurst Campus, Nottingham, UK.

Paul Worsfold, Department of Sports and Exercise Sciences, University of Chester, Chester, UK.

Takumi Yamamoto, National Defense Academy, Yokosuka, Japan.

Rene Zorn, Cognitronics and Sensor System Group, CITEC, Bielefeld University, Germany.

Preface

The first World Congress of Notational Analysis of Sport took place at Burton Manor, UK in 1992. Since then, eight further World Congresses have been held in Liverpool, UK (1994), Antalya, Turkey (1996), Porto, Portugal (1998), Cardiff, Wales (2001), Belfast, Northern Ireland (2004), Szombathely, Hungary (2006), Magdeburg, Germany (2008) and Worcester, UK (2012). It was at the Fourth World Congress in 1998, that 'performance analysis' was identified as being more appropriate than the term 'notational analysis' to better reflect the nature of research in the field and its practical application to sport. The overarching aim of each World Congress has been to bring together sport performance analysis academics, researchers, students, system providers and applied practitioners to disseminate cutting edge research and scholarly activity, to experience and exhibit new technologies and systems of analysis and to encourage mutual knowledge exchange between researchers and practitioners in the field.

The most recent World Congress of Performance Analysis of Sport IX (WCPAS IX) was hosted by the Institute of Sport & Exercise Science at the University of Worcester, UK, 25–28 July 2012, and exceeded all expectations in its aim to provide delegates with the opportunity to develop academic friendships and to promote cutting edge research and practitioner knowledge exchange in what has since been described as a 'boutique', friendly and social congress.

More than 200 abstracts were received for consideration for the scientific programme of WCPAS IX, resulting in 90 oral podium presentations and 120 poster presentations covering the broadest possible array of sport performance analysis themes including sports performance; analysis of referees; the coaching process; coach behaviour; biomechanics/analysis of technique; technical effectiveness; tactical evaluation/patterns of play; motor control; movement analysis in sport; motor learning and feedback; work rate and physical demands; performance analysis technology/systems; analysis of elite athletes and teams; effectiveness of performance analysis support; and performance analysis evidence of impact; and across a range of individual and team sports at many different levels of play. The delegate list included academics, researchers, students, applied practitioners and system developers from 36 countries from around the globe and as such confirmed the event as a truly *World* Congress. The abstracts for all of these presentations can be found in the *International Journal of Performance Analysis in Sport* 2012, **12**(3) pp. 643-839.

The scientific programme was completed with six keynote lectures with Professor Brian Dawson exploring movement patterns in team sports; Dr Tony Kirkbride evaluating media channels in performance analysis; Dr Wynford Leyshon recounting his experience of using performance analysis in the management of high-performance sport; Dr Vicky Tolfrey providing research and applied insight into the role of performance analysis during wheelchair team sport; Professor Jaime Sampaio examining the use of performance analysis in basketball for research and performance improvement; and Andy Scoulding and Dr Barry Drust delivering a joint keynote elucidating upon the roles of both the sport scientist and the performance analyst in an elite soccer club.

It would not have been possible to have achieved such a successful WCPAS IX without the dedication of the local organising and scientific committees as well as the support received from the Congress sponsors and without the participation of the Congress exhibitors. In particular, we would like to thank Donna Obrey and Andrea Bower in the Institute of Sport & Exercise Science Academic Support Unit for their time, effort and contribution to all aspects of the organisation and administration of WCPAS IX.

The podium and poster sessions were chaired by selected academics on a voluntary basis and our gratitude goes to Nic James, Michelle van Rooyen, Anita Hökelmann, Arnold Baca, Hyongjun Choi, Anna Volossovitch, Antonio Paulo Ferreira, Ricardo Duarte, Jaime Sampaio, Nuno Leite, Brian Dawson, Paul Canavan, Bruno Travassos, Paulo Vicente João, Martin Lames and Lucy Holmes. We wish to thank the following Congress sponsors for their support: FIBA Europe, Universitas; Cam*n*tech; Human Kinetics; Routledge; the International Society of Performance Analysis of Sport; the *Graduate Journal of Sport, Exercise & Physical Education Research*; *Basketball Research*; the Institute of Sport & Exercise Science's Motion & Performance Centre, and the University of Worcester. We would also like to extend our thanks to Sportstec, Kistler, S. Oliver Associates, and Alpha-Active for exhibiting at WCPAS IX.

Delegates presenting at WCPAS IX were offered the opportunity to submit extended chapters for consideration for inclusion in *Performance Analysis of Sport IX* as the first book of congress proceedings to be published by Routledge. All chapters submitted for consideration by the deadline underwent a peer review process, resulting in 41 chapters being accepted for inclusion in the book based upon their appropriate scope, quality, and their potential to raise the profile of, and interest in, performance analysis in their respective field or sport. The chapters selected fall into eight broad categories which form the sections of this book, these being Performance Analysis and Coaching; Soccer; Rugby; Team Games; Racket Sports; Individual Sports (including three equestrian papers); Systems; and Movement Analysis.

We are extremely grateful to the contributing authors for their effort in producing these chapters, conforming to the submission guidelines and addressing reviewers' comments when preparing the final versions of their manuscripts. Inspection of the contributor list reveals a truly international selection of papers incorporating an outstanding range of disciplines encompassed within sport performance analysis and representing an array of both well-established and less-often-researched individual and team sports.

We hope that you enjoy reading this book and that it inspires you to undertake your own sport performance analysis research. We also hope that you will be encouraged to join and play an active role in the International Society of Performance Analysis of Sport and we look forward to meeting you at the next World Congress of Performance Analysis of Sport in 2014!

Professor Derek M. Peters, PhD and Peter O'Donoghue, PhD

Part 1

Performance Analysis and Coaching

CHAPTER 1

The role of performance analysis in elite netball competition structures

Sara Horne

1.1 INTRODUCTION

Coaches at both the International and top domestic levels in netball have turned to performance analysis to assist in their decision making and provide reliable and accurate information to inform their coaching process (Jenkins *et al.*, 2007). The role of the performance analyst in this elite environment is to provide key objective information on performances which can be transformed into relevant feedback to facilitate learning and effect improvement. However, the coaching process and use of performance analysis to support the specific process are affected by the characteristics of the competition. Thus it is important to highlight the differences and constraints which occur as a result of the competition structure and identify how the challenges created impact the performance analyst and coaching process.

This chapter will focus upon the experience of the author working as performance analyst with the Netball Scotland squad in two distinct competition structures namely the Netball Superleague and International netball competitions. The Scotland squad competed as the Glasgow Wildcats within the Superleague, between 2008 and 2011, and compete as the Scottish Thistles in a range of International competitions. The Superleague comprised 16 matches played on consecutive weekends from January to May with some additional midweek, televised games. In comparison International competitions comprise multiple games over limited days. For example Test Matches generally consist of three games over 3–6 days and International competitions such as the Commonwealth Games and World Netball Championships consist of six games over 6–8 days. The current chapter will describe the development of the Scottish Thistles/Glasgow Wildcats squads coaching process and the use of performance analysis within this process. This will lead into a detailed discussion of the interactive feedback process implemented within the Scottish squads and the challenges faced in this process by the varying structures of competition.

1.2 OVERVIEW OF THE COACHING PROCESS

Figure 1.1 provides an operational model of the coaching process adopted by the Scottish netball squads (Scottish Thistles and Glasgow Wildcats). It is based on experience, knowledge and empirical evidence from best practice at the highest levels in netball and other team sports. The core elements of the process are a cycle of events, namely, perform, observe, analyse and train as suggested by current models (Cross and Lyle, 1999; Franks *et al.*, 1983). However, evaluation takes place throughout this process at each stage as relevant information is obtained. The information which supports this core process is provided by the performance analysis conducted. Hence objective information from video and statistics informs the evaluation of the performance. The coaches' subjective views combined with this objective information identify the performance strengths and weaknesses and are subsequently used to plan the necessary interventions. These interventions can occur in training, and through interactive feedback. In contrast to popular models for the coaching process this model reflects not only the interactive nature of the feedback of information between the coach, analyst and athletes but also the continual nature of this feedback which is provided as and when required throughout the coaching process.

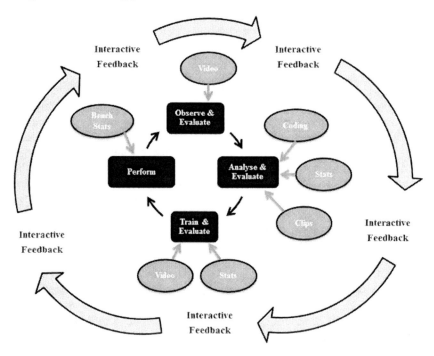

Figure 1.1 Operational model of the coaching process

1.3 INTERACTIVE FEEDBACK

The delivery of video-based performance analysis has been criticised as unstructured and reactive in nature with a focus on critical incidents (Groom *et al.*, 2011). Thus to provide a structure to the process of feedback with the Scottish netball squads, a model of the interactive feedback process has additionally been developed (See Figure 1.2). The feedback is driven by the process targets set prior to each performance, thus feedback is based upon whether the targets were achieved and the potential reasons for their achievement or non-achievement. Within this specific model the levels of feedback, divided into feedback within-match, post-match, analysis, train and pre-match, build upon each other to provide layers of information which are utilised to facilitate continued development and effect an improved performance.

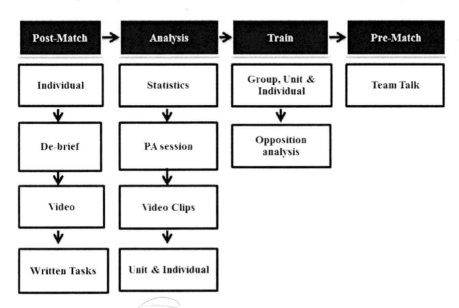

Figure 1.2 Model of the interactive feedback process

1.3.1 Within-match feedback

Within the match itself interactive feedback occurs between the coaches and athletes. The aim is to assist the athletes in achieving their pre-match targets in response to the particular opposition's abilities and strategies. The subjective views of the coaches are supported by the bench statistics which are the hand notated basic statistics recorded by the assistant coach and team manager. These statistics help the coaches' decision making within the game and can also be fed back to the athletes to provide the relevant evidence for necessary changes in behaviour. The accuracy of these bench statistics are ensured by the individual, experienced recorder before they are used within the match.

1.3.2 Post-match feedback

Directly after the match immediate individual feedback is provided by the coach to athletes who want to discuss elements of their performance. A whole squad debrief session follows, usually within 1–2 hours of the match after the cool-down, shower and refuel, where initial reflections, of the coaches and athletes, on the performance and the achievement of the specific targets take place. Statistical evidence is presented to inform the discussions and help identify strengths and weaknesses. Copies of the match are then provided on external hard drives and the coaches and athletes watch relevant parts or quarters directed by the debrief discussions. The athletes are then required to complete individual written feedback tasks answering relevant questions about the performance.

1.3.3 Feedback from performance analysis

The post-match feedback is subsequently combined with the quantitative performance analysis information of the key performance indicators and evaluated to determine the necessary interventions required. This evaluation then informs the content of the performance analysis session. The strengths and weaknesses in relation to the specific targets set are highlighted and relevant video clips are presented to the whole group. Subsequently specific unit and/or individual video clips are also viewed where required.

1.3.4 Feedback within training

The combined post-match and performance analysis feedback then informs the training session(s) which focus on the elements of the game identified as requiring further work. Within these sessions further group, unit and individual interactive feedback takes place as the athletes work to develop the weaknesses in technical and/or tactical elements of their game. Additional video and statistical information can also be provided within this environment to further support this development. Within the training stage of the process an assessment by the coaches and athletes is additionally made of the next opponent's play. Key strengths and weaknesses are identified, with support of statistical and video evidence, and relevant strategies are determined and trained.

1.3.5 Pre-match feedback

Before the next performance a team talk takes place where the targets for the game and strategies against the specific opposition are reinforced. Video clips can be used within these sessions to show evidence of the squad's previous, positive performance highlights to enhance confidence and motivation for the match ahead. The team talk is planned to allow sufficient time for the athletes to reflect on the game plan and their specific roles and allow discussion within the selected starting team and specific units.

A wealth of information is produced through the performance analysis process; however, it is the volume and when the information is delivered that determines whether performance improvements can be achieved (Hodges and

Franks, 2008). Thus it is important to provide the correct amount of feedback at the appropriate time, but not too much to overwhelm the athlete or make them overly dependent upon it (Hodges and Franks, 2008). A balance of positive and negative feedback is required to allow error correction while maintaining confidence and motivation (Dorrick, 1991). Understanding individual player needs and their preferred ways of learning are also important in ensuring an effective feedback process. However, the competition structures in which the Scottish squads perform provide challenges to this provision of feedback. Although there is flexibility to adapt and mould the Scottish squad's feedback process to the specific situation requirements, time constraints can cause significant challenge to the process.

1.4 CHALLENGES CAUSED BY COMPETITION STRUCTURE

The weekly match structure of the Netball Super league means there is sufficient time to conduct full team and individual analyses of the key performance indicators during and directly after the performances. Full statistical information, video of the whole match and specific video clips of team, unit and individual play can be provided within a day of the performance. Provision of both team and individual statistical and video feedback provides information which can be used to inform improvements in team performance and individual athlete development plans simultaneously. The competition schedule affords sufficient time for reflection, review and evaluation by the coach, analyst and players, time to view relevant aspects of video footage and conduct feedback tasks prior to three focused training sessions. This allows time to work on weaknesses in play identified from the previous match and assess the upcoming opponent's strengths and weaknesses. The game plan can then be constructed and specific strategies trained in preparation. Occasionally the coach and/or athletes will request further statistical information or video clips to inform the coaches' decision making, individual athlete learning and for confidence building and motivational purposes. The structure of this competition means there is time for such additional analysis to be conducted prior to the next game.

In contrast, the typical International competition structure of multiple games over a limited number of days significantly reduces the amount of time for the analyst to produce the necessary statistical results and video clips and for the feedback and training processes. A typical International schedule (e.g. Netball Europe) includes matches scheduled at 8pm, 4pm and 12pm on consecutive days with training sessions from 10am to 11am on the following mornings post matches 1 and 2. This leaves very limited time for the coding process so it becomes imperative to conduct real-time analysis. Consequently, to ensure quality of data collection the performance indicators which are coded are reduced to allow accurate feedback to be provided as quickly as possible. While additional coding can be conducted after the match, typically the key team performance indicators are produced during the match and the individual statistics, produced during the Superleague competition, are provided at a later stage after the International competition. Thus during International competitions individual feedback is largely qualitative in nature and provided as and when required within the time allowed with specific athletes. Individual quantitative feedback is provided post competition.

The timing of the elements of the feedback process (Figure 1.2) is significantly challenged within the International competition structure. The minimal time between matches means that the process must be flexible but still ensure that the feedback provided optimises the athlete's performances. As identified by Gasston (2004) the feedback of performance analysis during International competitions must also fit around set meals and training times, physiotherapy treatments and sufficient rest. Thus finding time to watch the match video and provide written feedback after an 8 pm match and before training at 10am the next morning can be difficult. In addition this specific timing means the performance analysis session, where specific video clips related to the statistical information are presented of the previous game, can only take place after the 10am training session. In this instance the match statistics are briefly fed back to the athletes at the start of the 1 hour training session so the team strengths and weaknesses and hence the focus of the training session is clear. With only 1 hour of training to concentrate on improving identified weak elements of play, and no training before the final match,   the performance analysis session then becomes an important non-physical extension of the training process. However, there is still a distinct lack of time to attend to both the squad's necessary improvements and the strategies required for the next opponents. Getting this balance right is a major challenge in this competition environment. Thus every opportunity is taken to gain relevant feedback. Hence the athletes watch at least two quarters of their opponent's games during the competition with the remit of providing specific details on the opposition's play within the performance analysis sessions. In an attempt to overcome some of these issues in International competition the Scotland squad's coaches focus the provision of feedback on "what can we fix now?" and "what requires more time to fix?". An assessment is made by coaches and athletes as to which tools, skills and strategies they have which have been trained and can be immediately implemented to effect an improvement. Conversely, assessment of the skills and strategies which require additional training post competition is also made. The relevant "what can we fix" information then becomes the focus of subsequent feedback in International competition. Hence, the most relevant information which results in performance improvements is prioritised.

1.5 SUMMARY

The diversity of the competition environments in which elite netball squads perform requires the specific coaching process and particularly the process of interactive feedback to be flexible and able to adapt to the environments' challenges. In particular the time constraints afforded by International competition structures require prioritising the most essential performance indicators. Producing the statistical and video information as soon after the match as possible then provides the most relevant feedback at the appropriate times for performance enhancement. The models used by the Scottish squads continue to evolve through regular reviews to ensure they allow the flexibility to adapt and change to athletes needs and facilitate continued development in all environments.

1.6 REFERENCES

Cross, N. and Lyle, J., 1999, *The Coaching Process*, (Oxford: Butterworth & Heinemann).

Dorrick P.W., 1991, Practical guide to using video in the behavioural sciences. In *Science and Football III*, edited by Reilly, T., Hughes, J. and Hughes, M. (London: E & FN Spon), pp. 267–278.

Franks, I.M., Goodman, D. and Miller, G., 1983, Analysis of performance: Qualitative or quantitative? *Science Periodical on Research and Technology in Sport*, March.

Gasston, V., 2004, Performance analysis during an elite netball tournament: Experiences and recommendations. In *Performance Analysis of Sport VI*, edited by O'Donoghue, P.G. and Hughes, M. (Cardiff: CPA Press UWIC), pp. 8–14.

Groom, R., Cushion, C.J. and Nelson, L., 2011, The delivery of video-based performance analysis by England youth soccer coaches: Towards a grounded theory. *Journal of Applied Sport Psychology*, **23**, pp. 16–32.

Hodges, N.J. and Franks, I.M., 2008, The provision of information. In *The Essentials of Performance Analysis: An Introduction,* edited by Hughes, M. and Franks, I.M. (London: Routledge), pp. 21–39.

Jenkins, R.E., Morgan, L. and O'Donoghue, P., 2007, A case study into the effectiveness of computerised match analysis and motivational videos within the coaching of a league netball team. *International Journal of Performance Analysis in Sport*, 7(2), pp. 59–80.

CHAPTER 2

Soccer match analysis: A qualitative study with Portuguese First League coaches

Hugo Sarmento, Antonino Pereira, Jorge Campaniço,
Maria T. Anguera and José Leitão

2.1 INTRODUCTION

Much of the activity of football coaches is embodied in the observation. Thus, it is important to clearly define the behavior which can be observed in a game (Carling *et al.*, 2009; Hughes, 2008), to produce an intervention to increase performance based on that information. However, despite a vast literature devoted to the game analysis (Carling *et al.*, 2009; Carling *et al.*, 2005; Hughes, 2008), there are few studies that focus on the characterization of the coach's thoughts about the observation of the game and his/her intervention before the information is collected. Thus, this study aims to understand what the coaches observe in the game and how they evaluate and make their intervention based on this observation.

2.2 METHODS

2.2.1 Participants

The participants in this study were eight expert high-performance Portuguese First League football coaches (denoted C1 to C8) with professional experience (as first coach) ranging from 2 to 30 years (14.9 ± 8.6 years). All of the coaches who were initially selected to participate in the study accepted the invitation, were involved in coaching at the time of the interviews, and worked at some time in their careers as first coaches within the Portuguese First League. Because of the in-depth character of each interview, the interpretational nature of the analysis, and the number of the teams in the First League (n = 16), eight coaches were considered representative and met the objectives of the study, as well as the criteria of expert selection.

2.2.2 Data collection

The methodology for collecting data in this study was the semi-structured interview (Bardin, 2008). The advantages of using this type of interview are diverse when compared with other methods of data collection (Ghiglione and Matalon, 2001). All the interviews were done by the first author.

The same format was used for each interview that began with general information about the purpose of the project. Next, the interviewer focused on background and demographic information. Finally, the knowledge elicitation took place using questions related to the purpose of the study, that are based mainly on the model of qualitative analysis of human movement proposed by Knudson and Morrison (2002). The interview schedule was designed to identify the issues most relevant to the coach and to focus on these issues in detail. The certification of the content validity of the interview was done according to the methodological recommendations of Ghiglione and Matalon (2001). None of the interviews were rushed, and the coaches always had time to clarify and reformulate their thinking. Each interview lasted between 1 and 2½ hours and was transcribed verbatim.

2.2.3 Data analyses

The objective of the analysis was to build an organizing system of categories that emerged from the unstructured data and that represented the organization and utilization of expert high-performance football coaches' knowledge.

Data analysis was performed using content analysis (Bardin, 2008). The construction of the categorical system was made *a priori* and *a posteriori*. The content analysis used was heuristic and confirmatory (Bardin, 2008). After the definition of the final system of classification of the material collected (properties), we analyzed the fidelity through the inter and intra codifier agreement. The software QSR NVivo 9 was used in coding the transcripts of the interviews.

2.3 RESULTS AND DISCUSSION

The objective of this study was to understand how the football coaches in Portugal prepare, observe and analyze the game and how they carry out their intervention based on the information they collected.

The analysis of the data allowed us to establish a model of qualitative analysis consisting of four dimensions: preparation; observation; diagnostic/ evaluation; intervention (see Figure 2.1).

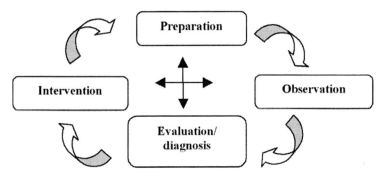

Figure 2.1 The coaching model in football

2.3.1 Preparation

We define the task of "preparation" in this study as being not only the set of procedures performed by the coaches in order to implement a strategy that allows them to effectively perform the observation and analysis of the game, but also the basic knowledge necessary to perform this procedure. The coaches interviewed consider that to perform an observation effectively it is essential to have a detailed knowledge of the game (16 pieces of qualitative evidence in the interviews support this point).

> Most important of all is the knowledge of the game (...) first you have to understand the game…
>
> (C6)

Moreover, coaches assigned significant importance to the procedures developed towards the definition/implementation of the observational strategy (n = 64). Within this category all coaches referred to the development/utilization of media technology (n = 27) as a valuable aid for the observation and analysis of the game, especially the use of video technology and specific software. However, this analysis assumes objective importance if the information is correctly selected. Aware of this premise, there are coaches who feel the need to adapt the technological means in order to make its use more practical and functional in accordance with its objectives.

> …we tried to develop a system that consists of the following: having an Ipad with the game matrix (the way we see the game), and a camera on the bench connected to a touchpad or a television in the dressing room. So it would be an integrated system in which the game was enough to identify something positive that was happening and we want to positively reinforce in half time. Touching the screen the pictures were captured five seconds before or five seconds after the relevant event (the same thing when something was not going well) and then just had to get there (dressing room), select and present, that is, we present and talk with the support of the footage.
>
> (C7)

The coaches also feel that the particular observer characteristics (n = 18) are essential in the process of watching the game. Thus, whenever they recruit an analyst to work in this area, they look for someone who has a similar understanding and sensitivity to the game that they themselves have.

> A good analyst, a good observer is one who sees the game not with his eyes, but with the eyes of the coach …
>
> (C3)

In order to minimize the effects that different sensitivities may exercise in the analysis of the observed aspects, the coaches opt for previously defining the items to watch in the game (n = 10), resulting in a standardized reporting instrument with pre-defined categories. Regarding the number of observations (n = 9) made of the opponents, we found they vary according to the coaches but especially according to the economic resources (2–6 games). Although much of the observation work is done by analysts, coaches reported that whenever possible they like to observe the opponents on the spot, because it allows them to have a more realistic perception of the intensity and rhythm of play beyond the observation of global team dynamics.

2.3.2 Observation

The second task of qualitative analysis consists in the observation of human movement. At this stage we tried to know what the coaches watch in a football game and what the key aspects which they should focus on are.

In this sense, we tried to know which aspects are observed before and during the game by the coaches that constitute our sample, and we conclude that they most often refer to the need to observe the overall dynamics of the teams (n = 18), the individual players' characteristics (n = 18), the tactical schemes (n = 14), the random/unpredictable aspects (n = 14) and the four moments of the game: offensive organization, defensive organization, offensive transition and defensive transition (n = 12).

> Essentially I observe dynamics and ways. Basically what I do is try to find solutions to any problems that the adversary creates for us, to find solutions to find ourselves, give clues for players to have a better performance.
>
> (C1)

> The tactical schemes, as we all know are very important (...) Then we have to find what is the randomness and unpredictability, i.e., how the team reacts in completely different, random and transient situations.
>
> (C2)

> ...basically we try to divide the game into four moments, to be easier to evaluate.
>
> (C4)

During the course of the game, while driving their teams, coaches are concerned primarily in observing the fulfillment of the game plan that was outlined (n = 11), and mainly focus their observation on their team (n = 10). We highlight the fact that coaches state that often their eyes are not directed to where the ball is but to spaces away from the center of the game, in order to decipher the dynamics that occur there.

They consider that the main factors that affect their observation are the psycho-emotional aspects (n = 18), the expectations (n = 16), the position on the bench (n = 9) and the referees' errors (n = 7). However, they acknowledge that the observation and analysis that they perform has evolved over the years, leading them to make more effective observations (n = 11) or to value aspects in the game that they did not previously value (n = 7). The factors responsible for the evolution of this observation are the accumulation of experience and a better knowledge of the game (n = 23), academic training (n = 6) and technical training (n = 5).

2.3.3 Evaluation and diagnosis

The third task consists of the evaluation that was observed in order to make a diagnosis that provides the development of an appropriate intervention plan in order to enhance performance. When evaluating the opposing teams coaches conduct an overall evaluation of the teams (n = 16) that enables them to identify strengths/weaknesses (n = 25), to allow them to "explore" these weaknesses, or in order to avoid any difficulties that the opposing team can place on the basis of its more positive aspects.

> ...try to understand where are the similarities, differences, which we can exploit, and what the opposing team can explore in our game, the more/less positive, stronger/weaker factors (...) what can create more imbalance in our team, and what we can do to imbalance the opposing team, according to what we see.
>
> (C4)

The assessment and diagnosis that coaches perform are based on a certain logic, i.e., a framework of ideals behind this process of evaluation/diagnosis, that we call logic of evaluation (n = 35). This logic that coaches follow in order to evaluate their own team or opposing teams is sustained, on the one hand, on a relation of antagonism toward the opposing teams, and on the other hand, on a referential that every coach has relative to his own game model.

> When I'm evaluating an opposing team, I have to know who my team is, to get a sense of what is important and more crucial in this vision of two antagonistic processes.
>
> (C4)

2.3.4 Intervention

The last task of qualitative analysis is the intervention that coaches perform, based on their interpretation of the data observed. The intervention is understood not only as the organization of training process, but also as a set of resources or techniques the coach uses to transmit effectively the information to his players.

The intervention of coaches is done during the micro cycle training (n = 43) or during the game (n = 35). During the micro cycle training, the intervention is sustained primarily on the adaptation/modification of training exercises (n = 26) depending on the diagnosis done based on the performance of own and opposing teams. However, this intervention is also done through meetings (n = 17) which are collective, individual or in small groups. Throughout the game, the coaches reported that half time is the most appropriate moment to perform their intervention (n = 12). However, they make use of other techniques such as the fact that they have a target player (n = 8) who they often use to transmit information so that it can get to their colleagues, the use of immediate feedback (n = 5) and the use of gestures (n = 3).

The coaches interviewed showed a great concern for making an appropriate intervention (n = 76). To do this, they carefully select the information they wish to convey to players (n = 20), resort to using images to enhance their feedbacks (n = 15), perform various meetings throughout the week with a short duration (n = 14), and attach particular importance to their body language (n = 7).

> ...much of this information we transmit to players; there is other that we will not pass, because they do not need to know everything. They just need to focus on what is essential, as we have all the information to understand some things that may have happened in the game.
>
> (C3)

2.4 CONCLUSIONS

In summary, the qualitative methodology used has led to a conceptualization of expert football coaches' knowledge. In fact, focusing on what Knudson and Morrison (2002) defined as the integrated model of qualitative analysis, the present study has adapted and systematized the different components and their links which appear to be central to the coaching process in football. The proposed model consists of four main tasks (preparation, observation, evaluation/ diagnosis, intervention).

However, the construction of this model is supported not only in a theoretical approach as some of the models that are presented in the literature (Carling *et al.*, 2005; Knudson and Morrison, 2002). On the contrary, it results from the analysis of the reports of high-performance coaches in this sport that daily face the reality of the practical application of their knowledge. Thus, it was possible to systematize in a detailed way the different tasks included in the process of qualitative analysis in football.

From this analysis we emphasize the rigor and systematization that characterize the preparation phase of the observation, beyond the fact that these coaches demonstrate similar concerns in respect to aspects to watch in a game. These are mainly characterized by the detection of regularities/patterns of behavior that emerge from the activity, from a qualitative perspective, rather than a data analysis of quantitative nature, which they consider to be less relevant in this context. The observed aspects are then evaluated taking as reference the specific game model of each coach who, based on that observation, carefully planned his intervention.

The underlying model of the process used by expert coaches to improve sport performance in football was an important basis for formalizing coaching knowledge. Indeed, a deeper understanding of each of the underlying tasks and appears to be necessary for obtaining a true understanding of coaching at any level of competition in football.

2.5 REFERENCES

Bardin, L., 2008, *Análise de conteúdo*, (Lisboa: Edições 70).
Carling, C., Reilly T. and Williams, A., 2009, *Performance Assessment for Field Sports*, (London: Routledge).
Carling, C., Williams, A. and Reilly, T., 2005, *The Handbook of Soccer Match Analysis*, (London: Routledge).
Ghiglione, R. and Matalon, B., 2001, *O inquérito: teoria e prática*, (Oeiras: Celta Editora).
Hughes, M., 2008, Notational analysis of soccer. In *Proceedings of the 5th International Scientific Conference on Kinesiology, Zagreb,* edited by Milanovic, D. and Prot, F. (Zagreb, Croatia), pp. 644–660.
Knudson, D. and Morrison, C., 2002, *Qualitative Analysis of Human Movement*, (New York: Human Kinetics).

CHAPTER 3

Coach behaviour analysis within elite youth soccer

Paul R. Worsfold

3.1 INTRODUCTION

Soccer clubs recruit talented youth players into their development programmes with the aim of nurturing their ability, and ultimately to develop them into professional soccer players (Carling *et al.*, 2012). Past talent identification and development research has identified that youth players who are then selected to play at higher standards of competition possess greater endurance capacity (Gil *et al.*, 2007; Reilly *et al.*, 2000), faster sprinting performance (Le Gall *et al.*, 2010), have faster dribbling performance (Huijgen *et al.*, 2009) and are generally more physically advanced in comparison to players of lower ability (Gravina *et al.*, 2008). In contrast to traditional measures, few studies have considered player development in relation to coach–player interaction.

There is general agreement that coaching is a process that primarily focuses on aiding athletes in achieving their peak performance (Woodman, 1993). Therefore, the way in which a coach facilitates learning through their words and actions, which is the core principle of the coach's instructional behaviour, can strongly impact upon an athlete's performance and progression, as well as their emotional well-being (Miller, 1992). Promoting a mastery climate, with equal opportunities and support for athletes, fosters group cohesion and reduces performance anxiety through the reduction of social pressures (Smith *et al.*, 2007). Despite the need for equality to promote cohesion throughout the team, differentiation between feedback provided to effective and non-effective team sport players has previously been identified. In many team sports, it has been suggested that coaches observe and interact more with effective players (based upon match time), provide more feedback (instructional, positive, and negative), and give more positive evaluations within training sessions when compared to non-effective players (Markland and Martinek, 1988; Wang *et al.*, 2001; Rosado and Mesquita, 2009).

To date no research has conducted a longitudinal assessment focusing on talent development and player progression through coach behaviour analysis within elite youth soccer. Therefore, the aim of the study was to objectively analyse coaching behaviour within three playing squads at an elite-level soccer club during two competitive seasons.

3.2 METHOD

3.2.1 Participants

Following ethical approval, one English professional soccer club agreed to participate in the study. Three coaches from different age group squads (Under 14, 15, 16 years) were analysed. From the three squads, 48 players were classified as effective (n = 26) and non-effective (n = 22) players based on their competitive match selection and playing time. An effective player was deemed to have played more than 65 per cent of the game time in more than 70 per cent of the competitive games during the research study.

3.2.2 Instrument

A customized analysis template, based around the 'Coach Analysis Instrument' (Franks *et al.,* 1988), was developed (Table 3.1) within SportsCode (Sportstec, Warriewood, NSW, Australia). Coach data for each age group were computed and analysed by the same analyst.

Table 3.1 Working definitions for coach behaviour indicators

	Key factors	
Direction	Individual	Directed at a single person
Focus	Skill related	Comments pertaining to skills (e.g. passing, technique, body position)
	Non-skill	Comments with no relevance to skills/technique
	Skill related	
Instruct		Explanation of the skill/drill
Correct		Feedback referring to skill performed correctly
Incorrect		Feedback referring to incorrectly performed skill
	Non-skill related	
Effort		Comment related to intensity of performance
Behaviour		Comment related to conduct of performers
Organizational		Comment related to function of practice
Non-specific		Comment with no specific emphasis
	Expression	
Positive		Encourage player
Negative		Criticize player

3.2.3 Procedures

To ensure coaches and players were not distracted during data collection, video cameras (Panasonic, AG-PVX100BE) recorded all coach and player behaviours from an elevated position in the stadia away from the training session. Each coach wore a wireless microphone (Sennheiser, EW100G2), which was synchronized to the video footage. Seventy-two training sessions, each lasting between 60 and 90 minutes, were recorded. All data collections were captured during 'typical' coaching sessions scheduled by the club. Coaches were informed that their coaching style was being assessed by the club, but were not made aware of the specific research question.

3.2.4 Reliability

Intra-operator reliability tests were conducted on two randomly selected coaching sessions within each age group (n = 6). Data were re-tested two months after they were originally analysed. The level of agreement for each performance indicator was assessed using Cohen's Kappa coefficient (κ). All assessed variables were identified as having either 'good' (0.6–0.8) or 'very good' agreement (>0.8) between tests.

3.2.5 Statistical analysis

Data for feedback type frequency per training session were initially analysed for violations of normality using the Kolmogorov-Smirnov test, and homogeneity using Levene's test. Independent-samples t-tests were used to calculate differences between effective and non-effective player feedback within each squad. Statistical significance was set at $P < 0.05$ for all variables. Data are reported as means and standard deviations ($\pm$) throughout and were analysed using SPSS (v.18, IBM Armonk, New York).

3.3 RESULTS

The analysis of coaching behaviour in relation to player status identified significant differences ($P < 0.05$) within 8 of the 12 measured variables across all age groups (Table 3.2).

The coaches provided more individual feedback to effective players during training sessions. Effective players received more comments based on skill and non-skill (focus-related) aspects of their play. This resulted in more feedback explaining the skill and more explanation of correct and incorrect techniques. Furthermore, effective players received more positive comments about their play but also more negative expressions. No differences were identified in the amount of non-skill related feedback given between players.

Table 3.2 Coach feedback frequencies per training session (mean ± SD)

Direction	U14 (24 sessions)		U15 (26 sessions)		U16 (22 sessions)	
	Effective	Non-effective	Effective	Non-effective	Effective	Non-effective
	(n = 8)	(n = 8)	(n = 9)	(n = 7)	(n = 9)	(n = 7)
Individual	112 ± 23*	85 ± 20*	109 ± 24*	84 ± 29*	104 ± 30*	88 ± 24*
Focus						
Skill	79 ± 18*	53 ± 13*	77 ± 16*	57 ± 15*	78 ± 19*	60 ± 17*
Non-skill	32 ± 12*	21 ± 9*	39 ± 10*	25 ± 9*	31 ± 11*	23 ± 13*
Skill-related comment						
Instruct	39 ± 15*	27 ± 19*	34 ± 14*	20 ± 9*	35 ± 12*	24 ± 10*
Correct	20 ± 11*	12 ± 13*	25 ± 10*	15 ± 7*	24 ± 10*	16 ± 8*
Incorrect	19 ± 9*	10 ± 5*	21 ± 8*	14 ± 9*	23 ± 11*	15 ± 7*
Non-skill related						
Effort	7 ± 9	6 ± 8	9 ± 6	6 ± 5	8 ± 6	6 ± 5
Behaviour	9 ± 6	10 ± 7	5 ± 5	5 ± 6	3 ± 5	4 ± 5
Tactical	11 ± 6	7 ± 6	10 ± 7	7 ± 6	14 ± 8	8 ± 6
Non-specific	9 ± 7	5 ± 6	7 ± 8	5 ± 4	5 ± 9	5 ± 8
Expressions						
Positive	48 ± 22*	37 ± 18*	55 ± 21*	41 ± 20*	51 ± 29*	39 ± 15*
Negative	42 ± 20*	33 ± 24*	42 ± 24*	31 ± 16*	50 ± 24*	35 ± 19*

*denotes a significant difference between effective and non-effective groups ($P < 0.05$)

3.4 DISCUSSION

It has been stated that the most successful team athletes are those who receive more tuition, encouragement and information from the coaches (Wuest *et al.*, 1986). Consequently, it is important that there are equivalent feedback and interventions from coaches with all players within developmental programmes. The results of the present study identified that in many facets of coaching, coach behaviour varied in relation to players' participation within the team. The findings support previous research (Markland and Martinek, 1988; Wang *et al.*, 2001; Rosado and Mesquita, 2009). Disparities between the type and quantity of coach feedback was identified across all age group squads, consequently the results cannot be considered an effect of an individual coach's style. The findings have implications for the effectiveness of talent identification and player development within the assessed youth programme. One could argue that the effective players would receive more instruction about tactics and formations as a consequence of them playing more regularly within the squad. However, with the aim of nurturing and developing players into professional soccer players, it can be hypothesized that coach feedback disparity should not exist within youth developmental programmes.

To date, elite youth soccer talent identification and development research has focused on biological maturation status, anthropometric and functional characteristic data (Carling *et al.*, 2012). In conjunction with traditional longitudinal talent research, an emphasis should be placed on further investigating the coaching process during the development cycle (player selection/contract offer/release/sale/senior team selection), as at present it is unclear what effect coaching disparities have on individual player progression.

3.5 REFERENCES

Carling, C., Le Gall, F. and Malina, R.M., 2012, Body size, skeletal maturity, and functional characteristics of elite academy soccer players on entry between 1992 and 2003. *Journal of Sports Sciences*, **11**, pp. 371–379.

Franks, I.M., Johnson, R.B. and Sinclair, G.D., 1988, The development of a computerised coaching analysis system for recording behaviour in sporting environments. *Journal of Teaching in Physical Education*, **8**, pp. 23–32.

Gil, S., Ruiz, F., Irazusta, A., Gil, J. and Irazusta, J., 2007, Selection of young soccer players in terms of anthropometric and physiological factors. *Journal of Sports Medicine and Physical Fitness*, **47**, pp. 25–32.

Gravina, L., Gil, S., Ruiz, F., Zubero, J., Gil, J. and Irazusta, J., 2008, Anthropometric and physiological differences between first team and reserve soccer players aged 10–14 years at the beginning and end of the season. *Journal of Strength and Conditioning Research*, **22**, pp. 1308–1314.

Huijgen, B.C., Elferink-Gemser, M.T., Post, W.J. and Visscher, C., 2009, Soccer skill development in professionals. *International Journal of Sports Medicine*, **30**, pp. 585–591.

Le Gall, F., Carling, C., Williams, M. and Reilly, T., 2010, Anthropometric and fitness characteristics of international, professional and amateur male graduate soccer players from an elite youth academy. *Journal of Science and Medicine in Sport*, **13**, pp. 90–95

Markland, R. and Martinek, T.J., 1988, Descriptive analysis of augmented feedback given to high school varsity volleyball players. *Journal of Teaching in Physical Education*, **1**, pp. 289–301.

Miller, A.W., 1992, Systematic observation behaviour similarities of various youth sport soccer coaches. *The Physical Educator*, **49**, pp. 136–143.

Reilly, T., Williams, A.M., Nevill, A. and Franks, A., 2000, A multidisciplinary approach to talent identification in soccer. *Journal of Sports Sciences*, **18**, pp. 695–702

Rosado, A. and Mesquita, I., 2009, Analysis of the coach's behaviour in relation to effective and non-effective players in basketball. *International Journal of Performance Analysis in Sport*, **9**, pp. 210–217.

Smith, R.E., Smoll, F.L. and Cumming, S.P., 2007, Effects of a motivational climate intervention for coaches on young athletes sport performance anxiety. *Journal of Sport and Exercise Psychology*, **29**, pp. 39–59.

Wang, J., Callahan, D. and Goldfine, B., 2001, Coaches' challenges working with substitute players of collegiate team sports. *Applied Research in Coaching and Athletics Annual*, **16**, pp. 110–124.

Woodman, L., 1993, Coaching: A science, an art, an emerging profession. *Sport Science Review*, **2**, pp. 1–13.

Wuest, D.A., Mancini, V.H., van der Mars, H. and Terrillion, K., 1986, The academic learning time-physical education of high-, medium-, and low-skilled female intercollegiate volleyball players. In *Olympic Scientific Congress Proceedings VI*, edited by Pieron, M. and Graham, G. (Champaign, IL: Human Kinetics Publishers), pp. 123–130.

CHAPTER 4

Performance Analysis in professional soccer: Player and coach perspectives

Rob Mackenzie and Chris Cushion

4.1 INTRODUCTION

Performance analysis (PA) is firmly positioned as an integral part of the coaching process (Hodges and Franks, 2002; Lyle, 2002; Stratton *et al.*, 2004; Carling *et al.*, 2005; Groom *et al.*, 2011). The application of video and computer technology in sport and the implementation of video review sessions into weekly training programmes (Guadagnoli *et al.*, 2002; Groom and Cushion, 2004) has led to the belief that PA "is now widely accepted among coaches, athletes and sport scientists as a valuable input into the feedback process" (Drust, 2010, p. 921). Moreover, the development of computer and video aided analysis systems (such as SportsCode, Warriewood, NSW, Australia; Focus X2, Elite Sports Analysis, Delgaty Bay, Fife, UK; ProZone, ProZone Sports Ltd, Leeds, UK and Sport Universal Process AMISCO Pro, Nice, France match analysis systems) has enhanced accessibility to resources in order to analyse sporting events objectively (Carling *et al.*, 2005), and as a result, research frequently utilises these data. For example, video analysis software has been used with a multitude of purposes in both individual and team based sports (Jenkins *et al.*, 2007; Di Salvo *et al.*, 2009).

However, PA research in soccer has tended to focus on the investigation of isolated key performance indicators. This has resulted in a consistent focus on descriptive research examining variables related to "successful performance", such as possession and passing patterns (e.g. James *et al.*, 2004; Hughes and Franks, 2005), score-box possessions (e.g. Tenga *et al.*, 2010a; 2010b) and shooting accuracy (e.g. Lago, 2007). There is, however, a significant lack of research that has investigated the role of PA in the complex, messy and dynamic coaching process (Cushion *et al.*, 2010). Moreover, research has often neglected the perspectives of practitioners who use PA in applied settings, such as professional soccer. The purpose of this study was to investigate the role of PA in the coaching process at a professional soccer club and the perspectives of both professional players and coaches in relation to its use.

4.2 METHODOLOGY

A case study approach was adopted (Yin, 2003) presenting both ethnographic data, in the form of participant observation and unstructured interviews (Hammersley and Atkinson, 1994) recorded over the period of one full season. Data were recorded at an English professional soccer club who were playing in the FA Championship by the primary researcher who occupied a dual role as First Team Performance Analyst and full time researcher during his time at the club. In addition, semi-structured interviews were conducted with both senior professional players (n = 8) and members of the senior management team (n = 3). The data were subjected to three levels of overlapping analysis using coding techniques (open, axial and selective) taken from grounded theory methodology (Strauss and Corbin, 1998). This allowed for the generation of descriptive themes and concepts relating to the use of PA at the club. A further level of analysis and abstraction allowed the introduction of wider theoretical perspectives. Four main concepts in relation to the use of PA were outlined: *PA as preparation*, *PA as reflection*, *PA as a disciplinary tool* and *PA as a learning resource*.

4.3 RESULTS AND DISCUSSION

Analysis revealed that the use of PA at the club was influenced by a number of sociological and cultural factors that until recently have been neglected within the PA literature (Stratton *et al.*, 2004; Groom *et al.*, 2012). Both players and coaches discussed pertinent issues relating to their perceptions of PA, both within the coaching process (Drust, 2010) and as a learning resource. Moreover, the results demonstrated that idealistic and unproblematic representations of PA within the coaching process (e.g. Hughes and Franks, 1997; 2008) are inaccurate as they do not consider confounding variables such as coaches' philosophies of practice (Nash *et al.*, 2008), the underlying culture at the club and perceptions of PA, players' learning preferences and group dynamics.

4.3.1 The culture

This research revealed that there was an underlying performance culture present at the club, in that the result of matches often influenced individuals' behaviour around the club as well as their perceptions of the value of PA in their practice and process of reflecting on their performance. For example, Player B revealed that if the team is successful, he would not reflect on his own performance and would not seek out PA support even if there were aspects of his performance that he was not happy about:

> It's like one of those where you can do something bad, and like I said earlier, if you win you just sweep it under the rug like "well that happens in football everyone is going to make mistakes" so I think like I say it's a lot of whether you've won or whether you've lost …
> I mean sometimes you play well and there's not … you know "Oh I give the ball away a couple of times." I'm not gonna watch a DVD to look at that, do you know what I mean?
>
> (Player B, age 22)

Similar sentiments were shared by Player E who described the emphasis that is placed on the result in his post-match evaluation of his own performance. He explained that if the team won the game the intensity with which he assesses his own contribution is diminished; leaving PA redundant in his post-match thoughts:

> That kind of self assessment is very, very important, but it depends … it really, really depends because we all know it's a results related, err, business, and it does depend on, on, on the results, how I do assess myself or not.
>
> (Player E, age 32)

Given the incentives associated with winning and the negative consequences associated with being unsuccessful in professional soccer it is perhaps unsurprising that the result has such an influence on individual's behaviour and reflective thinking (Dewey, 1933). When members of the coaching team were asked how PA was used when they were players, a similar theme emerged in that PA was only used with players by management following poor performances:

> My generation of players the only time you ever watched a game was when the manager said "Well I had to f****ng sit through it so you are" you have to watch the whole game and watch yourself so it used to be a tool to humiliate people but of course this generation of player now are much more open to it being a teaching tool because that's how we use it now, although some people I'm sure still use it as a big stick which is why we still get mixed reviews.
>
> (First Team Coach)

It could therefore be suggested that if players and coaches predominantly experience PA only in relation to poor performances, when the team is successful it is perhaps deemed as something that they do not necessarily have to engage in, given they achieved their pre-match aims. Moreover, the significance of a games' result appears to have resonated with the players, given that they reported a reluctance to actively reflect on their performances following a victory and did not perceive PA to be an integral resource to inform their future decision making. Subsequently, the environment in which PA is delivered and received is pivotal to how individuals perceive its role and function within their own role. This finding challenges the notion of PA being unproblematic, independent of the environment and unaffected by cultural stakeholders (e.g. Franks *et al.*, 1983; Robertson, 1999).

4.3.2 Player perspectives

Players referred to PA primarily being a feed forward mechanism (Dowrick, 1999) as opposed to a form of performance feedback (Hughes and Franks, 1997). While it could be argued that the club's distinctive culture may have influenced players' perceptions of PA's role at the club, it may also represent more common uses of

PA in the applied setting. For example, given players commonly referred to PA as having more of an effect prior to performance than post-performance, it may be that PA is received more positively when informing decision making before a game.   Subsequently, key stakeholders may use it more regularly prior to performance as opposed to following performance. Player A described that he valued pre-match presentations at the club more than the debrief (post-match) video sessions:

> Maybe the one before, erm, because I suppose it's more of a heads up to what's gonna happen, so, like I say, I can go into a game knowing who is their main header of the ball, who I'm marking is gonna spin round the back on a set piece and I know it's gonna happen, and I can sort of combat that to sort of prevent more chances and goal scoring opportunities.
>
> (Player A, age 22)

Similar preferences were described by Player G, who placed an emphasis on pre-match video-based PA sessions in his preparation in which information regarding opposing players' playing styles was presented:

> You know, you do PowerPoint presentations, you know, you know everything about the player before you've even ... stepped on to the pitch.   So you know before kick off, right, this guy's right-footed, he's gonna, he's gonna try and cut in and shoot with his right.   So it affects you where ... when you're in that level you don't, at the bottom, you don't know what they're gonna do, you know.
>
> (Player G, age 22)

When players were asked about how they perceived PA as a post-match evaluative resource, their responses revealed a club wide approach to PA following performance. Both players and coaches explicitly explained that they deemed video-based PA to be a checking mechanism that allowed them to confirm or dispute their initial interpretation and understanding of the situation that they had experienced:

> Interviewer: "For me, video at the minute, the way it's used seems to be as if it's a kind of checking mechanism, i.e. was I right or was I wrong in what I think?   So I think, 'Right, I should have just played that' and the only reason I'm looking at that is to see ..."
>
> Player: "Yeah."
>
> Interviewer: "Yeah I should have or no I shouldn't, and then I move on.   It's as if just by watching it again, I'm able to maybe get it clear in my head ..."

Player: "That's exactly how I use it, yeah, exactly. Like, I'll go back and I'll look at the goal and I think I probably could have done that, and then next time you, you know, that'll be it. I'd have gone 'I probably could have done that and I'll try and make sure that don't happen again.' Do you know what I mean? That'll be it, and then I'll go onto the next thing."

Interviewer: "Rather than sitting and critically analysing your own game."

Player: "Yeah, yeah, I'd say it was that, definitely."

With this in mind, players did not report on any novel learning experiences (Cushion *et al.*, 2010) based on critically revisiting their performance as they predominantly used PA to provide an alternative perspective to their initial experience during a predetermined event as opposed to observing their performance without an agenda. Subsequently, situations where players may have re-observed their performance in order to evaluate their performance and search for unnoticed critical incidents were not reported. In summary, analysis revealed a preference at the club towards using PA as a pre-performance resource in order to prepare specifically for the forthcoming opposition as opposed to as a post-performance evaluation method. Moreover, it was found that PA was used to consolidate initial responses to experiences as opposed to being used as a tool to create novel learning experiences (Cushion *et al.*, 2010).

4.3.3 Coach perspectives

Members of the management team made reference to a number of variables that influenced the delivery and use of video-based PA at the club. Despite the lack of research that has considered both cultural and sociological factors that may influence pedagogical practice (Stratton *et al.*, 2004), coaches discussed a number of elements that influenced their decision making. For example, the perceived needs of the group were always at the forefront of the First Team Coach's thinking and had a significant influence on how he delivered video-based PA to the group as well as whether sessions were actually provided for the players:

Any decisions that are ever made in terms of what we show them and what we don't show them and not because it's "I can't be bothered" it's about what has the best impact on the players and that's the reason why we ever do anything. It's about what's going to help them to play the next game and how we deliver it is about them, not about me or the coaches feeling good about ourselves and it's about what they need. It's always got to be about them.

(First Team Coach)

Subsequently, the dynamics of the group in terms of their personalities and relationships with each other as well as the mood of the players (often influenced by recent results) were considered when deciding upon how the video-based PA sessions would be delivered and the content of the presentations. As the Assistant Coach described, however, sometimes the potential for individual development would be compromised if the needs of the group outweighed the benefits of providing individual specific feedback in a group scenario:

> The games comes so thick and fast that sometimes you know you might have got beat 2–1 but played quite well and you want to talk about it in the debrief and there might be things in there that you feel as though there's an individual who can do better but collectively, you feel as though the group needs something different.
>
> (Assistant Coach)

Having established the cultural factors that influenced the decision making of the management team prior to presenting video-based PA to their players, it is important to acknowledge coaches' perceptions of PA itself as this may undoubtedly influence their choice of delivery (Groom *et al.*, 2011). The First Team Coach demonstrated an in-depth understanding of the inherent limitations associated with third party data analysis providers (such as ProZone, ProZone Sports Ltd, Leeds, UK and Sport Universal Process AMISCO Pro, Nice, France match analysis systems) and that this knowledge influenced the importance and emphasis he placed on it within the coaching process (e.g. Lyle, 2002; Cushion *et al.*, 2006). Specifically, with reference to the physical data that is provided by such companies, he cited a lack of specificity in the thresholds utilised to analyse a player's physical performance as a problem. Due to individual players having different sprint and high intensity thresholds that are not accounted for within the data he was aware that the data is somewhat incomparable and contributed to the lack of emphasis he placed on it within the coaching process:

> I actually think the players are interested in terms of distances and but again, unless you've got the individuality of the thresholds even that's flawed. You know so I understand it and I probably we know a bit more about it than a lot of people who use it and that's why I don't use it because you know we need to spend more time proving the players on the training field rather than showing them what they can't do and show what the opposition do do or can't do.
>
> (First Team Coach)

Similarly, the manner in which the information by third party data analysis providers is distributed to the club was an issue for the First Team Coach as he described the lack of flexibility in what could be analysed coupled with a rigid presentation format as being influential in his cautious approach to PA and its diminished role within his match assessment.

I want something different to what they are trying to do (third party data analysis providers). They are trying to show everybody in football what they do and then it's up to you now to f***ing make that work for you. Well actually its arse about face, it should be "this is what I want and what can they do for me?"

(First Team Coach)

It is evident that the First Team Coach of the club is acutely aware of the limitations inherent with PA presented by third party data analysis providers and this has contributed to his caution when using the information. This is in direct contrast to ignorance or a resistance to PA that may perhaps underpin other First Team Coaches' resistance to fully integrating PA within the coaching process. With this in mind, self-determined video-based PA has taken precedent over statistical PA in the First Team Coach's own coaching process (e.g. Lyle, 2002; Cushion *et al.*, 2006). His decision making relating to the delivery and content of video-based PA to the players is underpinned by a consideration of what is right for the players at that specific time point and may in some cases result in no video-based PA actually being presented. This finding further challenges previous representations within the literature of PA delivery and receipt being an unproblematic and linear process (e.g. Hughes and Franks, 1997; 2008).

4.4 CONCLUSION

This research sought to further an understanding of the role and function of PA within the coaching process at a professional soccer club. Moreover, the perspectives of both coaches and players were examined in an attempt to examine the impact of PA on their respective practice. The approach adopted in this study attempted to capture the role of PA within the "gritty reality" of the coaching process (Potrac and Jones, 2009, p. 561) within the confines and pressurised environment of a professional soccer club. The findings from this study revealed that the performance culture at the club, which focussed mainly on the results of matches, significantly influenced how key stakeholders perceived and used PA. It was found that players were reluctant to seek out PA following successful performances and although it was not reported by the players in this study, members of the coaching team made reference to their experiences of PA being primarily used as a disciplinary tool following poor performances. Players at the club did demonstrated a preference for PA as a preparatory tool in contrast to being a post-performance feedback mechanism and when players did describe instances where they had used PA following performances its primary role was to act as a checking mechanism to confirm or challenge their thoughts following their initial experience.

This study also revealed that a multitude of factors are considered by the club's management team when using PA with the club's players. Coaches explained that their interpretations of the players' needs underpinned every aspect of their practice and subsequently sociological factors such as the mood of the group; recent results and the characters within the group were considered prior to conducting video-based PA sessions with players. The First Team Coach's perception of the limitations associated with the third party service provider data contributed to its arguably negligible role in his coaching practice. This study has demonstrated the influence of sociological and cultural factors on the use and delivery of PA at a professional soccer club (Groom *et al.*, 2011). Consequently, future research focussing on the use and delivery of PA should seek to acknowledge these factors in their design and analysis. Furthermore, improved communication between researchers and practitioners (Bishop, 2008) is required in order to ensure that future research both furthers our knowledge and understanding but is also applicable and relevant to the needs of those working in the applied setting.

4.5 REFERENCES

Bishop, D., 2008, An applied research model for the sports sciences. *Sports Medicine*, **38**(3), pp. 253–263.

Carling, C., Williams, A.M. and Reilly, T., 2005, *The Handbook of Soccer Match Analysis*, (Abingdon: Routledge).

Cushion, C.J., Armour, K.M. and Jones, R.L., 2006, Locating the coaching process in practice: models "for" and "of" coaching. *Physical Education and Sport Pedagogy*, **11**(1), pp. 83–99.

Cushion, C., Nelson, L., Armour, K., Lyle, J., Jones, R., Sandford, R. and O'Callaghan, C., 2010, *Coach Learning and Development: A Review of Literature*, (Leeds: Sports Coach UK).

Dewey, J., 1933, *How We Think: A Restatement of the Relation of Reflective Thinking to the Educative Process*, (Boston: D.C. Heath and Company).

Di Salvo, W., Gregson, W., Atkinson, G., Tordoff, P. and Drust, B., 2009, Analysis of high intensity activity in Premier League soccer. *International Journal of Sports Medicine*, **30**, pp. 205–212.

Dowrick, P.W., 1999, A review of self-modeling and related interventions. *Applied and Preventive Psychology*, **8**, pp. 23–39.

Drust, B., 2010, Performance analysis research: Meeting the challenge. *Journal of Sports Science*, **28**(9), pp. 921–922.

Franks, I.M., Goodman, D. and Miller, G., 1983, Analysis of performance: Qualitative or quantitative? *Science Periodical on Research and Technology in Sport*, March.

Groom, R. and Cushion, C., 2004, Coaches perceptions of the use of video analysis: A case study. *Insight*, 7, pp. 6–58.

Groom, R., Cushion, C.J. and Nelson, L.J., 2011, The delivery of video-based PA by England youth soccer coaches: Towards a grounded theory. *Journal of Applied Sport Psychology*, **23**(1), pp. 16–32.

Groom, R., Cushion, C.J. and Nelson, L.J., 2012, Analysing coach-athlete "talk in interaction" within the delivery of video-based performance feedback in elite youth soccer. *Qualitative Research in Sport, Exercise and Health*, doi:10.1080/2159676X.2012.693525.

Guadagnoli, M., Holcomb, W. and Davies, M., 2002, The efficacy of video feedback of learning the golf swing. *Journal of Sports Sciences*, 20, pp. 615–622.

Hammersley, M. and Atkinson, P., 1994, *Ethnography: Principles in Practice*, (London: Routledge).

Hodges, N.J. and Franks, I.M., 2002, Modelling coaching practice: The role of instruction and demonstration. *Journal of Sports Sciences*, 20, pp. 793–811.

Hughes, M. and Franks, I.M., 1997, *Notational Analysis of Sport*, (London: E & FN Spon).

Hughes, M.D. and Franks, I.M., 2005, Analysis of passing sequences, shots and goals in soccer. *Journal of Sports Sciences*, 23, pp. 509–514.

Hughes M. and Franks, I.M., 2008, *The Essentials of PA: An Introduction*. (London: Routledge).

James, N., Jones, P. and Mellalieu, S.D., 2004, Possession as a performance indicator in soccer as a function of successful and unsuccessful teams. *Journal of Sports Sciences*, 22, pp. 507–508.

Jenkins, R.E., Morgan, L. and O'Donoghue, P., 2007, A case study into the effectiveness of computerised match analysis and motivational videos within the coaching of a league netball team. *International Journal of Performance Analysis in Sport*, 7(2), pp. 59–80.

Lago, C., 2007, Are winners different from losers? Performance and chance in the FIFA World Cup Germany 2006. *International Journal of Performance Analysis in Sport*, 7(2), pp. 36–47.

Lyle, J., 2002, *Sports Coaching Concepts: A Framework for Coaches' Behaviour*, (London: Routledge).

Nash, C.S., Sproule, J. and Horton, P., 2008, Sport coaches' perceived role frames and philosophies. *International Journal of Sports Science and Coaching*, 3(4), pp. 539–553.

Potrac, P. and Jones, R.L., 2009, Micropolitical workings in semi-professional Football. *Sociology of Sport Journal*, 26, pp. 557–577.

Robertson, K., 1999, *Observation, Analysis and Video*, (Leeds: The National Coaching Foundation).

Stratton, G., Reilly, T., Williams, A.M. and Richardson, D., 2004, *Youth Soccer: From Science to Performance*, (London: Routledge).

Strauss, A. and Corbin, J., 1998, *Basics of Qualitative Research: Grounded Theory, Procedures and Techniques*, (Newbury Park, CA: Sage).

Tenga, A., Holme, I., Ronglan, L.T. and Bahr, R., 2010a, Effect of playing tactics on achieving score-box possessions in a random series of team possessions from Norwegian professional soccer matches. *Journal of Sports Sciences*, 28(3), pp. 245–255.

Tenga, A., Ronglan, L.T. and Bahr, R., 2010b, Measuring the effectiveness of offensive match-play in professional soccer. *European Journal of Sport Science*, 10(4), pp. 269–277.

Yin, R. K., 2003, *Case Study Research, 3rd edn.*, (London: Sage Publications).

CHAPTER 5

Behaviour of academy soccer coaches during training sessions

Ceri Bowley, Wes Bodden and Peter O'Donoghue

5.1 INTRODUCTION

Systems used to analyse coach behaviour have followed advances in multimedia technology (More, 2008). Instructional sessions delivered by coaches as well as behaviour during competition can be observed and analysed. Video analysis systems allow coaches to reflect on their behaviour in the same way that players can reflect on their performances using a combination of quantitative and qualitative information, much of which can be obtained from video footage.

Coaching involves a range of behaviours, activities, interactions and processes (Lyle, 2002). Different coaching styles are suggested as more effective in different situations (Cratty, 1983) and can vary between sessions delivered by the same coach (Donnelly and O'Donoghue, 2008). Coaching style is influenced by individual coach philosophy (Abraham and Collins, 1998; Jones *et al.*, 2002), the type of sport (Massey *et al.*, 2002), the gender of the athletes (Lacy and Goldston, 1990; Millard, 1996), age of the athletes (Lacy and Darst, 1985; Miller, 1992), level of the athletes (Erle, 1981; Serpa *et al.*, 1991; Jones *et al.*, 1995) as well as coaching context, e.g. whether a training session is being conducted or if a competition is taking place (Chaumeton and Duda, 1988; Wandzilak *et al.*, 1988).

The Arizona State University Observation Instrument (ASUOI) has been used to analyse coach behaviour for almost 30 years (Lacy and Darst, 1984; Côté *et al.*, 1995; Trudel *et al.*, 1996). The ASUOI quantifies two dimensions of coaching; behaviour type and use of an athlete's first name. Behaviour type is a categorical variable of 14 named behaviours which are shown in Table 5.1).

The behaviour of coaches of youth soccer squads has been analysed using the ASUOI (Cushion and Jones, 2001; Smith and Cushion, 2006). Smith and Cushion (2006) analysed 6 current academy soccer coaches with soccer coaching qualifications and at least 5 years coaching experience. Four of these coaches were with academies at English FA Premier League clubs while the other two were at English FA Championship clubs. They presented the relative frequency of ASUOI behaviours during sections of 4 matches for each of the coaches. The most frequent behaviours were silence on task (30.3 per cent), praise (17.7 per cent) and concurrent instruction (12.8 per cent). The most recent study comparing coach behaviour during training and competition was by Trudel *et al.* (1996). The study of behaviour during competition done by Smith and Cushion (2006) is recent enough to be considered as relevant. However, there is a need for more up-to-date data on academy coach behaviour during training sessions. Therefore, the purpose of the current investigation was to analyse the behaviour of coaches within soccer academies, comparing coaches with different qualifications.

5.2 METHOD

The coaching behaviour dimension of the Arizona State University Observation Instrument (ASUOI) was implemented in Focus X2 (Elite Sports Analysis, Delgaty Bay, Fife, UK). Inter-operator reliability was established using video footage for a single coaching session delivered by one of the participants. The kappa (κ) statistic was computed for the proportion of session time when the two operators agreed on the behaviour of the coach adjusted for the proportion of time they would be expected to agree by chance. This revealed a good strength of inter-operator agreement ($\kappa = 0.712$). Seven coaches from different academies were observed during three or four training sessions each with sessions lasting 40–93 minutes. There were two Union of European Football Associations (UEFA) 'A' licence coaches, three UEFA 'B' licence coaches and two UEFA 'C' licence coaches. The participants coached athletes of different ages ranging from under 9 years to under 16 years. The sessions were all academy sessions and had similar content and broad structure. The first section of the sessions had a higher technical focus, concentrating on individuals' technical development. Later sections were focussed more on tactical areas finishing with small sided games of between six- and eight-a-side.

The percentage of time spent performing each behaviour within each session was determined and then the mean for each coach was determined. A series of Kolmogorov-Smirnov tests revealed that the percentage of time spent performing each behaviour was normally distributed ($p > 0.05$) except concurrent instruction ($p = 0.041$), negative modelling ($p = 0.035$), talking to an assistant ($p = 0.005$) and un-codable ($p = 0.002$). Levene's test revealed homogeneity of variances between the three levels of coaches for the percentage of time spent performing each behaviour ($p > 0.05$) except concurrent instruction ($p < 0.001$) and negative modelling ($p < 0.001$). A series of one-way ANOVA tests were used to compare the three groups of coaches for each of the 10 behaviours that satisfied the assumptions of the test. Where a p value of less than 0.05 was found a significant effect of coach qualification was indicated. The other four behaviours were not compared using inferential statistics because the distribution-free Kruskal Wallis H test requires at least five members of each group being compared.

5.3 RESULTS

Table 5.1 summarises the profile of behaviour of the coaches during the sessions. There was no significant difference between coaches of different levels for the percentage of session time spent performing any of the behaviours ($p > 0.05$).

Table 5.1 Percentage of time spent performing each behaviour (mean ± SD).

Behaviour	Level of licence held by coach			P (ANOVA)
	A (n = 2)	B (n = 3)	C (n = 2)	
Concurrent instruction	7.7 ± 0.6	6.9 ± 0.6	9.0 ± 4.9	
Humour	0.6 ± 0.2	0.5 ± 0.7	0.4 ± 0.2	0.933
Hustle	1.2 ± 0.5	3.3 ± 1.3	2.5 ± 0.9	0.195
Management	9.0 ± 10.2	14.2 ± 11.4	12.8 ± 15.8	0.900
Negative modelling	0.1 ± 0.0	0.0 ± 0.0	0.1 ± 0.2	
Positive modelling	1.3 ± 0.4	1.8 ± 1.9	1.0 ± 1.1	0.868
Post-instruction	5.7 ± 3.0	4.3 ± 1.6	3.4 ± 1.1	0.560
Praise	7.0 ± 2.0	7.2 ± 3.0	6.6 ± 1.3	0.956
Pre-instruction	8.1 ± 2.1	12.5 ± 1.9	7.6 ± 3.7	0.167
Questioning	2.7 ± 0.8	4.1 ± 3.1	0.7 ± 0.6	0.348
Scold	0.3 ± 0.4	0.4 ± 0.4	0.5 ± 0.2	0.919
Silent monitoring	47.6 ± 5.1	40.6 ± 19.6	51.7 ± 15	0.753
Talk to assistant	0.8 ± 1.1	1.9 ± 2.4	0.1 ± 0.1	
Un-codable	7.9 ± 9.0	2.3 ± 1.1	3.7 ± 0.2	

5.4 DISCUSSION

The current investigation did not find any significant differences in the percentage of time spent performing different behaviours between the three groups of coaches. One explanation for this is that all of the coaches were academy level coaches and their behaviours were dictated by the requirements at these age groups rather than what the coach is qualified to do at other levels. Another explanation is that between coach variability within some levels exceeded differences between mean behaviours for coaches of different levels. For example, there is large variance for management with coefficients of variation for two of the groups exceeding 100 per cent. Similarly, the standard deviation for silent monitoring within two of the groups exceeded the difference between the means of the groups performing the least and the most silent monitoring within sessions. Some of the differences between coaches may have been caused by the age groups of the players being coached. Indeed, Lacy and Darst (1985) and Miller (1992) state that age of players has an influence on coach behaviour.

The most common individual behaviour observed was silent monitoring. Silent monitoring can be a deliberate coaching strategy (Miller, 1992; Massey *et al.*, 2002), providing the opportunity to observe and reflect before intervening. Silent monitoring has been used within cycles of observation and feedback (Harry and O'Donoghue, 2012). Silence was usually followed by feedback or concurrent cues and was central to how the coaches delivered information since over-talking can dilute the quality of communication between coach and players.

Overall, instruction made up 21.9 per cent of the sessions observed (9.8 per cent for pre-instruction, 7.7 per cent for concurrent instruction and 4.4 per cent for post-instruction). This is a much lower volume of instruction than Cushion and Jones (2001) found for youth soccer coaches, where 29.7 per cent of session time was spent providing concurrent instruction. It is possible that coaches in soccer academies have video feedback technology available that allows some instruction, particularly post-instruction, to be provided outside session time. Such technology may be used to a much greater extent in academies today than in 2001 or before when Cushion and Jones collected their data. Smith and Cushion (2006) stated that seven behaviours within the ASUOI were directly related to the instructional process; pre-instruction, concurrent instruction, post-instruction, questioning, physical assistance, positive modelling and negative modelling. These behaviours accounted for 26.2 per cent of session time in the current investigation. Despite the current investigation looking at training sessions and Smith and Cushion's (2006) study looking at games, there were many similarities in the findings. The two studies agreed that there was a greater amount of pre-instruction than post-instruction, praise was used much more than scolding and there was a very low use of modelling. Praise is important as it can increase the confidence of young players (Smith and Cushion, 2006). There are also differences between the current findings for coach behaviour during training sessions and Smith and Cushion's (2006) findings for coach behaviour during competitive games. The current investigation found a greater volume of management behaviours but lower use of hustle and concurrent instruction than Smith and Cushion (2006) found in games. These differences are explained by the differences between training sessions and competitive games. There were some limitations to the current investigation, particularly the fact that the coaches coached players of different age groups, some had an assistant while others didn't and all coaches were observed undertaking the sessions they had planned rather than having a common session plan for the purpose of the research. In conclusion, qualification level had no significant influence on the behaviour of academy soccer coaches.

5.5 REFERENCES

Abraham, A. and Collins, D., 1998, Examining and extending research in coach development. *Quest*, **50**, pp. 59–79.

Chaumeton, N. and Duda, J., 1988, Is it how you play the game or whether you win or lose? The effect of competitive level and situation on coaching behaviors. *Journal of Sport Behavior*, **11**, pp. 157–174.

Côté, J., Trudel, P., Baria, A. and Russell, S.J., 1995, The coaching model: A grounded assessment of expert gymnastic coach's knowledge. *Journal of Sport and Exercise Psychology*, **17**, pp. 1–17.

Cratty, B.J., 1983, *Psychology in Contemporary Sport*, (Englewood Cliffs, NJ: Prentice-Hall).

Cushion, C.J and Jones, R.L., 2001, A systematic observation of professional top-level youth soccer coaches. *Journal of Sport Behaviour*, **24**, pp. 354–365.

Donnelly, C. and O'Donoghue, P.G., 2008, Behaviour of netball coaches of different levels. In *Performance Analysis of Sport VIII*, edited by Hokelmann, A. and Brummond, M. (Aachen, Germany: Shaker-Verlag), pp. 743–749.

Erle, F.J., 1981, Leadership in competitive and recreational sport. Unpublished master's thesis, (London, Canada: University of Western Ontario).

Harry, L. and O'Donoghue, P.G., 2012, Temporal aspects of coach behaviour, *International Journal of Performance Analysis in Sport*, **12**(3), p. 756.

Jones, D.F., Housner, L.D. and Kornspan, A.S., 1995, A comparative analysis of expert and novice basketball coaches practice planning. *Applied Research in Coaching Athletics Annual*, **10**, pp. 201–226.

Jones, R.L., Armour, K.M. and Potrac, P., 2002, Understanding the coaching process: A framework for social analysis. *Quest*, **54**(1), pp. 186–199.

Lacy, A.C. and Darst, P.W., 1984, Evolution of a systematic observation system: The ASU coaching observation instrument. *Journal of Teaching in Physical Education*, **3**, pp. 59–66.

Lacy, A.C. and Darst, P.W., 1985, Systematic observation of behaviour of winning high school head football coaches. *Journal of Teaching in Physical Education*, **4**, pp. 256–270.

Lacy, A.C. and Goldston, P.D., 1990, Behaviour analysis of male and female coaches in high school girls' basketball. *Journal of Sport Behaviour*, **13**(1), pp. 29–39.

Lyle, J., 2002, *Sports Coaching Concepts: A Framework for Coaches' Behaviour*, (London: Routledge).

Massey, C., Maneval, L., Phillips, J., Vincent, J., White, G. and Zoeller, B., 2002, An analysis of teaching and coaching behaviours of elite strength and conditioning coaches. *Journal of Strength and Conditioning Research*, 16, pp. 456–460.

Millard, L., 1996, Differences in coaching behaviours of male and female high school soccer coaches. *Journal of Sport Behaviour*, **19**(1), pp. 19–31.

Miller, A.W., 1992, Systematic observation behaviour similarities of various youth sport soccer coaches. *Physical Educator*, **449**, pp. 136–143.

More, K. (2008) Notational analysis of coaching. In *The Essentials of Performance Analysis: An Introduction*, edited by Hughes, M.D. and Franks, I.M., (London: Routledge), pp. 264–276.

Serpa, S., Patco, V. and Santos, F., 1991, Leadership patterns in handball international competition. *International Journal of Sport Psychology*, **22**, pp. 78–89.

Smith, M. and Cushion, C.J., 2006, An investigation of the in-game behaviours of professional, top-level youth soccer coaches. *Journal of Sports Sciences*, **24**(2), pp. 355–366.

Trudel, P., Côté, J. and Bernard, D., 1996, Systematic observation of youth ice hockey coaches during games. *Journal of Sport Behaviour*, **19**, pp. 50–65.

Wandzilak, T., Ansorge C.J. and Potter, G., 1988, Comparison between selected practice and game behaviours of youth sport soccer coaches. *Journal of Sport Behaviour*, **11**, pp. 78–88.

Part 2

Soccer

CHAPTER 6

Influence of environmental temperature on home advantage in Qatari international soccer matches

Franck Brocherie, Olivier Girard,
Abdulaziz Farooq and Gregoire P. Millet

6.1 INTRODUCTION

Soccer matches are often played in challenging environmental conditions where the ambient temperature can exceed 30°C, possibly with a high relative humidity. Such environments are known to be detrimental to a player's performance as it poses severe challenges to thermoregulatory control (Mohr *et al.*, 2012; Racinais *et al.*, 2012). Recently, the difficulties of playing in high temperatures were well illustrated during the final match of the 2008 Beijing Olympic Games, where air temperatures on the field reached 42°C (Maughan *et al.*, 2010).

With the announcement of the 2022 soccer World Cup to be held in Qatar, some participating countries' medical and technical teams have expressed concerns regarding the adverse impact the heat may have upon their players' performance and health. The climate in Qatar is a hot, arid and dry desert climate with an annual average temperature above 18°C and is classified as BWh (i.e. B: arid, W: desert and h: hot arid) in the Köppen-Geiger classification (Peel *et al.*, 2007). As an example, the average temperature is 19°C ranging from 13°C to 22°C in the coolest month (i.e. January) while in the warmest month (i.e. July) the average is 37°C (range 34–41°C). According to Maughan *et al.* (2010), all players are affected by the environmental conditions, but players who are accustomed to living, training and competing in temperate climates are placed at a particular disadvantage when a game is played in hot and/or humid regions against a local team acclimatised to those conditions. Recently, Mohr *et al.* (2012) showed that heat stress lowers the total match distance and high intensity running, by comparing two experimental games of 90 min (i.e. played in temperate (~21°C) vs. hot ambient conditions (~43°C)) with Scandinavian elite male players.

Home advantage is a worldwide phenomenon in soccer (Pollard, 2006) where venue influences the outcome of matches but varies considerably between countries and over time. Whilst several explanations including crowd support, travel effects, familiarity with local playing conditions, territoriality, referee bias, special tactics, psychological factors and altitude have been proposed to account for this diversity (McSharry, 2007; Pollard, 2006), no dominant factor influencing home advantage has been isolated. It is likely that the individual factors interact with each other in a manner yet to be established, and that home advantage is the result of their combined effect (Pollard, 2006). To our knowledge, no study has yet focused on potential environmental temperature influence on the home advantage phenomenon.

Thus, the present study examined the influence of environmental temperature on the existence of home advantage for the male national soccer team of Qatar for the last 40 years. It was hypothesised that the higher local environmental temperature (and the larger difference with the opponent) would lead to greater evidence for Qatar home advantage.

6.2 METHOD

6.2.1 Quantification of variables and sources of data

Average air temperature (°C) of the month preceding the matches was collected both in Qatar and in all opponents' countries for three different venues: home (H, played in Qatar) away (A, played in the opponent's country) or neutral (N, played neither at H nor at A), and then were expressed as temperature difference between opponents ($\Delta T_{opponent}$). Temperatures on the day for all match venues were also collected in order to determine the temperature difference between Qatar and the venue (ΔT_{venue}). These variables are zero when both home and away teams have the same temperature, are positive when Qatar team is warmer and negative when the Qatar team is cooler. In order to consider the relative strength of the opposition, the Fédération Internationale de Football Association (FIFA) ranking for Qatar and all opponents was noted and expressed as the difference ($\Delta Rank$). Reliable estimates of home advantage were calculated as the number of matches won (W) or lost (L) expressed as a percentage of the total number of matches for all the FIFA international matches played by the Qatar soccer team. The difference between the goals scored and the goals conceded was also calculated.

Two websites were selected from which relevant information could be extracted for meaningful worldwide comparisons. Temperatures were obtained from 'Weather Underground' website (1995) which centralised climatic data from weather stations owned by government agencies referenced by the World Meteorological Organization (WMO; http://www.wmo.int/pages/index_fr.html). Match results were collected on the official website of FIFA (1994). The total number of matches was 252. All matches were FIFA-recognised Olympic and A-team full international matches including 150 friendly and 102 official matches.

6.2.2 Statistical analysis

All data were coded and analysed in Statistical Package for Social Sciences (SPSS 19.0). A binary variable was created as 'favourable outcome' to categorise win vs. draw and loss. Chi-square test was used to test the hypothesis of no association between two categorical variables. Q–Q plots were used to assess normality of $\Delta T_{\text{opponent}}$ and $\Delta Rank$. Student t-test and Mann-Whitney U-test as appropriate were used to compare means of continuous variables between binary match outcome variables. To determine factors associated with favourable outcome, multiple binary logistic regression analysis was performed and Odds ratios with 95 per cent CI were reported. On the other hand, multiple linear regression analysis was done to assess predictors for goal difference. A p-value <0.05 was considered as cut-off for significance.

6.3 RESULTS

When playing at home, Qatar recorded 61.7 per cent wins compared to 40 per cent when playing away or on neutral ground ($p \leq 0.002$). In addition, as expected, $\Delta Rank$ was strongly associated with favourable outcome ($p < 0.001$). Interestingly, $\Delta T_{\text{opponent}}$ was significantly lower (unfavourable outcome, $p = 0.016$) in matches that resulted in wins (mean $4.7 \pm 7.0°C$; median $4.0°C$) when compared to lost matches (mean $7.0 \pm 8.0°C$; median $5.5°C$). Univariate analysis demonstrated home advantage, $\Delta T_{\text{opponent}}$ and $\Delta Rank$ as potential factors for match outcome.

The binary logistic regression showed that after adjustment for $\Delta T_{\text{opponent}}$ and $\Delta Rank$, Qatar appears to be 4 times more likely to have favourable outcome (Odds Ratio = 4.13, 95 per cent CI (1.93; 8.84), $p < 0.001$) when playing at home. When playing against an opponent with one rank lower, the favourable outcome increased by 2 per cent (Odds Ratio = 0.98, 95 per cent CI (0.96; 0.98), $p < 0.001$) after correction for home advantage and $\Delta T_{\text{opponent}}$. However, when temperature difference between Qatar and its opponent increased by one degree, favourable outcome tends to decrease by 1 per cent (Odds Ratio = 1.05, 95 per cent CI (1.00; 1.10)). But this association was not significant ($p = 0.055$).

Table 6.1 shows the results of multiple linear regression considering goal difference (difference between goals scored and goals conceded) as dependent variables using three different models. Parameter estimates with 95 per cent CI are shown. Temperature difference (Model 1) is a significant explanatory variable when used independently. When home advantage and $\Delta Rank$ (Model 2) are added, the effect of $\Delta T_{\text{opponent}}$ disappeared. Best fit is obtained when using ΔT_{venue}, which probably better reflects the impact of temperature on the match. In this case (Model 3), temperature difference between Qatar and venue was a significant ($p = 0.04$) determinant of outcome for the international matches played by the Qatar national soccer team after adjusting for difference in ranking and home advantage.

Repartition of the goals difference related to ΔT_{venue} is presented in Figure 6.1. The scatterplot clearly indicated that most of the largest goal differences were recorded with temperature difference ranging from approximately -5 to $+5°C$. However, when ΔT_{venue} ranged from $+10$ to $+20°C$, the goal differences were smaller; suggesting that increased ΔT_{venue} has a negative impact on performance.

Table 6.1 Parameters and diagnostics for each model of the probability of win in international matches

Variable	Generalised linear models†		
	Model 1	**Model 2**	**Model 3**
Intercept	0.259	1.739	2.061
$\Delta T_{opponent}$	−0.031* (−0.058; −0.004)	−0.017 (−0.043; 0.010)	
Home advantage		−0.958** (−1.374; −0.542)	−0.798** (−1.220; −0.376)
$\Delta Rank$		0.025** (0.020; 0.030)	0.025** (0.020; 0.030)
ΔT_{venue}			−0.037* (−0.071; −0.002)
R-squared	0.15	0.34	0.35
Adjusted Squared	0.12	0.33	0.34

† Model 1 = Intercept and temperature difference. Model 2 = Intercept, monthly temperature difference, home advantage and ranking difference. Model 3 = Intercept, home advantage, ranking difference and venue temperature difference. * P < 0.05 and ** P < 0.001.

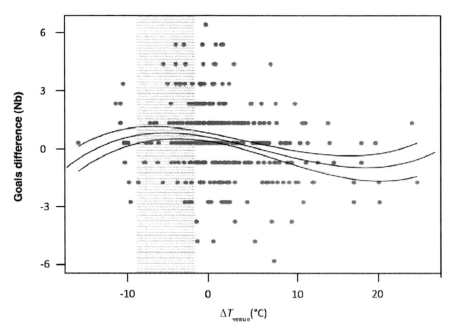

Figure 6.1 Effect of temperature difference between Qatar and match venue (ΔT_{venue}) on the repartition of goal difference (trend line with 95 per cent CI and optimal ΔT_{venue} range shown)

6.4 DISCUSSION

The results of this study suggest the existence of home advantage for the Qatar national soccer team. Favourable outcome was more likely when playing against a lower ranked team. In addition, the advantage when playing at higher temperature is to be expected given the environmental acclimatisation difference between Qatar and its opponents. However, the temperature difference between Qatar and its opponents in international soccer matches appears to significantly affect the outcome of matches. Thus, although not significant but very close (p = 0.055), an increasing temperature difference tends to impair the outcome for Qatar. This surprising result suggests that even accustomed to living, training and playing in hot condition, Qatari players also suffer from limited performance while playing in hot temperature. Maughan *et al.* (2010) already mentioned that severe heat stress is detrimental for all players' performance, whatever the acclimatisation status.

To further investigate impact of temperature, we calculated the temperature difference (ΔT_{venue}) between Qatar and the match's venue, in addition to the primary temperature variable ($\Delta T_{opponent}$). Mixed Model 3 clearly indicated that ΔT_{venue} is a better determinant for the goals difference during international matches played by the Qatar national soccer team. Based on this model, scatterplots were smoothed using a polynomial regression in order to reduce data fluctuation (Figure 6.1). The curve shape indicates that temperature difference between Qatar and its match venue had a significant negative impact on goal difference when it increased above a certain threshold (i.e. $\Delta T_{venue} \pm 10°C$) and confirms our findings previously mentioned. However, our results also indicate that goal difference is higher in a particular range of ΔT_{venue} which could be defined as optimal (Figure 6.1, tinted area) and could be the consequence of better exercise-heat acclimatisation for Qatari players than their opponents when temperature is hot but not extreme. It is important to note that all Qatari national team players are playing in their home country during the full season and are thus supposed to be well accustomed when they are exposed in countries with similar challenging climate. Similarly to runners, African and Middle East players (who most of them have African roots, e.g. Sudan, Nigeria) might have an advantage over Caucasian players. They might perform better in warm environments. Indeed, those athletes are usually thinner than Caucasians (smaller size and body mass index), producing less heat with lower rates of heat storage (Marino *et al.*, 2000). However, the comparison of the anthropometric characteristics of the different teams is required to confirm these assumptions.

The effect of temperature on soccer performance is complex to quantify, as many factors influence the outcome of a soccer match. By using a large soccer database, containing results of matches played at multiple environmental temperatures over a 40-year period, we attempted to reduce the effect of these factors. However, as Qatar did not play with better-ranked opponents during the hottest periods, more data from other countries with similar challenging environment are therefore needed. In addition, there are still other effects which could affect performance. Additional factors such as humidity, season and crowd support could influence the observations done in our sample.

In summary, this study shows a home advantage in Qatar which could be influenced by the temperature. Even if its proportion is still unclear, it is reasonable to postulate that exercise-heat acclimatisation can have an ergogenic effect (Racinais *et al.*, 2012) to limit the reduction in match running performance in hot (Sunderland *et al.*, 2008) but not extreme conditions. Thus, strategy to cope with playing on heat (for review, see Maughan *et al.*, 2010), will be an important component of the teams' preparation in perspective of the FIFA World Cup 2022.

6.5 REFERENCES

FIFA official website, 1994, available at http://www.fifa.com/worldfootball/statisticsandrecords/headtohead/index.html (accessed 22 February 2012).

Marino, F.E., Mbambo, Z., Kortekaas, E., Wilson, G., Lambert, M.I., Noakes, T.D. and Dennis, S.C., 2000, Advantages of smaller body mass during distance running in warm, humid environments. *Pflugers Archiv*, **441**, pp. 359–367.

Maughan, R.J., Shirreffs, S.M., Ozgunen, K.T., Kurdak, S.S., Ersoz, G., Binnet, M.S. and Dvorak J., 2010, Living, training and playing in the heat: Challenges to the football player and strategies for coping with environmental extremes. *Scandinavian Journal of Medicine and Science in Sports*, **20** (Suppl. 3), pp. 117–124.

McSharry, P.E., 2007, Effect of altitude on physiological performance: A statistical analysis using results of international football games. *British Medical Journal*, **335**, pp. 1278–1281.

Mohr, M., Nybo, L., Grantham, J. and Racinais, S., 2012, Physiological responses and physical performance during football in the heat. *PLoS One*, 7, p. e39202.

Peel, M.C., Finlayson, B.L. and McMahon, T.A., 2007, Updated world map of the Köppen-Geiger climate classification. *Hydrology and Earth System Sciences*, **11**, pp. 1633–1644.

Pollard R., 2006, Worldwide regional variations in home advantage in association football. *Journal of Sports Sciences*, **24**, pp. 231–240.

Racinais, S., Mohr, M., Buchheit, M., Voss, S.C., Gaoua, N., Grantham, J. and Nybo, L., 2012, Individual responses to short-term heat acclimatisation as predictors of football performance in a hot, dry environment. *British Journal of Sports Medicine*. **46**, pp. 810–815.

Sunderland, C., Morris, J.G. and Nevill, M.E., 2008, A heat acclimation protocol for team sports. *British Journal of Sports Medicine*, **42**, pp. 327–333.

Weather Underground Website, 1995, Internet weather service. Available at http://www.wunderground.com/history/ (accessed 22 February 2012).

CHAPTER 7

First goal and home advantage
at different levels of play
in professional soccer

Albin Tenga

7.1 INTRODUCTION

Soccer teams in balanced competitions achieving better results when playing at home than away from home, is a consistent finding. The mean home winning advantages of up to over 60 per cent have been reported to exist in international soccer (Pollard, 1986, 2006a). In addition, soccer's home advantage is known to differ according to long-term trends (Pollard and Pollard, 2005) and geographical variation (Pollard, 2006b). However, despite much research, the causes of home advantage are not yet fully understood. Different factors such as crowd support, familiarity, territoriality and special playing tactics (Nevill *et al.*, 2002; Pollard, 1986, 2006b; Tenga *et al.*, 2010) have been considered, but studies have so far failed to isolate a dominant factor explaining the home advantage in soccer. Pollard (2006a) suggested that the complexity of this phenomenon is due to the fact that many factors are associated with home advantage in soccer and that some of these factors seem to interact with each other.

Understanding the causes of home advantage is central to advancing knowledge, particularly regarding its prediction and intervention. This includes information on how home advantage occurs in soccer (i.e. mechanisms of home advantage). As a basis for intervention, detailed mechanisms of home advantage must be revealed in order to understand the causes of home advantage. At the moment, intervention studies on home advantage in soccer are lacking in the literature and one likely reason is the paucity of the evidence about the mechanisms of home advantage in soccer at different levels of play. Therefore, further knowledge on the mechanisms that lead to home advantage in soccer is needed. For example, in recent studies on NBA basketball (Jones, 2007) and NHL hockey (Jones, 2009) home advantage was revealed to be frontloaded, i.e. home advantage accumulated earlier rather than later on in the game. This is contrary to the current theories of home advantage which imply that home advantage would be mostly accumulated late in the game when the support from the home crowd is usually most intense at the same time the away team assumed to be more fatigued.

Psychological momentum is an alternative view advanced to explain a mechanism leading to high likelihood of winning a sport contest (Courneya,

1990). According to this view, it is a state of mind that makes winning more probable by mediating between early success in a game and advantage in subsequent play. For example, Courneya (1990) suggested that, regardless of home or away team, scoring first should serve as a strong predictor of winning the game through better performance in subsequent play. Apparently, this idea of better subsequent performance (e.g. more subsequent goals) from early success in a match (e.g. first scoring) needs support from the empirical evidence in order to qualify as a plausible mechanism behind high probabilities of winning matches.

Considering that home advantage is most pronounced in soccer among other team sports, it is therefore interesting to explore how front loadedness manifests itself in such a team sport. Thus, the purpose of the present study was to investigate whether home advantage in professional soccer is also frontloaded. Further, the effect of different levels of play and the hypothesis of psychological momentum will also be examined.

7.2 METHODS

The internet-based data on all goals scored in seasons 2009 (697) and 2010 (731) of Norwegian top professional league (NTL) and in seasons 2008/09 (942) and 2009/10 (1,053) of English Premier League (EPL) were used. Data were collected from the respective official soccer-league websites www.fotball.no and www.premierleague.com and reconfirmed in a commercial website www.altomfotball.no.

Home advantage may be expressed as home win percentage (HWP) using points or matches won, or home goal percentage (HGP) using goals scored (Pollard, 1986; Tenga *et al.*, 2010). To match the purpose of the present study, home advantage was calculated using goals scored and was expressed as home goal percentage (HGP). Home advantage was therefore defined as the proportion of goals scored at home compared to the proportion of goals scored away. Note that to obtain a true value of home advantage based on goals scored, home goal percentage for complete matches was calculated using goals scored from decided matches only. This means home advantage at the end of the match included goals from those matches won or lost by the home team and that all goals from matches ended up with a draw result were excluded.

Home advantage will be considered frontloaded if home advantage in first goals is larger than home advantage in subsequent goals and amounts to a large part of home advantage in complete matches (Jones, 2009). As for the hypothesis of psychological momentum, to be accepted or rejected will depend on whether or not scoring first led to more subsequent goals for home team as well as away team. The significance of the difference between two independent proportions was tested by a chi-square analysis. An alpha value of < 0.05 was used in all tests.

7.3 RESULTS AND DISCUSSION

A total of 1428 goals from NTL and 1995 goals from EPL were included in the present study. Of them, 852 (59.7 per cent) from NTL and 1177 (59.0 per cent) from EPL were scored at home. Further, 453 (31.7 per cent) goals from NTL and 686 (34.4 per cent) goals from EPL were registered as first goals, whereas 975 (68.3 per cent) goals from NTL and 1,309 (65.6 per cent) goals from EPL as subsequent goals. The distribution of first goals and subsequent goals scored in different 15-minute match periods throughout the match show similar patterns between the two levels of play. Nearly 80 per cent of all first goals were scored within the first half, while over 70 per cent of all subsequent goals were scored within the second half in both NTL and EPL.

The proportion of first goals scored at home (range = 58.9 per cent in EPL season 2008/09 to 61.6 per cent in NTL season 2010) was higher (P < 0.001) than those scored away in all four seasons in the two levels of play studied. The proportion of first goals scored at home (mean = 60.7 per cent in NTL; mean = 59.6 per cent in EPL) was consistently larger than the proportion of subsequent goals scored at home (mean = 59.2 per cent in NTL; mean = 58.7 per cent in EPL), but the difference was not significant (Table 7.1). In other words, home advantage in first goals was larger than home advantage in subsequent goals.

Table 7.1 Number of first goals (n = 453 in NTL; n = 686 in EPL) and subsequent goals (n = 975 in NTL; n = 1,309 in EPL) scored by home and away teams in the two seasons of Norwegian top level (NTL) (N = 1,428) and English Premier League (EPL) (N = 1,995)

Variable	NTL				EPL			
	Home team	Away team	HGP	P*	Home team	Away team	HGP	P*
First	275	178	60.7	0.602	409	277	59.6	0.702
Subsequent	577	398	59.2		768	541	58.7	

*Fisher's Exact Test.

Table 7.2 shows that the proportion of goals from all decided matches scored at home (mean = 62.4 per cent in NTL; mean = 60.9 per cent in EPL) was larger than those scored away. This means home advantage at the end of the match, i.e. in complete matches, was larger than home advantage in first goals in both NTL and EPL. These values of HGP are similar to those reported in previous studies for these two levels of play (Tenga *et al.*, 2010; Boyko *et al.*, 2007).

It can therefore be concluded that home advantage in professional soccer is heavily frontloaded, as home advantage in first goals comprises of over 85 per cent of the home advantage in complete matches. A contribution of home advantage in first goals to the home advantage at the end of the match was somewhat larger in EPL (88.5 per cent) compared to NTL (86.6 per cent). This difference is more attributed to the relatively small value of home advantage in complete matches rather than large value of home advantage in first goals in EPL.

Table 7.2 Number of goals scored by home and away teams in all decided matches in each of the four seasons of Norwegian top level (NTL) and English Premier League (EPL)

Season	N*	Home goals	Away goals	HGP	Season	N*	Home goals	Away goals	HGP
NTL					EPL				
2010	595	375	220	63.0	2009/10	871	554	317	63.6
2009	529	326	203	61.6	2008/09	780	451	329	57.8
Total	1124	701	423	62.4	Total	1651	1005	646	60.9

*Goals from matches with draw results are not included.

Lower values of frontloadedness (60 per cent and 50 per cent) than the current result were reported in NBA basketball (Jones, 2007) and NHL hockey (Jones, 2009), respectively.

The hypothesis of psychological momentum was rejected in both NTL and EPL. A similar result was found in NHL hockey (Jones, 2009). That means no evidence was found across all teams to support the idea that scoring first gives a team an advantage in subsequent play. Only home teams scored more subsequent goals when they scored first (462 goals in NTL; 496 goals in EPL) than when the away teams scored first (115 goals in NTL; 272 goals in EPL) (Table 7.3). The away teams scored fewer subsequent goals when they scored first (154 goals in NTL; 235 goals in EPL) than when the home teams scored first (244 goals in NTL; 306 goals in EPL) (Table 7.3).

Table 7.3 Number and percentage of subsequent goals scored when home team (n = 706 in NTL; n = 802 in EPL) and away team (n = 269 in NTL; n = 507 in EPL) scored first in the two seasons of Norwegian top level (NTL) (N = 975) and English Premier League (EPL) (N = 1,309)

Variable	Home team (%)	Away team (%)	P*	Home team (%)	Away team (%)	P*
	NTL			EPL		
Home first goal	462 (65.4)	244 (34.6)	<0.001	496 (61.9)	306 (38.2)	0.004
Away first goal	115 (42.8)	154 (57.2)		272 (53.6)	235 (46.4)	

*Fisher's Exact Test.

Home teams in both NTL (65.4 per cent) and EPL (61.9 per cent) scored subsequent goals in higher percentages of attempts (P < 0.001 and P = 0.004) when they scored a first goal than when away teams scored first (NTL = 42.8 per cent; EPL = 53.6 per cent) (Table 7.3).

The findings of the present study may have some practical implications for soccer teams seeking to take advantage of playing at home. As they prepare to play at home, soccer coaches and players should be aware that ideally a home team should score first. This is because if it allows the away team to score first, the percentage for them to score drops markedly from the advantage it had when the match started (mean = 62 per cent in NTL; mean = 61 per cent in EPL) to about 43 per cent in NTL and 54 per cent in EPL.

7.4 CONCLUSION

Home advantage in professional soccer was found to be heavily frontloaded, regardless of the level of play. In NTL (86.6 per cent) and EPL (88.5 per cent) the home advantage in first goals comprises of over 85 per cent of home advantage in complete matches. Home teams, but not away teams, scored more subsequent goals after they had scored a first goal compared to when the opponents scored first. In fact, the percentage of scoring a subsequent goal for a home team increased by 22 per cent in NTL and 8 per cent in EPL when they scored a first goal (NTL = 65 per cent; EPL = 62 per cent) compared to when the away team scored first (NTL = 43 per cent; EPL = 54 per cent). That home advantage in soccer was found to be not only a matter of playing at home but also about performing well early in a match (i.e. scoring a first goal), may be considered as a contribution to the search for the plausible mechanisms of home advantage.

7.5 REFERENCES

Boyko, R.H., Boyko, A.R. and Boyko, M.G., 2007, Referee bias contributes to home advantage in English premiership football. *Journal of Sports Sciences*, **25**, pp. 1185–1194.

Courneya, K.S., 1990, Importance of game location and scoring first in college baseball. *Perceptual and Motor Skills*, **71**, pp. 624–626.

Nevill, A.M., Balmer, N. and Williams, A.M., 2002, The influence of crowd noise and experience upon refereeing decisions in football. *Psychology of Sport and Exercise*, **3**, pp. 261–272.

Jones, M., 2007, Home advantage in the NBA as a game-long process. *Journal of Quantitative Analysis in Sports*, **3**, pp. 1–14.

Jones, M., 2009, Scoring first and home advantage in the NHL. *International Journal of Performance Analysis of Sport*, **9**, pp. 320–331.

Pollard, R., 1986, Home advantage in soccer: A retrospective analysis. *Journal of Sports Sciences*, **4**, pp. 237–248.

Pollard, R., 2006a, Home advantage in soccer: Variations in its magnitude and a literature review of the inter-related factors associated with its existence. *Journal of Sport Behavior*, **29**, pp. 169–189.

Pollard, R., 2006b, Worldwide regional variations in home advantage in association football. *Journal of Sports Sciences*, **24**, pp. 231–240.

Pollard, R. and Pollard, G., 2005, Long-term trends in home advantage in professional team sports in North America and England (1876–2003). *Journal of Sports Sciences*, **23**, pp. 337–350.

Tenga, A., Holme, I., Ronglan, L.T. and Bahr, R., 2010, Effects of match location on playing tactics for goal scoring in Norwegian professional soccer. *Journal of Sport Behavior*, **33**, pp. 89–108.

CHAPTER 8

Home advantage in derby and non-derby matches of the Premier Brazilian National Football League, played from 2007 to 2011 seasons

Anna Volossovitch, Jackson Cruz, António Paulo Ferreira and Ana Isabel Carita

8.1 INTRODUCTION

Home advantage is used as a term that describes the superior performance of teams playing at home comparatively to away teams. This phenomenon has been widely studied, particularly, in association football (Pollard, 1986; Clarke and Norman, 1995; Jacklin, 2005; Boyko *et al.*, 2007) and it has been explained by numerous factors related to game location (crowd and travel effect, familiarity), physiological states of players, coaches and referees, etc. (Carron *et al.*, 2005). However, the studies looking for cause-and-effect relationship did not provide a clear insight into a possible contribution of each of these factors on the team's home and away results.

Using multiple regression to examine the travel-related factors on the home advantage, Courneya and Carron (1991) and Pace and Carron (1992) verified only a small association between distance travelled and winning percentage of away teams in baseball and ice hockey, respectively. In turn, Brown *et al.* (2002) demonstrated that an increase in distance travelled was positively related to goals conceded and negatively with goals scores by visiting teams in association football.

Findings concerning the influence of crowd support on the home team's performance are not conclusive. Pollard (1986) and Clarke and Norman (1995) did not identify a significant relationship between crowd support and game outcome in the English Football Leagues. Likewise in ice hockey, Agnew and Carron (1994) did not find any significant effect of crowd size on the home team's performance, but registered a small positive effect of crowd density. At the same time, the results of Nevill *et al.* (1996) and Downward and Jones (2007) provided evidence that home advantage is significantly related to the game attendance until the crowd reaches a certain size.

To verify whether home game attendance influences the outcome of home teams, van de Ven (2011) compared the crowd effect at home match results in normal games played without attendance and in same-stadium derbies (games played between two local teams). In these latter matches the home team has always the greater crowd support given that they sell the tickets. No overall effect of crowd size on the home match outcomes was reported in the study. However, some aspects of the game, such as the referees' decisions that favoured the home team, seem to be influenced by match attendance. The author concluded that a crowd support is not necessary for the home advantage occurrence.

Although the matches played between local rivals generate great interest due to their large uncertainness, the study of van de Ven (2011) is one of very few that analysed teams' performances in derbies. To better understand how game location influences the teams' performance, it seems to be interesting to compare home advantage in derbies and non-derbies. In order to be plausible, this comparison should take into account the quality of teams, because a stronger team playing away may be expected to beat a weaker team playing at home.

Focusing on Brazilian professional football, the present study aimed 1) to assess home advantage effect on teams' performance in derby and non-derby matches and 2) to analyse the association between contextual variables and performance indicators of home and away teams in derby and non-derby matches. The match was considered to be a derby, when a game was played between two local teams without distinction between same-stadium and different-stadium derbies.

8.2 METHODS

The sample consisted of 1706 matches (111 derbies and 1595 non-derbies) of the Premier Brazilian National Football League, played in five seasons from 2007 to 2011. Data was collected from the www.ogol.com.br and www.cbf.com.br websites. In each match, the following teams' performance indicators were recorded: 1) match outcome; 2) goals scored; 3) goals conceded; and 4) yellow cards awarded. The context of each match was characterized by quality of opposition, game attendance and distance travelled by the visiting team (for non-derbies). The quality of opposition was determined by the difference between the latest rankings (RD) of the considered team and the opponent. A k-means cluster analysis was performed to identify a cut-off value of RD and classify the quality of opposition into two groups. The same method was used to classify the game attendance into three groups and distance travelled by visiting team into four groups (Table 8.1).

Home advantage has been quantified as percentage of games won at home and played under a balanced home and away schedule. To assess the existence of home advantage, the mean of home advantage values for five seasons was compared with a null value of 50 per cent (Gomez *et al.*, 2011) using a one-sample t-test. The independent-samples t-test was used to compare the magnitude of home advantage in derby and non-derby matches. Effect size (ES) was calculated using Cohen's d statistic. Pearson's chi-square analysis was performed to examine the home advantage effect in different competition contexts.

Table 8.1 Classes of contextual variables and performance indicators used in the study

Contextual variables	Classes
Quality of opposition	Better positioned opposite team (RD 1 to 19), worse positioned team (RD –19 to –1).
Game attendance	Less or equal to 12,906, from 12,915 to 26,084, more than 26,149.
Distance travelled	Less or equal to 800 km, from 801 to 1,707 km, from 1,708 to 2,678 km, more than 2,678.
Performance indicators	**Classes**
Match outcome	Win, draw, lost.
Goals scored	Less than 2, more than 2.
Goals conceded	Less than 2, more than 2.
Yellow cards	Less than 3, from 3 to 4, more than 4.

8.3 RESULTS

The results confirmed a slight, but significant ($p < 0.001$), home advantage effect in the Brazilian Professional Football League. Across the five-season period, the home teams won 51 per cent of matches. The home advantage was not consistent through the five seasons, varying from 54.6 per cent in 2008 to 47.1 per cent in 2010 season. The comparative analysis of home advantage in derbies and non-derbies, played from 2007 to 2011, has clearly pointed out the decreasing of home advantage magnitude in derbies comparatively to non-derbies ($p < 0.001$; ES = 5.5); see Table 8.2.

Chi-square tests have not revealed any significant association between contextual variables and performance indicators neither for home nor for away teams in derbies (Table 8.3). For non-derbies a significant interaction was found only between the game attendance and teams' performance.

Table 8.2 Home advantage in derby and non-derby matches of the Premier Brazilian National League (2007 to 2011)

	No. of matches	2007	2008	2009	2010	2011	Total
Derby	111	30.8	23.1	35.0	26.3	35.0	30.0
Non-derby	1,595	51.9	56.9	52	48.5	52.9	52.4
All matches	1,706	50.4	54.6	51.1	47.1	51.5	51.0

Table 8.3 Chi-square values for performance indicators and contextual variables of home and away teams in derbies and non-derbies

	Performance indicators	Quality of opposition		Game attendance		Distance travelled	
		Home	Away	Home	Away	Home	Away
Derby	Match outcome	0.33	3.233	1.900	1.900	-	-
	Goals scored	0.756	0.805	2.673	0.83	-	-
	Goals conceded	0.467	1.644	0.303	3.568	-	-
	Yellow cards	0.129	3.946	4.725	5.417	-	-
Non-derby	Match outcome	1.851	0.965	**10.189***	**9.719***	2.070	2.162
	Goals scored	0.790	0.194	0.855	9.532*	4.285	5.402
	Goals conceded	0.693	0.693	**9.445***	0.955	5.251	3.800
	Yellow cards	1.795	1.795	6.021	**16.658****	8.811	5.650

**p < 0.01; * p < 0.05.

Table 8.4 Significant adjusted standardized residuals (above 1.96) for game attendance and performance indicators of home and away teams in non-derbies

Performance indicators		Game attendance					
		Less than 12,906		12,915 to 26,084		More than 26,149	
		Home	Away	Home	Away	Home	Away
Match outcome	Lost	2.2	−2.8	-	-	-	2.1
	Draw	-	-	-	-	-	-
	Win	−2.9	2.1	-	-	-	-
Goals scores	<2	-	−2.9	-	-	-	-
	2-3	-	2.4	-	-	-	-
	>3	-	-	-	-	-	-
Goals conceded	<2	−2.9	-	2.0	-	-	-
	2-3	2.4	-	-	-	-	-
	>3	-	-	-	-	-	-
Yellow cards	<3	-	2.0	-	-	-	−3.0
	3-4	-	−3.0	-	-	-	3.4
	>4	-	-	-	-	-	-

The analysis of adjusted standardized residuals, presented in Table 8.4, showed that small crowd size did not favour the home match result in non-derbies. There was a significant positive association between the small crowd size and lost matches at home, as well as a negative association between the small crowd size and won matches on the road. In matches with small crowd size, home teams conceded significantly more goals.

For away teams, the results were opposite. Playing away in non-derbies with large game attendance, teams lost significantly more matches, but scored more goals in matches with small game attendance. A significant positive association was found between the crowd size and the number of yellow cards awarded to the away teams in non-derbies (Table 8.4). In matches with large game attendances, referees' awarded significantly more yellow cards against the away team.

8.4 DISCUSSION AND CONCLUSION

The home advantage in matches of the Brazilian National Football League, quantified as a home winning percentage (excluding drawn games from consideration), was higher than registered in English football (Jacklin, 2005). This finding is in line with results of Pollard *et al.* (2008), analysing home advantage in Brazilian football for five seasons from 2003 to 2007 and concluded that it was higher than in the major football leagues of Europe. This difference in home advantage magnitude was explained by the large geographical size of Brazil that could intensify the effect of travel factors and climate influences. The significant difference between home win percentages in derbies and non-derbies, observed in our study, seems to corroborate this conclusion.

The analysis of quality of opposition and game attendance on performance indicator values of home and away teams in derbies did not identify any significant interaction. These results might be explained by small ranking differences between the opposing teams in Brazilian derbies, as far as by the fact that five teams share the same home stadium (Botafogo, Flamengo and Fluminence from Rio de Janeiro, as well as Atlético Mineiro and Cruseiro from Belo Horizonte). Similar findings were reported by van de Ven (2011), who compared the home advantage in Italian same-stadium derbies with home advantage in non-derbies, where teams played against equal quality opponents. No home advantage was observed in matches where away teams were as familiar with the stadium as the home team was, even when faced with the large opponent crowd support.

However, some studies supported the need to consider the team's ability in home advantage assessment (Nevill and Holder, 1999; Pollard *et.al.,* 2008), our data suggests no significant association between quality of opposition and match outcome, as well as other performance indicators of home and away teams in non-derbies. These findings could be explained by two main reasons: 1) the weak differentiating power of quality of the opposition variable that included only two classes and 2) the way of assessment of home and away teams' performances applied to whole competitions, rather than to individual teams. Problems with this measure were discussed in the studies of Clarke (2005) and Pollard *et al.* (2008). It seems reasonable to justify the same cause for the absence of a significant interaction between distance travelled and away teams' performances in non-derbies. Therefore, further research should identify home advantage for individual teams taking into account team ability for quality of opposition.

Findings of this study provide some evidence that game attendance is significantly associated to teams' performances in non-derbies of the Brazilian National Football League, contributing to home advantage. According to our results, which support the conclusions of Nevill *et al.* (1996), small crowd size favours the performance of the visiting team, while the large crowd size is positively associated with better performances for home teams. The results also suggest that crowd size influences the referees' decisions related to awarded yellow cards, as already shown by Nevill *et al.* (2002), Boyko *et al.* (2007) and Downward and Jones (2007). A higher number of yellow cards awarded against visiting teams in matches with large game attendance confirms that referees' decisions are influenced by the presence of fans and crowd noise (e.g., Unkelbach and Memmert, 2010) and in turn may amplify home advantage (e.g., Boyko *et al.,* 2007). To better understand the home advantage phenomenon, it is necessary to assess the individual teams' home and away performances in relation to factors that influence the context of the match. Particular attention should be given to the different aspects of game attendance effect (noise, size and density). Further research needs to use complex and more accurate methods with recourse to continuous, rather than categorical data.

8.5 REFERENCES

Agnew, G.A. and Carron, A.V., 1994, Crowd effects and the home advantage. *International Journal of Sport Psychology*, **25**, pp. 53–62.
Boyko, R.H., Boyko, A.R. and Boyko, M.G., 2007, Referee bias contributes to home advantage in English Premiership football. *Journal of Sports Sciences*, **25**, pp. 1185–1194.
Brown, T.D., Van Raalte, J.L., Brewer, B.W., Winter, C.R., Cornelius, A.E. and Andersen, M.B., 2002, World Cup Soccer home advantage. *Journal of Sport Behavior*, **25**, pp. 134–144.
Carron. A.V., Loughhead. T.M. and Bray. S., 2005, The home advantage in sport competitions: Courneya and Carron's (1992) conceptual framework a decade later. *Journal of Sports Sciences*. **23**, pp. 395–407.
Clarke, S.R., 2005, Home advantage in the Australian Football League. *Journal of Sports Sciences*, **23**, pp. 375–385.
Clarke, S.R. and Norman, J.M., 1995, Home ground advantage of individual clubs in English soccer. *Statistician*, **44**, pp. 509–521.
Courneya K.S. and Carron, A.V., 1991, Effects of travel and length of home stand/road trip on the home advantage. *Journal of Sport Exercise and Psychology*. **13**, pp. 42–49.
Downward, P. and Jones, M., 2007, Effects of crowd size on referee decisions: Analysis of the FA Cup. *Journal of Sports Sciences*, **25**, pp. 1541–1545.
Gomez, M.A., Pollard, R. and Luis-Pascual, J.C., 2011, Comparison of the home advantage in nine different professional team sports in Spain. *Perceptual and Motor Skills*, **113**, pp. 150–156.

Jacklin, P.B., 2005, Temporal changes in home advantage in English football since the Second World War: What explains improved away performance? *Journal of Sports Sciences*, **23**, pp. 669–679.

Nevill, A.M. and Holder, R.L., 1999, Home advantage in sport: An overview of studies on the advantage of playing at home. *Sports Medicine*, **28**, pp. 221–236.

Nevill, A.M., Newell, S.M. and Gale, S., 1996, Factors associated with home advantage in English and Scottish soccer matches. *Journal of Sports Sciences*, **14**, pp. 181–186.

Nevill, A.M., Balmer, N.J. and Williams, A.M., 2002, The influence of crowd noise and experience upon refereeing decisions in football. *Psychology of Sport and Exercise*, **3**, pp. 261–272.

Pace A. and Carron, A.V., 1992, Travel and the home advantage. *Canadian Journal of Sport Sciences*, **17**, pp. 60–64.

Pollard, R., 1986, Home advantage in soccer: A retrospective analysis, *Journal of Sports Sciences*, **4**, pp. 237–248.

Pollard. R., Silva. C.D. and Medeiros. N.C., 2008, Home advantage in football in Brazil: Differences between teams and the effects of distance traveled. *The Brazilian Journal of Soccer Science*, **1**, pp. 3–10.

Unkelbach, C. and Memmert, D., 2010, Crowd noise as a cue in referee decisions contributes to the home advantage. *Journal of Sport and Exercise Psychology*, **32**, pp. 483–498.

van de Ven. N., 2011, Supporters are not necessary for the home advantage: Evidence from same-stadium derbies and games without an audience. *Journal of Applied Social Psychology*, **41**, pp. 2785–2792.

CHAPTER 9

Regular patterns of play in the counter-attack of the FC Barcelona and Manchester United football teams

Hugo Sarmento, António Barbosa, Maria T. Anguera,
Jorge Campaniço and José Leitão

9.1 INTRODUCTION

Traditionally, the frequency of occurrence of events (e.g., number of passes made in a certain area of the field or how many times a team committed an error) have been used as indicators of performance. Studies based on the analysis of frequency of certain performance parameters provide important information for coaches and athletes, enabling advances in training processes. However, the game of football is characterized by great complexity that makes it difficult to objectify its observation and analysis.

The expression "playing style" is now commonly used by the fans, coaches and in academic settings. However, this is a complex concept that is influenced by many factors, like the strategy or philosophy of the playing style (i.e., a plan of how a team should play), the tradition, identity and history of the club, as well as the specific environment that characterizes the game (e.g., quality of opposition, match status). Determining which style of play is more effective has long been disputed by soccer performance analysts including match-performance researchers. Initially the published data advocated a direct approach to goal (Reep and Benjamin, 1968) which has created much debate and rebuttal for those who suggest possession as a key indicator of success (Hughes and Franks, 2005).

Trying to predict future performance on the basis of previous performances is an important goal for notation analysts. Typically, the basis for any prediction model is that performance is repeatable, to some degree. In other words events that have previously occurred will occur again in some predictable manner. This type of prediction is based on the principle that any performance is a consequence of factors like prior learning, inherent skills and situational variables (James, 2012). In order to detect regular structures of behavior, T-patterning has been already been used to establish playing patterns in football. The basic premise here is that the interactive flow or chain of behavior is governed by structures of variable stability that can be visualized by detecting these underlying T-patterns.

Thus, the aim of the present study is to demonstrate the potential of the software THÈME 5.0, for the detection of behavior temporal patterns (T-patterns) in the football game, more specifically, in the actions of counter-attack of the FC Barcelona and Manchester United football teams.

9.2 METHODS

The sample included 24 games (12 per team) from the sporting season 2009/2010 of the FC Barcelona and Manchester United teams. The design used in the present study was based on an observational methodology. The matches were analyzed through systematic observation using a specific instrument to observe the offensive process (Sarmento *et al.* 2010). The reliability of data was calculated by the intra- and inter-observer agreement (Cohen's Kappa), and values above 0.90 were achieved for all criteria:

    i Type of attack (0.99, 0.97, intra-observer agreement and inter observer agreement, respectively);
    ii Start of the offensive process (0.94, 0.91);
    iii Development of the OP (0.99, 0.98);
    iv End of the OP (0.96, 0.95);
    v Area where the action was performed (0.96, 0.93);
    vi Interactions contexts in the centre of the game (0.93, 0.91).

The following criteria were used in this study:

    1 Type of attack;
    2 Start of the offensive process (OP);
    3 Development of the OP;
    4 End of the OP;
    5 Area where the action was performed (Figure 9.2);
    6 Interactions contexts in the centre of the game.

To analyze the interaction context, we used the concept of the centre of the game (Castelo, 1992), that is defined as the zone of the field where the ball moves at a certain instant, through a context of cooperation and opposition of the influential players in the game, in the specific zone where the player that is in the possession of the ball is.

For the detection of temporal patterns, we used the software THÈME 5.0, and the following criteria were used: the minimum number of times a pattern must occur to be detected was set at 3 and the level of significance was set at 0.05. In this context, the software THÈME, as a program that detects temporal patterns, assumes a particular importance. The temporal patterns recognized are based on an algorithm described in several publications (e.g., Magnusson, 2000) that was developed and extensively tested in non-sporting contexts. We can characterize this algorithm based on the assumption that the flow of complex human behavior (e.g., sports performance) is based on sequential structure as a function of the time, has a discrete nature that is not fully detectable without the use of standardized statistical methods, as well as by the use of behavioral analysis techniques (Borrie *et al.*, 2002). In the analysis of actions in football, if we have this registration done in a systematic way, taking into account the successive units in which it breaks down the flow of practice runs, it is possible to evidence that there are repetitive temporal patterns of behavior (T-pattern) (Anguera, 2004).

The most valuable contribution of T-patterns arises from the possibility of detecting particular types of temporal structures (Borrie *et al.*, 2002). Given that patterns facilitate the detection of hidden structures, they are of significant importance in the analysis of the football game. This technique of analysis allows the representation of a specific diagram (Figure 9.1), which corresponds to the actions that occur in the same order, with distances (relatively to the number of frames) that remain relatively invariant, always within the critical interval time (Anguera, 2004).

9.3 RESULTS AND DISCUSSION

The data analysis revealed the existence of 787 different T-patterns in the team of FC Barcelona, ranging from a minimum of one level to a maximum of six levels and a minimum of two events to a maximum of nine events. We selected eight T-patterns (four per team), in relation to different phases of the counter-attack that were analyzed in a detailed way (each pattern occurs at least three times). Initially we present the diagram of the software together with the respective graphical representation of the obtained T-pattern. Subsequently we will put only the visual representations of the T-patterns obtained.

The first pattern (Figures 9.1a and b) represents an incomplete T-pattern (it does not include the end of the offensive process) in relation to the start of a counter-attack sequence (this pattern occurred three times). This counter-attack:

1. was initiated by an interception of the ball in the left corridor (zone 6) in an interaction context of numerical superiority,
2. followed by a short pass (diagonally forward) in the central defensive midfield (zone 5) in a context of numerical superiority;
3. a player performed the reception/control of the ball (zone 9) in a interaction context of numerical equality,
4. and then, the sequence developed through a short pass (diagonally forward) performed in zone 5 (numerical inferiority);
5. this pass is followed by a reception/control of the ball by a colleague in zone 8 (numerical superiority).

In a general way, there is a similar feature in the selected FC Barcelona T-patterns (Figures 9.1a and b, 9.2, 9.3 and 9.4), i.e., the sequences start through an interception of the ball in the left corridor (zone 6) in terms of numerical superiority, after that, there was a quick transfer of the game centre, from the right to the left side, trying to take advantage, probably, of the imbalance of the opposing defensive structure (numerical equality). The sequences are developed through actions like the conduction of the ball with the intention of displacing the centre of the game in the field of the game, to the areas close to the penalty area. Analysis of the sequences that end through a shot with a scored goal allowed us to understand (beyond the fact that these sequences are developed by the left corridor) that these shots are performed in the central zone of the offensive sector (zone 11) in conditions of numerical inferiority. All the presented patterns are repeated at least three times.

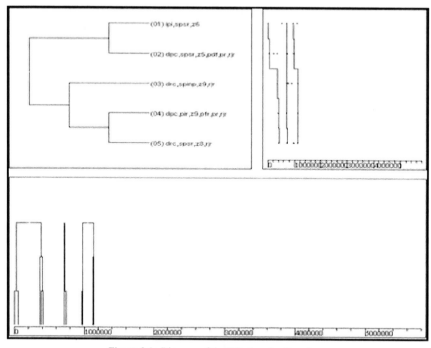

Figure 9.1a Diagram of the T-Pattern 1 – Barcelona

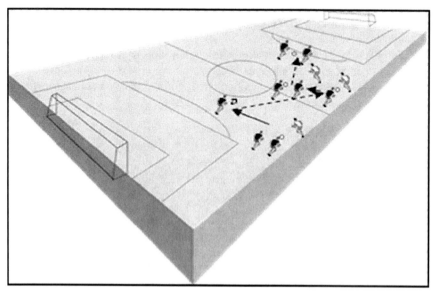

Figure 9.1b T-Pattern 1 – Barcelona

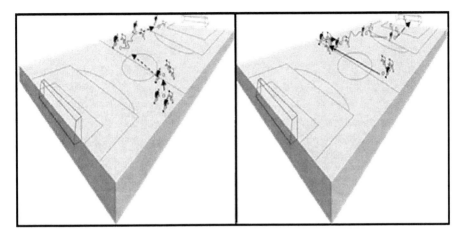

Figure 9.2 T-Pattern 2 – Barcelona   **Figure 9.3** T-Pattern 3 – Barcelona

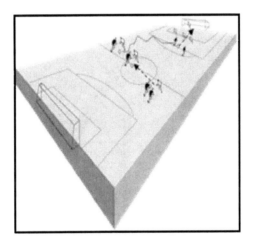

Figure 9.4 T-Pattern 4 – Barcelona

Relating to the Manchester United team, the data analysis revealed the existence of 118 different T-patterns (Figures 9.5, 9.6, 9.7 and 9.8), ranging from a minimum of one level to a maximum of five levels and a minimum of two events to a maximum of eight events.

In a similar way to the patterns found with the FC Barcelona team, the selected Manchester United T-patterns showed that the sequences of the counter-attacks start in the central zone of the defensive midfield (zone 5), in a context of numerical superiority, and are developed in the left corridor through actions like the short pass forward, the diagonal pass forward, and reception/control of the ball, in contexts of numerical equality. The last pass came from the left corridor (zone 7), and the sequences finished in the central zone of the offensive midfielder (zone 8 and 11), through a shot inside or a shot with a scored goal.

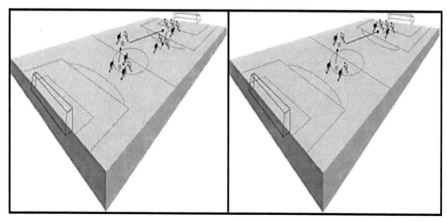

Figure 9.5 T-Pattern 5 – Manchester Utd   **Figure 9.6** T-Pattern 6 – Manchester Utd

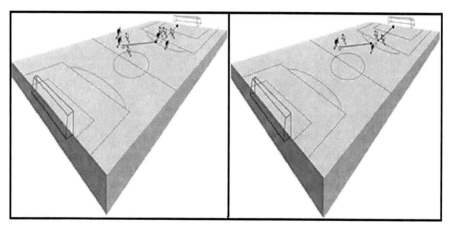

Figure 9.7 T-Pattern 7 – Manchester Utd   **Figure 9.8** T-Pattern 8 – Manchester Utd

When we analyzed the obtained results for the two studied teams, we observed that many more patterns were detected for the team of Barcelona (n = 787) compared with the Manchester United team (n = 118). This suggests that the offensive sequences of Barcelona have a more defined temporal and sequential structure than the sequences of counter-attack of Manchester United, which seem to reveal a greater variability of the behaviors performed by this team.

On the other hand, when we analyzed the patterns presented above jointly, we found that there are similar aspects. Although these counter-attack sequences begin in the central zone (Manchester United) or right zone (Barcelona) of the defensive midfield in situations of relative numerical superiority, they developed subsequently in the left side of the offensive midfielder. However, while the players of the Barcelona team used actions like conduction of the ball and dribble to progress through the field of play, the players of the Manchester team make it through the use of short passes. In both teams, the effectively ending sequences (e.g., goal, shot defended by the goalkeeper, etc.) are preceded by actions (reception/control of the ball, shooting) in the central sector of the offensive sector (zone 11) in interaction contexts of numerical inferiority.

9.4 CONCLUSIONS

The results show that many temporal patterns exist in soccer, namely in the teams of FC Barcelona and Manchester United. The number (787 and 188, respectively), frequency (at least three repetitions for each of the previously mentioned patterns) and complexity (ranging from one to six and one to five levels, respectively) of the detected patterns indicate that sport behavior is more synchronized than the "human eye" can detect.

This type of analysis allows us to know and to characterize the regular structures of offensive sequences in football teams. The T-patterns detected in these successful teams allowed us to study how that process is developed in an effective way. This information is relevant, on the one hand for the team itself because it makes it possible to conceive training exercises in order to increase this efficiency, and on the other hand it allows, for example, the opposing coaches to develop strategies to prevent the Barcelona and Manchester United teams performing these transitions effectively.

Through the use of this methodology, the coaches can have a new tool to analyze the game that is different from the tools currently available. Now they can analyze the patterns of play that most often lead to the effectiveness or ineffectiveness of their team or opposing teams. It becomes thereby possible to complement in a scientific way the analysis that usually is performed through "the naked eye".

9.5 REFERENCES

Anguera, T., 2004, Hacia la búsqueda de estructuras regulares en la observación del fútbol: Detección de patrones temporales. *Cultura, Ciencia y Deporte*, 1(1), pp. 15–20.

Borrie, A., Jonsson, G.K. and Magnusson, M.S., 2002, Temporal pattern analysis and its applicability in sport: An explanation and exemplar data. *Journal of Sports Sciences*, 20(10), pp. 845–852.

Castelo, J., 1992, Conceptualização de um modelo técnico/tático do jogo de futebol: Identificação e caraterização das grandes tendências evolutivas do jogo das equipas de rendimento superior. *Tese de Doutoramento*, (Lisbon, Portugal: Universidade Técnica de Lisboa).

Hughes, M. and Franks, I., 2005, Analysis of passing sequences, shots and goals in soccer. *Journal of Sports Sciences*, 23(5), pp. 509–514.

James, N., 2012, Predicting performance over time using a case study in real tennis, *Journal of Human Sport and Exercise*, 7(2), pp. 421–433.

Magnusson, M., 2000, Discovering hidden time patterns in behavior: T-patterns and their detection. *Behavior Research Methods, Instruments and Computers*, **32**, pp. 93–110.

Reep, C. and Benjamin, B., 1968, Skill and chance in association football. *Journal of the Royal Statistical Society, Series A*, **131**, pp. 581–585.

Sarmento, H., Anguera, M.T., Campaniço, J. And Leitão, J., 2010, Development and validation of a notational system to study the offensive process in football. *Medicina (Kaunas)*, **46**(6), pp. 401–407.

CHAPTER 10

The influence of manipulating the defensive playing method on collective synchrony of football teams

Ricardo Duarte, Bruno Travassos,
Duarte Araújo and Michael Richardson

10.1 INTRODUCTION

Successful performance in Association Football is typically viewed as an expression of a purposeful collective synergy between the individual performances within each team (Duarte *et al.*, 2012a). Indeed, the collective performance of football teams needs to be regarded as more than the sum of individual aggregated performances. Evidence is beginning to reveal that the player's motion dynamics on the field can functionally influence the spatial-temporal movement characteristics of neighbouring teammates and opponents, creating a purposeful aggregation during specific performance sub-phases (Passos *et al.*, 2011; Duarte *et al.*, 2012b). Some performance constraints, however, such as strategic behaviours related with the playing methods, are likely to influence the way teammates synchronise their on-field behaviours (Travassos *et al.*, 2012). For example, the differences found on interpersonal coordination observed for lateral and longitudinal displacements between basketball (Bourbousson *et al.*, 2010) and futsal players (Travassos *et al.*, 2011) can be grounded on the distinct defensive playing methods used in each study.

The aim of this study was, therefore, to analyse how the manipulation of the defensive playing method influences the collective synchrony of football players during performance.

10.2 METHODS

10.2.1 Participants

Twelve, U-17 Portuguese youth elite football players (16.2 ± 0.6 years; 1.75 ± 0.04 m; 67.0 ± 3.5 kg; 5.6 ± 1.5 years of competition engagement) were recruited to participate in this study. All the participants voluntarily agreed to participate in the study and appropriate informed consent was gathered.

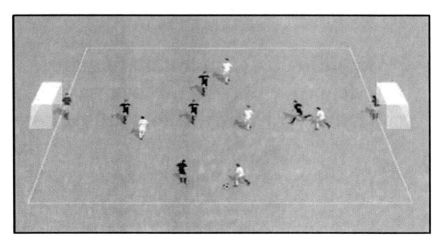

Figure 10.1 Scheme of the GK+5 vs. 5+GK small-sided games used as *in situ* experimental task

10.2.2 Field procedures

The *in situ* experimental task consisted of a Gk + 5 vs. 5 + Gk small-sided game, with pitch dimensions of 40 m × 42 m. The footballers were divided in two balanced teams by the coach, with a Gk + 1 + 3 + 1 diamond shape formation, with players assigned to their common field positions. Two games were performed, with 10 minutes duration each, interspersed with 8 minutes of passive recovery. In the first condition/game, both teams used zone defence. In the second condition/game, players were paired in attacking–defending dyads and both teams used man-to-man defence. Positional data (2D) from the 10 outfield players were gathered using a global positioning system (GPSports SPI Elite system, GPSports, Canberra, Australia) with a sample rate of 15 Hz (Gray *et al.*, 2010). The goalkeepers were not monitored during the games but were included in order to maintain the representativeness of the ecological performance constraints.

10.2.3 Cluster phase method

The collective synchrony of the movement displacement trajectories of players was assessed using the cluster phase method. This method was recently proposed to analyse synchrony within systems with a small number of oscillating components (Frank and Richardson, 2010). The cluster phase is based on the Kuramoto order parameter (Kuramoto and Nishikawa, 1987), which describes the collective phase synchronisation of oscillatory movement components (e.g., team players' movement displacement trajectories) in a single collective parameter:

$$\dot{r}(t_i) = \frac{1}{n}\sum_{k=1}^{n}\exp(i\theta_k(t_i)) \tag{10.1}$$

$$r(t_i) = \mathrm{atan2}(\dot{r}(t_i)) \tag{10.2}$$

Frank and Richardson (2010) have adapted this model and showed its applicability using a rocking chair paradigm of only six oscillatory units (i.e., six individuals coordinating rocking chair movements). Based on the cluster (equations 10.1 and 10.2) and individual phases, it is possible to determine the relative phase between each player and his team's movement synchronisation (see equation 10.3):

$$\phi_k(t_i) = \theta_k(t_i) - r(t_i) \tag{10.3}$$

Besides, a specific measure of collective synchrony – the cluster amplitude – was obtained, which captured how players collectively synchronised their movement displacement trajectories on-field:

$$\rho_{group}(t_i) = \left| \frac{1}{n} \sum_{k=1}^{n} \exp\{i(\phi_k(t_i) - \bar{\phi}_k)\} \right| \tag{10.4}$$

The reader is directed to Frank and Richardson (2010) and Strogatz (2000) for further understanding on the mathematical equations of the method.

10.3 RESULTS

The players' collective synchrony within each team suggested a mean tendency to superior values in lateral (side-to-side) movement displacements than in the longitudinal (goal-to-goal) direction (see upper and bottom panels of Figure 10.2, respectively).

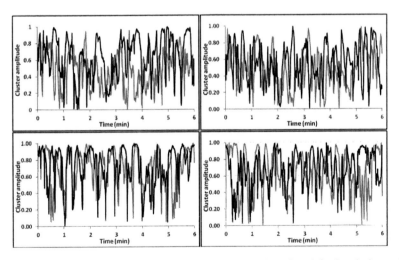

Figure 10.2 Collective synchrony of both teams is shown as a function of the defensive playing method used by teams. Panels show longitudinal/goal-to-goal movements (top) and lateral/side-to-side movements (bottom), for team A and B in left and right panels, respectively

Table 10.1 Mean, standard deviation and correlation values of the collective synchrony of teams as a function of the defensive playing method

Playing method	Direction	Team A	Team B	Correlations
Zone defence	Goal-to-goal	0.63 ± 0.24	0.55 ± 0.23	0.05, n.s.
	Side-to-side	0.74 ± 0.22	0.68 ± 0.21	0.43, p < 0.05
Man-to-man defence	Goal-to-goal	0.47 ± 0.21	0.48 ± 0.21	0.01, n.s.
	Side-to-side	0.70 ± 0.21	0.64 ± 0.24	0.74, p < 0.05

In addition, correlation values showed significant positive values between the movement synchronisation of both teams in the lateral (side-to-side) movements but not in longitudinal ones.

To evaluate the space–time coordination tendencies between each individual player and his team as a whole, we used relative phase analysis (e.g., Travassos *et al.*, 2012). Overall frequency histograms (see Figure 10.3) reinforce previous data, showing important differences in the way individual players synchronised their movement displacement trajectories with the whole team. Adopting a man-to-man defence implied less attraction for any specific mode of relation and large spread for the entire spectrum of coordination possibilities. Conversely, adopting zone defence implied higher attraction for relative phase values near in-phase mode of coordination (62.9 per cent between –30 and 30 degrees).

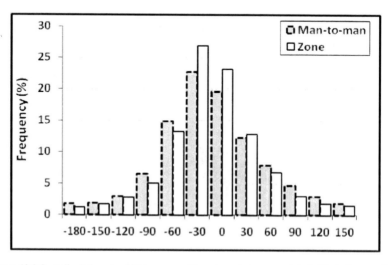

Figure 10.3 Overall relative phase histograms with analyses between each individual player and the team movement synchronisation

10.4 DISCUSSION

The present study demonstrated that the defensive playing method adopted during small-sided games practices exert an influence in the collective synchronisation of football players. The interpersonal interactions established by the small groups of competing players were, collectively, more synchronised when teams adopted zone defence strategic behaviours.

Data indicated that zone defence implied more cohesiveness within a team, especially in the lateral displacements of players. It suggests that when the defending team is between the attacking team and his own goal, the lateral movement synchronisation contributes to defensively stabilise the opponent forward movements intended to create attacking perturbations (Travassos *et al.*, 2011). This interpretation is strengthened by the correlation values found, which indicated a tendency for a simultaneous increase and decrease in the two teams' synchronies in the lateral movements.

Frequency histogram analyses demonstrated important differences in the way individual players synchronised their movement displacement trajectories with the whole group. Adopting a man-to-man defence implied less attraction to any specific mode of relation and more spread for the entire spectrum of coordination possibilities. Also, we observed a slight shift for negative values compared with the zone defence condition, which suggested a lead–lag relation attributed to the individual players' movements. This means that the player tends to move slightly more at first than the increments in team synchrony. On the contrary, adopting a zone defence strategy promoted higher attraction to relative phase values near in-phase mode of coordination, which means that the individual players are near-perfectly increasing and decreasing their movements at the same time of team synchrony. As suggested in the literature, this data indicated that structural and functional performance constraints imposed with zone defence influenced the players to be more synchronised with the collective movements of the team (Duarte *et al.*, 2012a).

From a functional perspective, the data reported here showed that distinct ecological constraints imposed on team players may change the emergent individual and collective behaviours associated with performing as a synchronised social unit. These findings revealed that by adopting zone defence strategies, team players are more likely to achieve stable relations with teammates, creating a purposeful aggregation expressed by the specific collective behaviours of the teams such as stretching and contracting space on the field (Duarte *et al.*, 2012a, 2012b). Future research needs to assess the relation between the collective movement synchronisation and the emergence of perturbations leading to successful outcomes such as goals scored and shots on goal.

10.5 REFERENCES

Bourbousson, G., Sève, C. and McGarry, T., 2010, Space-time coordination dynamics in basketball: Part 1. Intra- and inter-couplings among player dyads. *Journal of Sports Sciences*, **28**, pp. 339–347.

Duarte, R., Araújo, D., Correia, V. and Davids, K., 2012a, Sports teams as superorganisms: Implications of sociobiological models of behaviour for research and practice in team sports performance analysis. *Sports Medicine*, **42**(8), pp. 633–642.

Duarte, R., Araújo, D., Freire, L., Folgado, H., Fernandes, O. and Davids, K., 2012b, Intra- and inter-group coordination patterns reveal collective behaviours of football players near the scoring zone. *Human Movement Science*, **31**(6), pp. 1639–1651.

Frank, T.D. and Richardson, M.J., 2010, On a test statistic for the Kuramoto order parameter of synchronization: An illustration for group synchronization during rocking chairs. *Physica D*, **239**, pp. 2084–2092.

Gray, A.J., Jenkins, D., Andrews, M.H., Taaffe, D.T. and Glover, M.L., 2010, Validity and reliability of GPS for measuring distance travelled in field-based team sports. *Journal of Sports Sciences*, **28**(12), pp. 1319–1325.

Kuramoto, Y. and Nishikawa, I., 1987, Statistical macrodynamics of large dynamical systems: Case of a phase transition in oscillator communities. *Journal of Statistical Physics*, **49**, pp. 569–605.

Passos, P., Milho, J., Fonseca, S., Borges, J., Araújo, D. and Davids, K., 2011, Interpersonal distance regulates functional grouping tendencies of agents in team sports. *Journal of Motor Behavior*, **43**, pp. 155–163.

Strogatz; S.H., 2000, From Kuramoto to Crawford: Exploring the onset of synchronization in populations of coupled oscillators. *Physica D*, **143**, pp. 1–20.

Travassos, B., Araújo, D., Vilar, L. and McGarry, T., 2011, Interpersonal coordination and ball dynamics in futsal (indoor football). *Human Movement Science*, **30**(6), pp. 1245–1259.

Travassos, B., Araújo, D., Duarte, R. and McGarry, T., 2012. Spatiotemporal coordination patterns in futsal (indoor football) are guided by informational game constraints. *Human Movement Scienc*, **31**(4), pp. 932–945.

CHAPTER 11

Effect of small-sided games on the physical performance of young football players of different ages and levels of practice

Luís Barnabé, Anna Volossovitch and António Paulo Ferreira

11.1 INTRODUCTION

Small-sided games (SSGs) are less structured than traditional fitness training methods, but represent very popular specific training drills for players of different levels (Hill-Haas *et al.*, 2011). In football, SSGs are used to train physical, technical and tactical aspects of performance in a way similar to match play (Dellal *et al.*, 2011; Randers *et al.*, 2010). Previous studies have pointed out that SSGs represent an efficient training tool that increases players' game practice time and induces the specific physiological responses within a major technical and tactical involvement (e.g., Duarte *et al.*, 2009; Hill-Haas *et al.*, 2009; Katis and Kellis, 2009). Coaches and researchers assume that the time spent in these types of activities can be defined as deliberate practice experience and should play an important role in youth football training programs.

Several studies have analyzed the effects of SSGs on physiological (Owen *et al.*, 2004; Rampinini *et al.*, 2007), physical and motor responses (Hill-Haas *et al.*, 2009; Casamichana and Castellano, 2010) of adult (Rampinini *et al.*, 2007) and young football players (Jones and Drust, 2007; Hill-Haas *et al.*, 2009). In general, there is a broad consensus about the influence of the game format on players' performance profile (Katis and Kellis, 2009; Hill-Haas *et al.*, 2011).

Jones and Drust (2007) studied the physiological and technical demands of four-a-side vs. eight-a-side games in elite youth football players. Their results demonstrated the heart rate responses, total distance covered and distance covered by players at different speeds did not alter significantly according to SSG format. The number of players participating in each SSG format only significantly influenced technically related actions of young footballers. These findings are in contrast with the results of Rampinini, *et al.* (2007), which revealed that three-a-side games provoked more intense physiological responses in adult players than four- and five-a-side games; while the last two game formats induced more intense responses of three physiological measures (heart rate, blood lactate concentration and rating of perceived exertion) comparatively to six-a-side games. Using the same physiological measures of intensity and analyzing time–motion characteristics, Hill-Haas *et al.* (2009) verified that, when SSGs performed by young football players decrease in size maintaining the relative pitch area constant, there is an increase in physiological and perceptual demands of the game.

Several studies confirmed that, in the scope of a constraints-led approach, the game format (pitch size, number of players and rules modifications) has implications on the individual and collective actions performed by players (Duarte, *et al.*, 2010; Ford and Williams, 2012). Nevertheless, it is still not clear how players of different ages and playing experience behave in analogous practice tasks, if their performances are similar and, if not, how the differences could be explained.

Therefore, to better understand the behavior of young players in different SSGs formats, this study aimed to analyze the combined effects of age and deliberate practice experience on physical performance and heart rate responses of football players of three different age groups in two SSGs formats 3 vs. 3 + GKs (SSG1) and 5 vs. 5 + GKs (SSG2). First, the responses of players from the same age group to SSGs format alteration were evaluated; second, the performances of players from different age groups in the same SSG format were compared.

11.2 METHODS

Thirty six young male football players of three different age groups (under-16 (U16), under-17 (U17) and under-19 (U19)) participated in the study. Each group was constituted by 12 players (10 players and 2 goalkeepers), whose characteristics are shown in Table 11.1.

Table 11.1 Characteristics of study participants (mean ± SD)

Team / group	Age (years) mean ± SD	Height (m) mean ± SD	Weight (kg) mean ± SD	Body mass index (kg.m^{-2}) mean ± SD	Playing experience (years) mean ± SD
U16	15.2 ± 0.4	1.74 ± 0.03	62.6 ± 4.2	20.7 ± 2.2	6.0 ± 1.8
U17	16.3 ± 0.5	1.78 ± 0.04	67.5 ± 4.1	21.3 ± 1.9	7.0 ± 1.4
U19	17.4 ± 0.5	1.80 ± 0.07	69.0 ± 5.8	21.1 ± 2.1	8.7 ± 2.8

The selection of players to participate in the study was carried out according to the criterion for technical and tactical evaluation previously stipulated in the club. Each group was divided into two balanced teams. One goalkeeper, two defenders, three midfielders and one forward participated in the six-a-side games; as well as the same goalkeeper, one of the defenders, one of the midfielders and the same forward took part in the four-a-side games. The game system, the teams' formation and the playing positions of the participants were conserved across the three experimental sessions and also respected the positions normally used by players in training and competition.

The three groups of participants completed three independent sessions separated by one-week intervals. In each session, the three groups performed two SSGs formats – four-a-side (3 vs. 3 + GKs) and six-a-side (5 vs. 5 + GKs) games – during 8-minute periods interspersed with 5 minutes of passive recovery. The players participated in 12 SSGs (i.e., three four-a-side games and three six-a-side games per group). In each session the games were presented in a random order. The pitch size was set according to the following references: 23 m × 40 m for SSG1 and 33 m × 60 m for SSG2. The relative space, available for each player (ratio of pitch area per player), as well as the pitch length and width relationship were similar in both game situations. All the official rules of soccer have been implemented with the exception of the offside rule.

The players' actions have been recorded using the global positioning system (GPS) – (SPI PRO tracking system, GPSports, Canberra, Australia).

The physical performance of players was characterized by following variables: 1) distance covered (D); 2) average speed (Sp_{avg}); 3) maximum speed (Sp_{max}). Heart rate minimum (HR_{min}), heat rate maximum (HR_{max}) and heart rate average (HR_{avg}) have also been recorded.

One-way and two-way mixed-model ANOVA tests were used to analyze the effect of SSG format, as well as chronological age and level of practice on the physical performance and heart rate responses of young football players.

11.3 RESULTS

Table 11.2 shows the results of performance indicators that characterize the physical performance and heart rate (HR) responses of young football players according to their ages and levels of practice in SSG1 and SSG2.

Table 11.2 Performance profile of three groups of players in SSG1 and SSG2 (mean ± SD)

	SSG1			SSG2		
	U16	U17	U19	U16	U17	U19
	Mean ± SD	Mean ± SD	Mean ± SD	Mean ± SD	Mean ± SD	Mean ± SD
D	$957 \pm 91.6^{**\#\#}$	$881.4 \pm 64^{**}$	$853.3 \pm 63^{\#\#}$	$988 \pm 114^{**\#\#}$	$981 \pm 74.2^{**}$	$956 \pm 68.8^{\#\#}$
Sp_{max}	$24.1 \pm 1.7^{\#}$	22.9 ± 2.3	$22.3 \pm 1.9^{\#}$	$23.6 \pm 2.04^{\#}$	23.4 ± 2.02	$24.1 \pm 2.1^{\#}$
Sp_{avg}	$6.96 \pm 0.6^{**\#\#}$	$6.4 \pm 0.47^{**}$	$6.3 \pm 0.4^{\#\#}$	$7.12 \pm 0.8^{**\#\#}$	$7.02 \pm 0.52^{**}$	$6.94 \pm 0.53^{\#\#}$
HR_{max}	185.6 ± 15.13	186.3 ± 7.2	178.6 ± 14.3	184.8 ± 11.12	181.6 ± 9.6	178.1 ± 7.99
HR_{avg}	$168.9 \pm 20.2^{\#}$	167.9 ± 9.6	$156.9 \pm 10.9^{\#}$	$160.1 \pm 14.5^{\#}$	161.4 ± 13.07	$154.3 \pm 9.3^{\#}$
HR_{min}	$120.4 \pm 14.5^{\#}$	111.1 ± 1.05	$107.4 \pm 14.3^{\#}$	$105.9 \pm 18.4^{\#}$	104.6 ± 14.9	$101.7 \pm 13.9^{\#}$

** significant difference between U16 and U17 (p < 0.01); \# significant difference between U16 and U19 (p < 0.05); \#\# significant difference between U16 and U19 (p < 0.01).

The significant differences between players' performances in SSG1 and SSG2 were observed for D – U17 (p < 0.05) and U19 (p < 0.001); Sp_{avg} – U16 (p < 0.05), U17 (p < 0.05) and U19 (p < 0.001); HR_{min} – U16 (p < 0.05). For smaller game format, total distance covered by older and more experienced players was significantly less than for larger game format; the average speed of players from all groups was higher in larger game format. The minimum heart rate was significantly higher in smaller game format for players from group U16.

The significant differences between performances of U16 players and players from other groups in SSG1 were observed for D – U17 ($p < 0.01$) and U19 ($p < 0.01$); Sp_{avg} – U17 ($p < 0.01$), U19 ($p < 0.01$); Sp_{max} – U19 ($p < 0.05$); HR_{avg} – U19 ($p < 0.05$); HR_{min} – U19 ($p < 0.05$); and in SSG2 for D – U17 ($p < 0.01$) and U19 ($p < 0.01$); Sp_{avg} – U17 ($p < 0.01$), U19 ($p < 0.01$); Sp_{max} – U19 ($p < 0.05$); HR_{avg} – U19 ($p < 0.05$); HR_{min} – U19 ($p < 0.05$).

Results clearly show that older and more experienced players demonstrated less intensive performance in both game formats. Although no significant differences were observed between performances of U17 and U19 groups, it can be argued that the change of SSG format had diverse impact on the physical performance and HR responses of young football players of different ages and levels of practice.

11.4 DISCUSSION

The analysis of players' responses from the same age group in SSG1 and SSG2 showed that, when the size of SSG increased and the relative pitch area remained constant, the average speed of players of all age groups raised. However, only the players from older and more experienced groups (U17 and U19) covered significantly more total distance in the six-a-side game. The significant differences in HR responses, according to SSG format, were observed only for the youngest group of players (U16) and for the minimum values of HR. Therefore, higher average speed of players, registered in the six-a-side game, was not reflected by the HR responses of players, except of the U16 group. Partially, these results are in line with findings reported by Jones and Drust (2007), which analyzed eight football players from under-8 group and also did not observe any significant alterations in their heart rate responses in SSGs according to the number of players. The authors also found greater distance covered by jogging in the larger game format. The higher intensity running observed in SSG1 compared to SSG2, as well as the greater distance covered by players from the two oldest groups, could be explained by a superior time of individual ball possession observed in larger game formats, as has been suggested by Rampinini *et al.* (2007).

Our findings demonstrate that players of different ages and level of practice do not react in the same way to the game format modification. Several studies reported that changing of the number of players and the pitch dimensions lead to the alteration of the technical and physiological demands of game (Owen *et al.*, 2004; Hill-Haas *et al.*, 2009); the results of our study pointed out that to better understand these demands' alteration, the age and practice level of players should be taken into account.

A comparison of performances of players from different age groups in the same SSG format allows us to conclude that, in both formats of SSG, younger players had significantly higher workload intensity, compared to older and more experienced players. These results seem to indicate that age and playing experience have a substantial influence on how the players manage the functional space and their playing actions during the SSG. An additional explanation may be that more experienced players use more collective actions, compared to their younger colleagues, who solve the game's situations using predominantly individual actions. Thus, the lower effort of older and more experienced players is a result of more evolved tactical behavior with obvious effects on the physical performance of players.

Despite the considerable number of studies concerned with analysis of SSG demands, the knowledge about the physical, technical and tactical responses of young players to the alteration of players' number, pitch area and game type constraints is still incomplete. This study is one of very few (Duarte *et al.*, 2010) that reported the physical and HR responses of players of different ages and practice experience to the SSG format changing.

Our findings clearly suggest that the alteration of players' number, pitch area and individual playing area do not induce the same responses of players of different age groups. Therefore, choosing a particular SSG format the coach needs to take into account not only the objectives of the training process, but also the age and level of practice of players. As far as the main aim of soccer drills is to enable players to increase their technical and tactical competencies (Casamichana and Castellano, 2010), further research should analyze the tactical and technical responses of young players caused by different SSG formats, considering the players age and practice experience.

11.5 REFERENCES

Casamichana, D. and Castellano, J., 2010, Time–motion, heart rate, perceptual and motor behaviour demands in small-sides soccer games: Effects of pitch size. *Journal of Sports Sciences*, **28**, pp. 1615–1623.

Dellal, A., Lago-Penas, C., Wong, D.P. and Chamari, K., 2011, Effect of the number of ball contacts within bouts of 4 vs. 4 small-sided soccer games. *International Journal of Sports Physiology and Performance*, **6**, pp. 322–333.

Duarte, R., Batalha, N., Folgado, H. and Sampaio, J., 2009, Effects of duration and number of players in heart rate responses and technical skills during futsal small-sided games. *The Open Sports Sciences Journal*, **2**, pp. 37–41.

Duarte, R., Araújo, D., Fernandes, O., Travassos, B., Folgado, H., Diniz, A. and Davids, K., 2010, Effects of different practice task constraints on fluctuations of player heart rate in small-sided football games. *The Open Sports Sciences Journal*, **3**, pp. 13–15.

Ford, P.R. and Williams, A.M., 2012, The development activities engaged in by elite youth soccer players who progressed to professional status compared to those who did not. *Psychology of Sport and Exercise*, **13**, pp. 349–352.

Hill-Haas, S.V., Dawson, B.T., Coutts, A.J. and Rowsell, G.J., 2009, Physiological responses and time-motion characteristics of various small-sided soccer games in youth players. *Journal of Sports Sciences*, **27**, pp. 1–8.

Hill-Haas, S.V., Dawson, B., Impellizzeri, F.M. and Coutts, A.J., 2011, Physiology of small-sided games training in football: A systematic review. *Sports Medicine*, **41**, pp. 199–220.

Jones, S. and Drust, B., 2007, Physiological and technical demands of 4 v 4 and 8 v 8 games in elite youth soccer players. *Kinesiology*, **39**, pp. 150–156.

Katis, A. and Kellis, E., 2009, Effects of small-sided games on physical conditioning and performance in youth soccer players. *Journal of Sports Science and Medicine*, **8**, pp. 374–380.

Owen, A., Twist, C. and Ford, P., 2004, Small-sided games: The physiological and technical effect of altering pitch size and player numbers. *Insight*, 7, pp. 50–53.

Rampinini, E., Impellizzeri, F.M., Castagna, C., Abt, G., Chamari, K., Sassi, A. and Marcora, S.M., 2007, Factors influencing physiological responses to small-sided soccer games. *Journal of Sports Sciences*, **25**, pp. 659–666.

Randers, M.B., Nybo, L., Petersen, J., Nielsen, J.J., Christiansen, L., Bendiksen, M., Brito, J., Bangsbo, J. and Krustrup P., 2010, Activity profile and physiological response to football training for untrained males and females, elderly and youngsters: Influence of the number of players. *Scandinavian Journal of Medicine and Science and Sports*, **20**, pp. 14–23.

Part 3

Rugby

CHAPTER 12

Scoring team performance in rugby union

Ed Burt, Mike Hughes and Nic James

12.1 INTRODUCTION

Performance indicators (PIs) are widely regarded as a means of objectively measuring sporting performance in terms of success (Hughes and Bartlett, 2002). However, their use assumes that performance can be understood, described and, by inference, improved through their measurement (Lames and McGarry, 2007). Whilst some sports have identified a correlation between frequency-based performance indicators and match outcome, e.g. basketball (Csataljay *et al.*, 2009) and squash (Vučković *et al.*, 2009), no consistent relationship has yet been identified for rugby union (Vaz *et al.*, 2011). This may not be a surprise given the complex nature of rugby union and the variety of techniques and tactics that teams can choose to deploy from one match to the next. For example, van Rooyen *et al.* (2010) studied ruck frequency in the 2007 World Cup and found that different styles of play between the pool and knock-out stages of the competition led to winning. However, research in rugby union has suggested key PIs such as set-pieces (Jackson and Hughes, 2001; Ortega *et al.*, 2009; Sasaki *et al.*, 2007) and territorial gains and losses (Hughes and Franks, 2004; Correia *et al.*, 2011). However, very few attempts have been made to combine this information into a performance model, with the exceptions of Bracewell *et al.* (2003) and Jones *et al.* (2008). Potential weaknesses of these models are that they compare performance to a historic average and are subject to issues of volatility and the influence of confounding variables.

The aim of this study, therefore, was to design and test a new methodology for analysing rugby union matches using a combination of frequency of actions, quality of action, territory gain and pitch location so that each passage of play could be assigned a numerical value where high values indicated good and low values poor performance. On this basis "highlights" could be identified through a simple identification of high value passages of play. On this basis, if coaches agree with the utility of the identified passages of play, then the key performance indicators, at the individual match level, will be identified. If this methodology can be shown to be valid then further work is required to develop a robust system for use in both applied and academic settings.

12.2 METHODS

12.2.1 Software, coding and algorithms

Commercial notation packages such as Sportscode and Focus X2 lack the programming functionality required to manipulate and transform variables without recourse to other software packages. It was therefore decided to use Visual Basic for Applications within Microsoft Excel 2010, running on a Windows 7 64-bit platform, to capture, process and output all variables.

A rugby-specific notational template was designed, based upon operational definitions agreed through a combination of expertise from the three authors (as players, coaches and analysts of rugby union) and input from UKCC-qualified RFU coaches. For example, a quick ruck was defined as one where the ball was passed or carried away less than 3 seconds from the ruck forming, an average ruck between 3 and 6 seconds and a slow ruck greater than 6 seconds. Each action variable comprised a single top-level descriptor and one or more sub-level descriptors in addition to a quality rating, territory gained and pitch location information. For example, when a maul occurred the codes used were: maul; the duration notated as (long, medium or quick); whether the maul was won, lost, whether or not it was incomplete; the quality scored as (high, normal or low); information regarding making the gain line (positive, equals, negative or line break) and pitch location (red, amber, green and blue).

12.2.2 Type of action

A total of 56 different action variables were defined and weighted values (available from the first author) agreed between authors and coaches with respect to published literature. For example Ortega *et al.* (2009) conducted a univariate analysis on the differences in game statistics between winning and losing teams across the 2003–2006 Six Nations Championships and found that scrums lost, line-outs lost, mauls won, line breaks, possessions kicked, tackle completion and turnovers had a significant difference between winning and losing teams. This implied that these variables should receive relatively high weightings. Having utilised the available literature in this way and after much debate and refinement a starting point for weighting action variables was achieved. At this stage of development of this algorithm, no attempt is made to academically justify the weightings; rather they are presented as a proof of concept.

Since scoring is the most significant action in rugby (tries, conversions and penalties) it would have been easy to award these actions very high values and hence passages of play that resulted in scoring would have received high values. This would have meant that the algorithm would have identified outcomes (scoring) well but processes (actions not including scoring) may not have been. To avoid this scenario the action of scoring a try was awarded a very low value (one point) thus ensuring that if the algorithm identified tries as being significant passages of play it would be because of the processes involved prior to the try being scored.

The value of penalty kicks at goal and drop-kicks were calculated based upon how far from the posts the kick was, on the assumption that the further away a kick is, the harder it is complete successfully. The horizontal position within a zone was also considered, to reflect that a kick in front of the posts is considerably easier than one on the edge of the pitch.

12.2.2.1 Quality

Quality was assessed on the execution of actions with three levels defined. High was awarded for exceptional skill, either as a result of performing under extreme pressure or for creating an opportunity that would not have reasonably been expected. Neutral (default value) was the expected value for most actions commensurate with players at this level of participation. Low quality denoted the inadequate execution of skill by a player that typically resulted in an unexpected loss or disruption of possession or a loss of territory.

12.2.2.2 Territorial gain

In order to maintain the relevance of this methodology for rugby coaches and players, the territorial gain categories were based on those routinely used within rugby union, i.e. gain line –ve, gain line, gain line +ve and line break. As rugby is a game in which the ball is passed backwards whilst players run forwards a more circumspect view of territorial gains and losses was required. Gain line +ve and gain line –ve were defined by comparing the location of the previous place of contact between the defence and attack with the current position. To negate the effect of the different ways in which players can position their bodies at the breakdown, an action was deemed to have had a respective +ve or –ve gain in territory if the entire body of the ball carrier and the ball were beyond the offside line at the point at which the next action took place. A line break was defined as when an attacker in possession of the ball managed to get behind the defence, thereby causing them to turn. Simply running into a defender and pushing him backwards would be a gain line +ve.

Territorial gain does not just involve assessments of running with the ball since players will often kick the ball during open play. This was judged by comparing the location of the kick with the location of where the kicking team next legally gained possession. The difference between these two locations was used in the calculation of the "territorial gain" parameter.

12.2.2.3 Pitch location

The pitch was divided into 4 sections (red, amber, green, blue) with red being between a team's try line and their 22m line, amber from the 22m line to the half-way line, green half-way line to opposition 22m line and blue the opposition 22m line to the opposition try line. Based on logic and previous research it was hypothesised that positive actions were worth more the closer they were to the opposition try line. Similarly, mistakes made further away from one's own try line were regarded as of less magnitude as errors nearer one's own try line. Hence values 1, 2, 3 and 4 were assigned to red, amber, green and blue zones for positive actions and 4, 3, 2, 1 for errors.

12.2.3 Calculating values for each action variable

In order to assign a numerical value for each action variable, where high values indicated good and low values poor performance, weightings had to be calculated for each descriptor for every action variable. Thus a score was calculated for each action variable using the formula:

*Type of action * quality * territorial gain * pitch location*

Sequences of action variables were linked together to form phases and sequences of phases linked to form a passage of play, which equated to an individual team possession (Figure 12.1). Whenever possession changed between teams a new passage of play began thereby creating a timeline of the match in the database. It should be noted that if the game was stopped this only signalled a new passage of play if the possession changed. For example, if a team was awarded a penalty and opted to kick the ball to touch, the subsequent line-out would form part of the original passage of play, as possession had not changed. Ultimately, a single team score was calculated by adding together all of the possession scores.

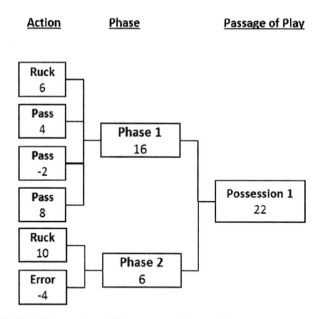

Figure 12.1 Combining action variables to create phases and phases to create passages of play

Once a match had been input, data could be extracted at whichever level of detail was required. For example, using the example in Figure 12.1, if rucks were selected for analysis in isolation, the software would only extract the values 6 and 10. Alternatively, how effectively a team used the ball after each ruck could be evaluated by the software extracting all phase data that began with a ruck, the values of 16 and 6 from Figure 12.1. The same principle could be applied at the match level, for example extracting the passages with the highest scores, lowest scores or whatever type of query the coach or analyst felt was of value.

12.2.4 Matches analysed

Matches from two distinct population groups were analysed. Group one comprised (n = 26) home and away matches from a single team in the RFU National 3 League in the 2011/2012 season. Matches were videoed used a tripod-mounted camera located in an elevated position as close to the half-way line as possible. Written permission was obtained from the rugby club for the use of these videos in this project. The second group (n = 13) comprised International matches played in 2012, with ten chosen at random from the 2011/2012 Six Nations Competition and three Test Matches from the England tour to South Africa in June 2012. All International matches were coded using recordings of broadcast transmissions and were provided by the RFU. Since the two groups had very different skill levels it was felt this would reduce sampling bias (Thomas *et al.*, 2005) and improve the validity of the methods.

12.2.5 Reliability

An intra-rater reliability study was conducted by recoding two matches from each group with a minimum gap of two weeks between coding. An overall reliability rating of <5 per cent difference was found between matches at the level of data input and so the coding process was deemed sufficiently reliable for the purpose of this preliminary study.

12.2.6 Validity

Across all (n = 39) matches, over 22,000 lines of notation data, each containing 8–14 fields, were processed. Hughes *et al.* (2012b) argue that using match outcome as the sole independent variable to differentiate between significant and insignificant on-field activities can compound the effect of confounding variables. However, as the purpose of this study was to identify performance indicators within a match, rather than across matches, it is valid to use match outcome as a prediction of validity. Other methods such as expert evaluation and corroboration will be used at later stages.

The algorithm's calculated match outcome (the team with the highest overall calculated score was deemed to be the winner) matched the actual result in 24 out of 26 matches (92 per cent) at National 3 level and 9 out of 13 matches (69 per cent) at International level. Two International matches were drawn and so removing these matches would have increased this to 82 per cent. It should be noted that tries were deliberately given low values for this version of the algorithm and consequently only 17.62 per cent ± 0.12 per cent of total scores awarded for National 3 games and 10.19 per cent ± 0.10 per cent in International games were for passages of play resulting in a try being scored. This meant that the algorithm was predominately assessing the quality of performance using non-try-scoring passages of play. However, 72.6 per cent of tries at National 3 level and 86.8 per cent at International level were above the 80th percentile of passages of play ranked in order of magnitude for total score.

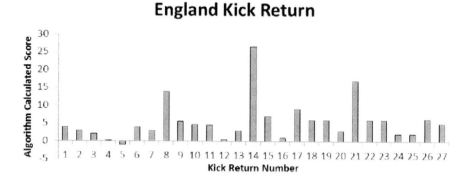

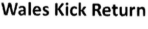

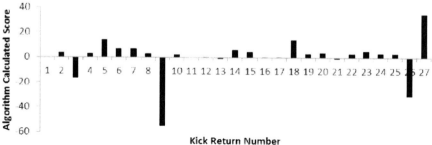

Figure 12.2 England and Wales kick return scores

12.3 RESULTS

Having established a value for each action, a more contextual analysis of action variables could be completed than is possible with a frequency-based analysis and a variety of visual coaching aides could be produced without any further coding. For example, examining kick returns in the match between Wales and England using a traditional frequency-based analysis would have showed that Wales successfully caught 24/27 (89 per cent) of kicks whilst England caught 26/27 (96 per cent) kicks, suggesting reasonably similar performances. By contrast, the algorithm scores highlight that England scored a total of 150 points at an average of 5.5 per kick return compared to Wales' total of 20.5 points at an average of 0.76 points per kick return. Thus the inclusion of qualitative and pitch location information used by the algorithm has suggested that England were far more effective in the use of the ball at the kick return compared to Wales. Furthermore, presenting this information as a graph enables players and coaches to quickly and easily identify passages of play of interest.

Key moments in a match (both highlights and lowlights) can be automatically presented to the coach by sorting algorithm scores for passages of play into descending numerical order. Then, using percentiles, the top X per cent can be presented as highlights and the bottom Y per cent as lowlights. Using the Wales vs. England match the bottom 15th percentile of plays for Wales included five "errors" of which four occurred after a slow ruck and three of these following a pass to the right which occurred immediately after a kick return.

12.4 DISCUSSION

This study used a combination of actions performed, quality of action, territory gain and pitch location to analyse rugby union matches identifying key passages of play. This method produced qualitatively based performance indicators that were suggested to highlight aspects of performance that would not necessarily be detected using more traditional frequency-based measures. It also answers the call from Hughes *et al.* (2012a) that performance analysis should move away from predetermined frequency based performance indicators across matches and towards qualitatively based performance indicators within matches. This approach may also help to overcome some of the issues of bias inherent in predetermining what we are looking for (Balague and Torrents, 2005). Using the key principles of rugby union to devise a computer-based algorithm approach to analysis also satisfies Perl's (2005) argument that computerised systems are of little value to sport if their underlying understanding of the sport is poor.

This methodological approach has been tested and has shown good reliability and validity measures. However, it is a work in progress and it is hoped that further developments will improve the algorithm. First, the accuracy of the algorithm may be improved by factoring in the role of defence. Second, beyond a categorical indication of ruck and maul duration, the algorithm does not yet account for the duration of actions, phases or passages of play and subsequently the time spent in different parts of the pitch by each team. Factoring time into the equations could provide an indication of team efficiency that may prove useful. Furthermore, linking individual players to actions could be used to construct player contribution scores, which could then aid player profiling (O'Donoghue, 2005; Heasman *et al.*, 2008; Hughes *et al.*, 2001). Finally, and most critically, further work is required to justify the underlying assumptions on the weightings applied at each stage of the formula.

12.5 CONCLUSION

Whilst the algorithm presented in this study is embryonic, it outlines a practical way forward for applied performance analysis in rugby union. It is hoped that this work encourages the sport to move beyond its historic obsession with counting and reporting on frequencies, which whilst interesting, have largely been unable to explain what happens on the pitch. Further work is required to develop the algorithm and address its current limitations, not least around the calculation of weighted values and the interaction of attacking and defensive systems, which is currently ignored.

12.6 REFERENCES

Balague, N. and Torrents, C., 2005, Thinking before computing: Changing approaches in sports performance. *International Journal of Computer Science in Sport*, **4**(1), pp. 5–13.

Bracewell, P.J., Meyer, D. and Ganesh, S., 2003, Creating and monitoring meaningful individual rugby ratings. *Res. Lett. Inf. Math. Sci.*, **4**, pp. 19–22.

Correia, V., Araújo, D., Davids, K., Fernandes, O. and Fonseca, S., 2011, Territorial gain dynamics regulates success in attacking sub-phases of team sports. *Psychology of Sport and Exercise*, **12**(6), pp. 662–669.

Csataljay, G., O'Donoghue, P.G., Hughes, M.D. and Dancs, H., 2009, Performance indicators that distinguish winning and losing teams in basketball. *International Journal of Performance Analysis in Sport*, **9**, pp. 60–66.

Heasman, J., Dawson, B., Berry, J. and Stewart, G., 2008, Development and validation of a player impact ranking system in Australian football. *International Journal of Performance Analysis in Sport*, **8**(3), pp. 156–171.

Hughes, M., Caudrelier, T., James, N., Donnelly, I., Kirkbride, A. and Duschesne, C., 2012a, Moneyball and soccer: An analysis of the key performance indicators of elite male soccer players by position. *Journal of Human Sport and Exercise*, **7**(2), pp. 402–412.

Hughes, M., Hughes, M.D., Williams, J., James, N., Vučković, G. and Locke, D., 2012b, Performance indicators in rugby union. *Journal of Human Sport and Exercise*, **7**(2), pp. 383–401.

Hughes, M.D. and Bartlett, R.M. (2002). The use of performance indicators in performance analysis. *Journal of Sports Sciences*, **20**, pp. 739–754.

Hughes, M.D., Evans, S. and Wells, J., 2001, Establishing normative profiles in performance analysis. *International Journal of Performance Analysis in Sport*, **1**, pp. 4–27.

Hughes, M.D. and Franks, I.M., 2004, Sports Analysis. In *Notational Analysis of Sport, 2nd edn*, edited by Hughes, M.D. and Franks, I.M. (Abingdon, Oxford: Routledge), pp. 107–117.

Jackson, N. and Hughes, M.D., 2001, Patterns of play of successful and unsuccessful teams in elite women's rugby union. *Proceedings of the 5th World Congress of Performance Analysis in Sport*, edited by Hughes, M. (Cardiff, UK: CPA Press, UWIC), pp. 111–118.

Jones, N., James, N. and Mellalieu, S., 2008, An objective method for depicting team performance in elite professional rugby union. *Journal of Sports Sciences,* **26**(7), pp. 691–700.

Lames, M. and McGarry, T., 2007, On the search for reliable performance indicators in game sports. *International Journal of Performance Analysis in Sport,* **7**(1), pp. 62–79.

O'Donoghue, P.G., 2005, Normative profiles of sports performance. *International Journal of Performance Analysis in Sport,* **5**(1), pp. 104–119.

Ortega, E., Villarejo, D. and Palao, J.M., 2009, Differences in game statistics between winning and losing rugby teams in the Six Nations Tournament. *Journal of Sports Science and Medicine,* **8**, pp. 523–527.

Perl, J., 2005, A computer science in sport: An overview of present fields and future applications (part 2). *International Journal of Computer Science in Sport,* **4**(Part II), pp. 36–45.

Sasaki, K., Furukawa, T., Murakami, J., Shimozono, H., Nagamatsu, M., Miyao, M. and Yamamoto, T., 2007, Scoring profiles and defense performance analysis in Rugby Union. *International Journal of Performance Analysis in Sport,* **7**(3), pp. 46–53.

Thomas, J., Nelson, J. and Silverman, S., 2005, *Research Methods in Physical Activity, 6th edn,* (Champaign, IL: Human Kinetics).

van Rooyen, M.K., Diedrick, E. and Noakes, T.D., 2010, Ruck frequency as a predictor of success in the 2007 Rugby World Cup Tournament. *International Journal of Performance Analysis in Sport,* **10**(1), pp. 33–46.

Vaz, L., Mouchet, A., Carreras, D. and Morente, H., 2011, The importance of rugby game-related statistics to discriminate winners and losers at the elite level competitions in close and balanced games. *International Journal of Performance Analysis in Sport,* **11**(3), pp. 130–141.

Vučković, G., Pers, J., James, N. and Hughes, M.D., 2009, Tactical use of the T area in squash by players of differing standard. *Journal of Sports Sciences,* **27**(8), pp. 863–871.

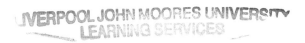

CHAPTER 13

Tackling effectiveness in professional rugby league

Nimai Parmar and Nic James

13.1 INTRODUCTION

It has been suggested that tackling is one of the most arduous and challenging aspects of rugby league (Austin *et al.*, 2011) with tackling effectiveness identified as an important skill related, in part, to the success of rugby league games (Gabbett *et al.*, 2010; Austin *et al.*, 2011). Gabbett *et al.* (2011) found that an average of 300 tackles are made within a professional rugby league match, with forwards making approximately 39 tackles per game and backs a slightly lower average of 16 tackles per game (Gissane *et al.*, 2001; Gabbett *et al.*, 2010). Wheeler *et al.* (2011) further demonstrated the importance of defence through their analysis of ball-offloading strategies in rugby league, showing that the defending team's ability to employ the right tackle technique could be effective in preventing offloads by the ball carrier. This paper will investigate the different factors involved in determining the success or failure of a tackle, as just one missed tackle or offload by a team can lead to a try that could win or lose a game of rugby league.

13.2 METHODS

13.2.1 Data gathering

Ten London Broncos RLFC games (known as Harlequins Rugby League at the time) were randomly selected from the 2011 Engage Super League season with a balanced win–loss record. Games were coded using the Focus X2 software (Elite Sports Analysis, 2002). Action variables were defined to analyse and identify how the number of defending players involved in a tackle and the technique used in the tackle influence the successfulness of tackles and whether this relates to winning or losing in professional rugby league. Each tackle was coded for this study according to the number of defenders committed to the tackle (one, two or three or more); the tackle technique (standard, chop or flop) and the tackle outcome (tackle completed, player put onto back, error forced, offload, missed tackle, penalty/error).

The tackling techniques were defined as '*standard*' when one or two players made the initial contact either low (below waist) or high (above waist) to complete the tackle. A '*chop*' tackle occurred when the initial contact was high by one or two players but an additional player came in low to complete the tackle. The '*flop*' tackle occurred when the initial contact was high by one or two players but an additional player came in high to complete the tackle. Hence chop and flop tackles require two or more defending players involved whereas the standard tackle can involve a minimum of one player. Similarly the tackle outcomes were defined with three successful and three unsuccessful definitions. A tackle was deemed successful if the attacking player was stopped (*tackle completed*). If the ball-carrying player was also turned onto his back or his position changed on the ground then this was deemed a better tackle and coded as '*player put onto their back*'. Finally '*error forced*' was used when the ball carrier committed an infringement or turnover. The fail definitions were used when the ball carrier was able to make an offload (a pass to a teammate during the tackle) and coded as '*ball-carrier offload*', the ball carrier was not stopped '*missed tackle*' and when an infringement was committed '*penalty/error*'.

13.2.2 Reliability and data analysis

An intra-observer reliability test was carried out through percentage error tests, calculated by using the formula; '$(\Sigma(abs[V1-V2])/Vmean)*100$ per cent; where $\Sigma=$ sum of; abs = absolute value; V1= analyst 1; V2= analyst 1 recode; Vmean= mean of all variables' (Hughes *et al.*, 2002, p. 19). This test found a percentage error of <5 per cent, which was deemed an acceptable rate of reliability. Data was analysed using the Mann-Whitney U test and the chi-square test for independence (to determine if ratios of related data changed) to compare winning and losing performance using the IBM SPSS Statistics package (v19, SPSS Inc, 2010).

13.3 RESULTS

There were 24.8 per cent of tackles that involved one defending player and was therefore the standard tackle, whereas 41.0 per cent involved two players and 34.2 per cent three or more, and were therefore any of the three forms of tackle. Mann-Whitney U tests showed that the frequency of standard, chop and flop tackles did not differ between winning and losing matches (p = .22, .69 and .69) although a chi-square test indicated that the proportionate frequency of standard tackles was higher for winning matches compared to losing (Figure 13.1) with chop and flop tackles used more frequently in losing matches.

The success rate for tackling when using the standard tackle was significantly lower (U = 247192, p < 0.001) in losing matches (65.3 per cent) compared to winning matches (76.6 per cent). However there were no differences between tackling success rates when the chop tackle ($\approx$ 97 per cent, U = 5317, p = 0.95) and flop tackle ($\approx$ 98 per cent, Mann-Whitney = 4562.5, p = 0.09) were used.

Analysis of the successful chop and flop tackles revealed high proportionate rates for putting the ball carrier on his back (70.50 per cent chop and 62.10 per cent flop; Figure 13.2). In comparison the standard tackle only achieved this 33.6 per cent of the time in winning matches and 35.5 per cent in losing matches (Figure 13.3)

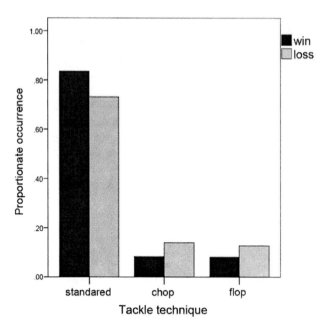

Figure 13.1 The proportionate occurrence of different tackle techniques for matches won and lost

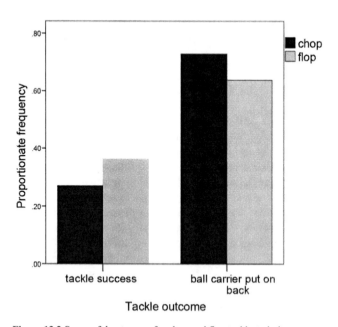

Figure 13.2 Successful outcomes for chop and flop tackle techniques

Figure 13.3 suggests that for standard tackles there were less missed tackles (U = 3.0, p = .056) in winning matches than in losing matches, which would

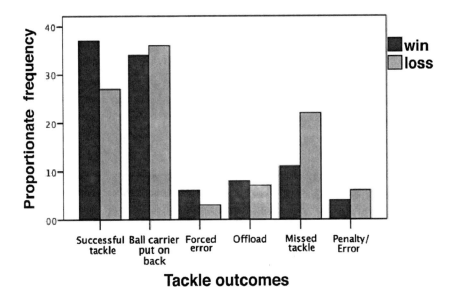

Figure 13.3 Tackle outcomes for the standard tackle technique in winning and losing games

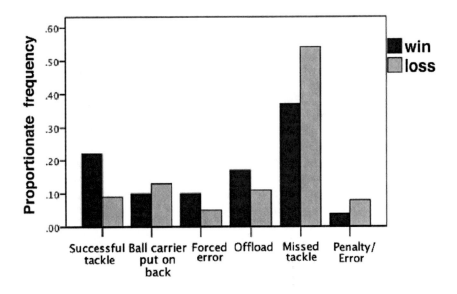

Figure 13.4 Tackle outcomes for the standard tackle technique (only one defender committed) in winning and losing games

largely account for the higher proportionate frequency of successful tackles in the winning matches. However, this analysis assessed tackle outcomes without considering the number of defenders committed to the tackle.

Figure 13.4 shows that when only one defender was committed to the standard tackle success rates decreased markedly in comparison to Figure 13.3 (which included all standard tackles irrespective of the number of defenders involved). Particularly evident was the high frequency of missed tackles, which was also higher ($U = 2.5$, $p < .05$) in losing matches (54.4 per cent) in comparison to winning ones (36.8 per cent)

13.4 DISCUSSION

It was evident that the analysed team used the same proportion of standard (≈ 78 per cent), chop (≈ 11 per cent) and flop (≈ 11 per cent) tackles for both winning and losing matches. The chop and flop tackles were very successful (≈ 98 per cent) resulting in the best outcome, the ball carrier on his back (75 per cent chop, 62 per cent flop) irrespective of match outcome. The success rate for standard tackles was significantly lower in losing matches (65.3 per cent) in comparison to winning matches (76.6 per cent) suggesting that this could be deemed a performance indicator. It seemed that in winning matches there were less missed tackles than in losing matches but this was not significant and did not account for the number of defending players involved in the tackle. When standard tackles with only one defender involved were examined it was clear that success rates were markedly lower in comparison to when the analysis did not distinguish the number of defenders involved. It was evident therefore that the majority of errors occurred when only one defending player was involved in the tackle, this resulted in a high frequency of missed tackles, which was significantly higher in losing matches (54.4 per cent) in comparison to winning ones (36.8 per cent).

The clear advantage of using the chop and flop techniques over the standard technique was evident due to the increased success rate of this tackle, in particular the frequency of the ball carrier being put on their back. This has the effect of slowing the attacking team down as it takes longer to get the next play going thus enabling the defensive line to retreat 10 metres, re-align and adjust their formation and identify attacking opportunities (Eaves and Broad, 2007). However, these tackles need more than one player to be committed to the tackle and as the analysis of the standard tackle showed, having less than two defending players involved in a tackle seems to be a main cause of lower success rates. Eaves and Broad (2007, p. 61) confirmed this by suggesting that sending more players into the tackle area will aid tackle outcomes, in particular by slowing down the opposition. Hence, it can be seen that the tackle outcome is highly determined by the number of defending players committed and the technique used is less important for achieving success although better outcomes, i.e. the ball carrier ends up on his back, are associated with the chop and flop techniques.

13.5 CONCLUSION

Clear evidence is provided to promote the use of more than one defender into a tackle in rugby league on the basis of better tackle outcomes and the reduction of missed tackles. In this study about a quarter of all tackles involved only one defending player and a reduction in this would likely improve the defensive capabilities of the team. This could be achieved if the coach and the players recognise the importance of committing more than one defending player to the tackle and identify the necessary training drills, match strategies and fitness components to enable a reduction in the match. It appears that when a team is not able to commit more than one defending player to the tackle the only option is the standard tackle whose outcomes are significantly worse in losing matches than winning ones. Future studies should try to better understand the factors involved in determining which tackling technique is used and try to ascertain strategies for increasing the number of players committed to a tackle and this may also promote more use of the flop and chop techniques.

13.6 REFERENCES

Austin, D., Gabbett, T. and Jenkins, D., 2011, Tackling in professional rugby league. *Journal of Strength and Conditioning Research*, **25**(6), pp. 1659–1663.
Eaves, S. and Broad, G., 2007, A comparative analysis of professional rugby league football playing patterns between Australia and the United Kingdom. *International Journal of Performance Analysis in Sport*, 7(3), pp.54–66.
Elite Sports Analysis Ltd. 2002, *Focus X2 Help Manual*, (Fife, Scotland: Elite Sports Analysis Ltd).
Gabbett, T.J., Jenkins, D.G. and Abernethy, B., 2010, Physiological and anthropometric characteristics of junior elite and sub-elite rugby league players. *Journal of Strength and Conditioning Research*, **24**, pp. 2989–2995.
Gabbett, T.J., Jenkins, D.G. and Abernethy, B., 2011, Correlates of tackling ability in high performance rugby league players. *Journal of Strength and Conditioning Research*, **25**(1), pp. 72–79.
Gissane, C., White, J., Kerr, K. and Jennings, D., 2001, Physical collisions in professional super league rugby, the demands on different player positions. *Cleveland Clinic Journal of Medicine*, **4**, pp. 137–146.
Hughes, M., Cooper, S.M. and Nevill, A., 2002, Analysis procedures for non-parametric data from performance analysis. *International Journal of Performance Analysis of Sport*, **2**, pp. 6–20.
SPSS Inc., 2010, IBM SPSS Statistics 19 Brief Guide, (Champaign, IL: SPSS Inc).
Wheeler, K., Wiseman, R. and Lyons, K., 2011, Tactical and technical factors associated with effective ball offloading strategies during the tackle in rugby league. *International Journal of Performance Analysis in Sport*, **11**, pp. 392–409.

CHAPTER 14

Defence performance analysis of rugby union in Rugby World Cup 2011: Network analysis of the turnover contributors

Sasaki Koh, Takumi Yamamoto, Jun Murakami and Yuichi Ueno

14.1. INTRODUCTION: TRENDS FROM IRB GAME ANALYSIS

Despite the 2009 rules amendment for advantage to the attacking side (severe limitations on the defensive side in the tackle), the number of try scores per match in the Rugby World Cup has decreased (6.9 tries in 2003, 6.2 tries in 2007 and 5.5 tries in 2011) (IRB, 2011). It is suggested that defensive capabilities have improved. Various performance profiling techniques have been proposed to represent typical performances of individuals and teams (O'Donoghue, 2005; James *et al.*, 2005). Common and individual behaviours would be needed for a more accurate representation of players' contributions to performance (James *et al.*, 2005) to raise evidence relating to defence. The current study focused on defensive turnover situations in the game and applied social network analysis to organizational strategy. Figure 14.1 shows the starting point of tries scored in the Rugby World Cup in 2007 and 2011. The frequency of the tries where possession started between the try line and opposition 10 m line has decreased from 63 per cent of tries at the 2007 World Cup to 54 per cent in 2011. There were 55 per cent of the tries of the New Zealand team, who had the highest number of tries, where possession started in the remainder of the pitch. The team with the second highest number of tries was Wales who scored 58 per cent of their tries from possessions commencing outside the opposition last 10 m. This characteristic might suggest that such tries progressed with high level fitness during the offensive game and also with high level defensive performance as a crucial factor.

	2007 RWC	2011 RWC	(NZL)	(WAL)
Try-line – Oppose10m-line	63% →	54%		
Oppose – 10m-line – Own Half	37% →	46%	(55%)	(58%)
	(296 tries)	(262 tries)	(40 tries)	(29 tries)

Figure 14.1 Start of a possession that leads to a try in Rugby World Cup 2011 comparing 2007

For understanding defence performance towards the final score difference, a regression analysis was done (independent variables; 'tackle success ratio: 0–100 (per cent)', 'frequencies of the missed tackles', and 'frequencies of crucial turnover get', dependent variable; 'final score difference'). This allowed comparison of results with past study (Sasaki *et al.*, 2005). High regression values were obtained in this analysis ($R^2 = 0.77$, SE = 221.34, F = 17.75, $p < 0.01$). The findings presented in Table 14.1 indicate that the three independent variables of defensive performance were contributing factors for final score difference. A 1 per cent increase in the 'tackle success ratio' (for example: 79 per cent to 80 per cent) could contribute positively 1.43 points in the final score difference. An increase of 1 in the frequency of 'missed tackles' could contributes negatively 2.28 points to the final score difference. Increasing the frequency of the crucial 'turnover get' by 1 could contribute positively 9.23 points to the final score difference. Furthermore, a statistically significant correlation was found between the independent variable 'frequencies of turnover get' and the dependent 'final score difference'. Practically speaking, the index of 'turnover get' compared with tackle situations (tackle success or not, missed tackle or not) would have a more positive effect towards the final score difference. So the next focus of our research effort was on tackle turnover situations. After the 2009 rules amendment giving advantage to the attacking side, the discussion about the defence should include the greater physical intensity of cooperation between team-mates. Greenwood (2003, p. 281) pointed out that the defensive team-mates must move up as one man and make pressure through balanced aggression. However, there has been little descriptive research about two man tackle turnovers which would be part of an aggressive defence.

Table 14.1 Regression equation between 'score balance' and the defence performances in 2011 Rugby World Cup

Score Balance = 1.43*TS − 2.28*MT + 9.23*TOG − 116.43			
S => (2.16)	(1.88)	(2.89)	(205.69)
t => (0.66)	(−1.21)	(3.20)**	(−0.56)
$R^2 = 0.77$, SE = 221.34, F = 17.55**, **$p < 0.01$			

TS; Tackle success Ratio, MT; Missed Tackle, TOG; Turnover Get

14.2 METHODS

Network analysis has been developed in communication-network studies as a graph theory within mathematics. The network has a structure of both the vertex (players' positions) and the edge line (cooperation between team-mates in match; two man tackle turnover) and network analysis presents a descriptive index of the graph structure with supporting statistics for which position plays a central role of two man tackle turnover.

Data were derived from 20 matches of close and balanced scores (under 20 points between the two teams with results from cluster analysis according to game final score differences of the 40 pool matches) referring to past study structure (Vaz *et al.*, 2011). Network analysis in the current study would clarify the evidence of dynamic balance mechanism of defensive cooperation of team-mates in close and balanced matches. The proportion of the two man tackle turnovers was 31 per cent (204/660) of all tackle turnover situations. To understand the two man positional relation structure, the frequencies of two man tackle turnovers were plotted in the adjacent matrix (15 × 15). The density centrality by the frequencies of turnover and eigenvector centrality by the intimacy relationship within positional cooperations were calculated. The calculation and making the networking map program was done by a computer program tool 'R'. The weighting process used Jaccard coefficients which are defined as the intersection divided by the sample numbers.

$$J(A,B) = \frac{|A,B|}{|A \cup B|} \qquad (14.1)$$

Degree means the frequency of links incident upon a position (vertex) and calculated for all the vertexes in an adjacency matrix. The network map was completed by the degree centrality of a vertex '*v*'. Degree centrality is as follows:

$$C_D = \frac{\sum_{i=1}^{V}\left[C_D(v*)-C_D(v_i)\right]}{(n-1)(n-2)} \qquad (14.2)$$

where C_D is degree centrality, $v*$ is vertex with highest degree centrality, v_i is actual degree centrality, i is vertex number, V is total vertexes, $(n-1)(n-2)$: the maximum value occurs when the graph contains one central vertex to which all other vertexes are connected (a star graph).

14.3 RESULTS AND DISCUSSION

The map layout was calculated by the Fruchterman-Reingold Algorithm (Fruchterman and Reingold, 1991) which is a force-directed layout algorithm for centralization of the double tackle contributors' positioning. The purpose was to position the vertexes of a graph in a two-dimensional space so that all the edges were of more or less equal length and there were as few crossing edges as possible (Eades, 1984; Kamada and Kawai, 1989; Inoue *et al.*, 2012). The force-directed algorithms achieved this by assigning forces among the set of vertexes and the set of edges. The forces were applied to the vertexes, pulling them closer together or pushing them further apart. This was repeated iteratively until the system comes to a state of equilibrium. Main double tackle contributors which mapped centrally in the team positions graph were '8', '6', '2', '12', and '7'. Defensive pressure to opposition is generated by the front three of backs (fly half and centre three-quarter backs) and the back row of the forwards to deny the opposition the initiative (Greenwood, 2003, p30). These five positions might have been frequent occurrences in 'double tackle turnover' in the Rugby Union World Cup 2011. When playing in a rugby union game, these positions would be expected to be comparatively key to 'break-downs' (high values for the frequency of fighting for ball contests and play continuity of possession not only by oneself but also with partners, i.e. double tackle situation).

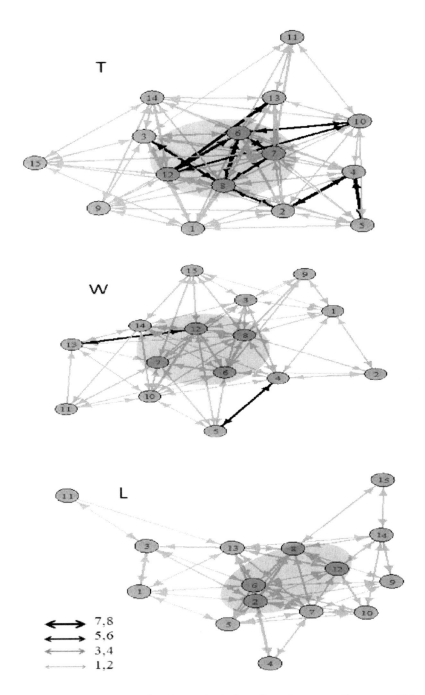

Figure 14.2 Double tackle contributor's mapping by force-directed placement (degree centrality) at 2011 Rugby World Cup close games in pool matches (T: total, W: winners, L: losers, bold black lines: more than 5 times double tackle turnover partners)

Table 14.2 Degree and eigenvector centrality scores

Position	Total		Winning side		Losing side	
	D	EVC	D	EVC	D	EVC
1	28	0.51	18	0.39	10	0.49
2	**42**	**0.80**	20	0.49	**22**	**1.00**
3	34	0.64	24	0.50	10	**0.77**
4	40	0.54	**34**	0.59	6	0.34
5	30	0.46	18	0.39	12	0.36
6	**64**	**0.92**	**42**	**0.92**	**22**	**0.74**
7	**56**	**0.73**	**38**	**0.81**	18	0.54
8	**72**	**1.00**	**52**	**1.00**	20	**0.87**
9	26	0.41	16	0.39	10	0.35
10	40	0.57	28	**0.60**	12	0.44
11	19	0.25	16	0.38	3	0.08
12	**54**	**0.78**	**40**	**0.80**	14	**0.58**
13	40	0.54	25	0.56	**15**	0.45
14	35	0.40	23	0.44	12	0.31
15	18	0.24	14	0.28	4	0.09

D: degree, EVC: eigenvector centrality scores; bold figures indicate 5 high score indices

The graph of the T (total) and the W (winning sides) might show the stable structure by existence of multiple bold relations with double tackle partners. Comparing the losing side's with winning side's characteristics, the former's were suggested to sometimes be out of the balanced networking systems because less bold relations of double tackle pairs occurred.

The tendency of the differences between the winning and losing sides would be observed in the eigenvector centralities (Table 14.2). Eigenvector centrality means an index of adjacency of vertexes by using the first eigenvector and would also be seen as a weighted sum of not only direct connections but also indirect connections of every vertex (Bonacich and Lloyd, 2004). It is the solution to the following matrix equation: $Av = \lambda v$ (A: adjacency matrix, λ: scalar, v: non-zero eigenvector).

Network analysis (graph theory) using some centrality indices would present a practical evaluation for positional functions in team sport and organizations. Centre three-quarter backs (position '12' and '13') in rugby union play a central and balanced role of the other backs positions. The back row forwards (position '6', '7' and '8') and the hooker (position '2') play a linking role between forwards and backs to fill a gap, to deny the opposition the initiative, to harry them into confusion and, if possible, to get a turnover (Greenwood, 2003, p. 30). These positive defensive tactics would be performed through team-mates' cooperation, successive pressure, cover and communication. It would also present some kind of strategic and tactical knowledge for planning the game, practice and the communication situations concerning team/game centrality.

It is a future task to describe a more clear and detailed dynamic equilibrium (Fukuoka, 2009; Inoue *et al.*, 2012) between positions by applying various network force-directed approaches.

14.4 REFERENCES

Bonacich, P. and Lloyd, P., 2004, Calculating status with negative relations. *Social Networks*, **26**, pp. 331–338.

Eades, P., 1984, A heuristic for graph drawing. *Congressus Numerantium*, **42**(11), pp. 149–160.

Fruchterman, T.M.J. and Reingold, E.M., 1991, Graph drawing by force-directed placement. *Software: Practice and Experience*, **21**(11), pp. 1129–1164.

Fukuoka, S., 2009, *Dynamic Equilibrium*, (Tokyo, Japan: Kirakusya).

Greenwood, J., 2003, *Total Rugby*, (London, UK: A&C Black).

International Rugby Board (IRB), 2011, Rugby World Cup 2011 statistical review and match analysis. http://www.irb.com/mm/document/newsmedia/mediazone/02/06/06/64/111026irbgameanalysis2011irbrugbyworldcupstatisticalreview.pdf

Inoue, K., Shimozono, S., Yoshida, H. and Kurata, H., 2012, Application of approximate pattern matching in two dimensional spaces to grid layout for biochemical network maps. *PLoS ONE*, 7(6), e37739.

James, N., Mellalieu, S.D. and Jones, N.M.P., 2005, The development of position-specific performance indicators in professional rugby union. *Journal of Sports Science*, **23**, pp. 63–72.

Kamada, T. and Kawai, S., 1989, An algorithm for drawing general undirected graphs. *Information Processing Letters (Elsevier)*, **31**(1), pp. 7–15.

O'Donoghue, P., 2005, Normative profiles of sports performance. *International Journal of Performance Analysis in Sport*, **5**(1), pp. 104–119.

Sasaki, K., Murakami, J., Simozozno, H., Furukawa, T., Miyao, M., Saito, T., Yamamoto, T., Nakayama, M., Hirao, S., Hanaoka, N., Katuta, T. and Kono, I., 2005, Defence performance analysis of Rugby Union: The turnover-play structure, In *Science and Football V*, edited by Reilly, T., Cabri, J. and Araújo, D. (London, UK: Routledge), pp. 243–246.

Vaz, L., Mouchet, A., Carreras, D. and Morente, H., 2011, The importance of rugby game-related statistics to discriminate winners and losers at the elite level competitions in closed and balanced games, *International Journal of Performance Analysis in Sport*, **11**, pp. 130–141.

CHAPTER 15

Tackling in Super 15 Rugby 2011

Michele van Rooyen

15.1 INTRODUCTION

In rugby matches, players are frequently exposed to multiple physical contacts and tackles and, as a result, good defensive and tackling skills are required. Success in rugby has also been linked with tackle frequency and tackling proficiency (Ortega et al., 2009; van Rooyen et al., 2008; Vaz et al., 2011).

The purpose of the tackle is to stop the attacking team from moving forward and to create opportunities for the defending team to contest possession of the ball (Takarada, 2003; IRB, 2011). The tackle is both a key component to successful defense and a platform for potential counter-attacks (Fuller et al., 2007).

Research into the tackle has found that professional rugby matches contain over 200 tackle situations (Fuller et al., 2007; Quarrie and Hopkins, 2007; 2008), with the forwards making the majority of the these contacts (Quarrie and Hopkins, 2008; Smart et al., 2008; van Rooyen et al., 2008). Statistics have shown that winning teams miss fewer tackles than losing teams although this did not always reach the level of significance ($P < 0.05$) and small to moderate size effects were observed (Jones et al., 2004; Ortega et al., 2009; Vaz et al., 2011). Studies that have combined data from several seasons of matches (Ortega et al., 2009; Vaz et al., 2010) and, in the case of Vaz et al. (2010), with multiple tournaments, have not taken into account potential inter-season or intra-competition performance variations.

It is important to understand how the effects of tackle situation influences performance and match outcome of a single season of a rugby competition (Duthie et al., 2005). This study was designed, therefore, to investigate the influence different playing positions have on tackling performance and how this affects the match outcome.

15.2 METHODS

Data for this comparative study were collected from statistics supplied by Verusco Sport's Advanced Rugby Analysis System (Verusco, 2012) after the 2011 Super 15 rugby competition. The log matches (n = 118.5 of 120; match 11 Hurricanes vs. Crusaders, match not played and match 46 Western Force vs. Melbourne Rebels data incomplete) and the five knockout games were studied. The data collected were: number of points conceded; points difference; number of tackles 'attempted' and 'made'; and the tackle completion rate. Additional information was calculated from these raw data: percentage of tackles 'made' and 'missed' per positional group; percentage of missed tackles per team; and the percentage of tackles 'attempted' (the percentage of tackles 'made' plus the percentage of tackles 'missed') per positional group. The data from the substitutes (n = 7 max and n = 0 min) were incorporated into the appropriate positional groups. Mann-Whitney and Kruskal-Wallis tests were conducted to determine the variation in the data. Significance was set at P = 0.05. The normality of the data was determined using the procedure defined by Hughes *et al.*, (2001). Correlations were calculated using the Spearman Rank Order method.

15.3 RESULTS

A total of 38,807 tackle situations were recorded during the 123.5 analyzed matches. There were 88.6 per cent (34,395) of these were tackles 'made' and 11.3 per cent (4,412) were tackles 'missed'. This equates to an average of 139 (±34 SD) tackles 'made' per team per match or 278 tackles (±48 SD) 'made' per game. There was an average of 18 'missed' tackles (±7 SD) recorded per team per match. These data (tackles 'made' and tackles 'missed' and thus tackles 'attempted') although the variance was insignificant, were found to be less consistent than the normalized counterparts according to the profiling technique of Hughes *et al.*, (2001), so the remaining tackle data presented is normalized to percentage frequency.

The percentage contribution of the back row forwards was significantly higher than the percentage contribution of the other five positions (P < 0.0001) for tackles 'attempted', tackles 'made' and tackles 'missed'. It was also noted that the three forward positional groups (props and hookers, locks and back row) all significantly varied from the three back groups (scrumhalf/flyhalf, centre and fullbacks/wings) for both tackles 'attempted' and tackles 'made'. Individual group comparisons were also found to show large size effects.

By combining the data into the two gross positional groups, forwards (n = 8) and backs (n = 7) it was discovered that forwards contributed to 64.4 per cent (±6.1 SD) of the team tackles 'made' per match whereas the backs only contributed 35.6 per cent (±6.1 SD). These data are not significantly different across the teams and matches (P > 0.05) but they show a large size effect when compared with each other that also reached the level of significance (P < 0.05).

To determine whether these data were genuinely different from each other or whether this observation was simply a result of the differing numbers of group members, the data were further normalized per player and this was compared to the hypothetical chance (100 per cent/15) that the percentage of tackles each player makes are equal. The significant differences observed between the back row (9 × 3 = 27) and the wings/fullbacks (3 × 3 = 9) were a genuine difference in tackle performance rather than being primarily related to group size. The data when corrected for group size found that the forwards group (8.0 per cent ± 0.76 SD per player) and the backs group (5.1 per cent ± 0.87 SD per player) continued to show a large size effect and a significant difference (P < 0.0001).

The data for the percentage of 'missed' tackles, when corrected for the number of players within each group show that both the forwards (6.7 ± 1.7 per cent) and the backs (6.7 ± 1.9 per cent) had an equal probability of contributing to the percentage of team 'missed' tackles.

The forwards made an average 11 per cent greater contribution to the percentage of tackles 'made' than the tackles 'missed' although this was not a significant difference (P > 0.05) there was a large size effect. The reverse was true for the backs, with this group making an 11 per cent greater contribution to the tackles 'missed' (P < 0.001). The balance of the contributions (63 per cent for the forwards vs. 36 per cent for the backs) to the tackles 'made' showed that there was a 1.2 times greater probability of a forward successfully completing a tackle than would occur by chance and a 1.8 times greater probability a forward would successfully execute a tackle than a back.

Repeating the analysis of the data when it was expressed according to match outcome, win or lose (n = 119 matches) found that the differences between the specific playing groups and the gross playing groups (forwards and backs) were insignificant (P > 0.05) and not related to match outcome for 'attempted' and 'made' tackles. The mean number of points conceded for winning teams was almost 2 tries fewer (13 points) when compared to the points conceded for losing teams (17 ± 8 vs. 30 ± 9 points conceded for winning and losing teams respectively). It was interesting to note than when the size of the points difference (1–7 vs. 8 and above) was taken into account there was a 'stronger' correlation between the percentage of 'missed' tackles and points conceded for the winning teams (R^2 = 0.29 for winning (P = 0.04) compared to R^2 = 0.10 for losing (P = 0.47)) than for losing teams when the difference was 7 or less.

When the tackle data was categorized as either more 'missed' tackles or less 'missed' tackles, the team that 'missed' the fewest tackles won a greater number of matches (n = 68 or 55 per cent), even though the difference between the winning and losing teams was only 1 per cent. The average percentage of 'missed' tackles per team per match was 10.8 per cent (±3 per cent SD) for winning and 11.8 per cent (±4 per cent SD) for losing teams.

Examination of the data by the final log placing identified that an average of 60 per cent of matches were won with fewer 'missed' tackles by the top six teams compared with an average of only 41 per cent by the remaining 9 teams (Table 15.1). This trend was reversed when the matches lost by a smaller percentage of 'missed' tackles were taken into account. An average of 41 per cent of matches were lost with a lower percentage of 'missed' tackles by the 9 lower placed teams than the 28 per cent of matches observed by the top 6 teams. The data for the tackles 'missed' did show a difference between the winning and losing teams. The forwards from winning teams 'missed' on average fewer tackles than the forwards from losing teams (P = 0.74). The backs from winning teams, however, 'missed' a greater number of tackles than the backs from losing teams (P = 0.06) with a small effect size.

15.4 DISCUSSION

The average tackle completion rate found in this study was 88 per cent for the matches analyzed (n = 124). This figure is consistent with other findings, 90 per cent (Quarrie and Hopkins, 2008) and 89 per cent (Ortega *et al.*, 2009) from matches between the early 1990s and present times.

The forwards made a significantly greater contribution to the tackles 'attempted' and 'made' than the backs by 2:1. These findings underline the differentiated roles of the forwards and backs documented during rugby matches and especially in contact situations (Duthie *et al.*, 2005, Quarrie and Hopkins, 2008; Gabbett *et al.*, 2011).

The distribution of the percentage of 'missed' tackles was similar between the forwards and the backs, when the number of players per group was accounted for (a player, irrespective of position would 'miss' 6.7 per cent of the tackles 'attempted' (P = 0.75)). However, the significance of this only became apparent when the match outcome was taken into consideration.

The team that made the smallest percentage of 'missed' tackles won on average 55 per cent of the matches analyzed. When these data were contextualized according to team and the final position in the league table, it was found that the 'top six' won 60 per cent of their matches by 'missing' fewer tackles than their opposition. The remaining nine teams on the other hand won only 41 per cent of their matches by 'missing' tackles less frequently than their opponents. This would tend to indicate that the percentage of 'missed' tackles a team made was related to the final result of the game and thus the final log position at the end of the conference stage of the tournament.

These data indicate that there were fluctuations in the percentage contribution that the forwards and the backs make to the final team's percentage 'missed' tackles and this also affected the outcome of the match. Specifically for the top six finishing teams as their tackle completion rate was marginally worse (87 per cent) than the rate for the remaining nine teams (88 per cent) when they lost the match. It is also possible to infer that the 1 per cent increase in the tackles 'missed' was due to the forwards rather than the backs because in the majority of cases when the backs 'missed' a greater percentage of their tackle 'attempts' the team still recorded a positive match outcome. This suggestion was based on the simple categorization of 'win' vs. 'lose' and 'more' missed tackles versus 'less' missed tackles and provided no indication of the magnitude of the differences in tackle performance between the teams because when values were assigned to the tackles, the variation in the data obscured potentially important differences.

Winning teams were more susceptible to conceding points through 'missed' tackles than the losing teams when the point's difference between the two teams was ≤7. This was more apparent during 'derby' matches, were two teams from the same nation played each other or when the teams where within five positions of each other in the log table. A reason for this could be the adoption of more expansive attacking strategies in order to either increase a team's lead or reduce the current score deficit at the cost of their defensive structure and so when possession of the ball is lost the winning team were less able to execute their tackles effectively.

Table 15.1 Summary data for the whole Super 15 Tournament showing the number of matches played, matches won, lost or drawn and the number of matches won or lost with a lower percentage of tackles 'missed' (matches won/lost with lower % 'missed' tackles as a percentage of the individual team's matches won/lost)

Whole tournament	Played	Matches won (>7 points diff)	Matches lost (≤7 points diff)	Matches drawn	Matches won with smaller % 'missed' tackles	Matches lost with smaller % 'missed' tackles
Reds	18	15 (7)	3 (1)	0	11 (73%)	0 (0%)
Stormers	17	12 (9)	5 (3)	0	6 (50%)	2 (40%)
Crusaders [1*]	18	13 (9)	5 (3)	0	12 (92%)	2 (40%)
Blues	18	11 (6)	6 (4)	1	5 (45%)	2 (33%)
Waratahs	17	10 (7)	7 (3)	0	8 (80%)	3 (43%)
Sharks	17	10 (6)	6 (1)	1	2 (20%)	0 (0%)
Vodacom Bulls	16	10 (5)	6 (3)	0	4 (40%)	3 (50%)
Highlanders	16	8 (3)	8 (3)	0	3 (38%)	4 (50%)
Hurricanes [1*]	15	5 (1)	9 (5)	1	3 (60%)	4 (44%)
Chiefs	16	6 (2)	9 (4)	1	4 (67%)	5 (56%)
Toyota Cheetahs	16	5 (5)	11 (7)	0	3 (60%)	2 (18%)
Western Force [2*]	15	5 (2)	8 (5)	2	3 (60%)	3 (38%)
Brumbies	16	4 (3)	11 (4)	1	3 (75%)	5 (45%)
MTN Lions	16	3 (1)	12 (5)	1	1 (33%)	8 (67%)
Melbourne Rebels [2*]	15	2 (1)	13 (2)	0	0 (0%)	8 (62%)
Total	123	119 (67)	119 (52)	4 (3%)	68 (55%)	51 (43%)

Key:
* Represents missing match data for 2 of the 125 matches played. - - - - - Separation point between the teams that qualified for the knockout stages of the competition and the remaining 9

These data only reflect the findings of the first year of the Super 15 competition so the addition of subsequent season's data will help to verify these findings. Future studies that incorporate the location on the field where the 'attempted' tackle occurs and relate this to the time in the match would add a valuable dimension to statistical tackle data.

This study has provided insight into the information that can be obtained from a more in-depth analysis of statistical reports. However, it is only a starting point to determining the effect defending has on match outcomes and has generated more questions that require further investigation. Two practical implications from this study are: i) the need for continued development of specific match-related exercises to condition players more effectively for the demands of tackling within a rugby match, and ii) the importance of effective defensive structures need to be instilled into the players especially when leading closely contested matches.

15.5 REFERENCES

Duthie, G.M., Pyne, D.B. and Hooper, S.L., 2005, Time motion analysis of 2001 and 2002 super 12 rugby. *Journal of Sports Sciences*, **23**(5), pp. 523–530.

Fuller, C.W., Brooks, J.H.M., Cancea, R.J., Hall, J. and Kemp, S.P.T., 2007. Contact events in rugby union and their propensity to cause injury. *British Journal of Sports Medicine*, **41**(12), pp. 862–7; discussion 867.

Gabbett, T.J., Jenkins, D.G. and Abernethy, B., 2011, Correlates of tackling ability in high-performance rugby league players. *Journal of Strength and Conditioning Research/National Strength and Conditioning Association*, **25**(1), pp. 72–79.

Hughes, M.D., Evans, S. and Wells, J., 2001, Establishing normative profiles in performance analysis. *International Journal of Performance Analysis in Sport*, **1**, pp. 4–27.

International Rugby Board (IRB), 2011, *Rugby Ready*. Available at: http://www.irbrugbyready.com/pdfs/rugby_ready_book_2011_en.pdf (accessed 27 June 2012).

Jones, N.M.P., Mellalieu, S.D. and James, N., 2004, Team performance indicators as a function of winning and losing in rugby union. *International Journal of Performance Analysis in Sport*, **4**(1), pp. 61–71.

Ortega, E., Villarejo, D. and Palao, J.M., 2009, Differences in game statistics between winning and losing rugby teams in the Six Nations Tournament. *Journal of Sports Science and Medicine*, **8**, pp. 523–527.

Quarrie, K.L. and Hopkins, W.G., 2007, Changes in player characteristics and match activities in Bledisloe Cup rugby union from 1972 to 2004. *Journal of Sports Sciences*, **25**(8), pp.895–903.

Quarrie, K.L. and Hopkins, W.G., 2008, Tackle injuries in professional Rugby Union. *The American Journal of Sports Medicine*, **36**(9), pp. 1705–1716.

Smart, D.J., Gill, N.D., Beaven, C.M., Cook, C.J. and Blazevich, A.J., 2008, The relationship between changes in interstitial creatine kinase and game-related impacts in rugby union. *British Journal of Sports Medicine*, **42**(3), pp.198–201.

Takarada, Y., 2003, Evaluation of muscle damage after a rugby match with special reference to tackle plays. *British Journal of Sports Medicine*, **37**, p. 4.

van Rooyen, M.K., Rock, K., Prim, S. and Lambert, M., 2008, The quantification of contacts with impact during professional rugby matches. *International Journal of Performance Analysis in Sport*, **8**(1) pp. 113–126.

Vaz, L., van Rooyen, M.K. and Sampaio, J., 2010, Rugby game-related statistics that discriminate between winning and losing teams in IRB and Super twelve close games. *Journal of Sports Science and Medicine*, **9**, pp. 51–55.

Vaz, L., Mouchet, A., Carreras, D. and Morente, H., 2011, The importance of rugby game-related statistics to discriminate winners and losers at the elite level competitions in close and balanced games. *International Journal of Performance Analysis in Sport*, **11**, pp. 130–141.

Verusco, 2012, http://www.verusco.com/verusco_stats_portal.php?compid=1 &yearid=1&weekid=0&gameid=0.

CHAPTER 16

The effect of game location on positional profiles of a professional rugby union team during a competitive season

John Francis and Gareth Jones

16.1 INTRODUCTION

Since the International Rugby Board's decision to turn the sport professional in 1995, staff and players have evolved and developed rapidly. A variety of performance analysis tools and other technological advances are now being utilised by teams and individuals to gain a competitive advantage by half a per cent, a second or a millimetre (Mellalieu *et al*. 2008). One area in particular has received considerable interest, with the aim of investigating the use of profiling to predict future performance (Mellalieu *et al*. 2008).

To date, a small number of rugby union studies have investigated positional specific profiles; however, these studies have used a variety of participants and positional clusters, consequently discovering a variety of results. Most recently, James *et al*. (2005) developed a valid and reliable methodology for creating individual playing position profiles within rugby union. The study identified that positional decision making skills and styles of play varied, confirming that intra-positional differences existed. This, therefore, suggested that various positional profiles are required to gain a further understanding of the positional-skill demands, such as game location.

Thomas *et al*. (2008) identified that an overall statistically significant ($p < 0.05$) home advantage of 61 per cent existed when 120 Six Nations Rugby Union matches were analysed between 2000 and 2007. Morton (2006) also discovered that home teams demonstrate an attacking style of play, scoring an average of 20.9 points in comparison to 13.4 points when playing an away fixture, when teams adopted a more defensive approach. Utilising this information, the aims of this study were therefore twofold; first, to investigate the effect of game location on positional specific profiles in professional rugby union; second, to investigate how positional specific profiles can be utilised by coaches in professional rugby union.

16.2 METHOD

16.2.1 Data collection

Match footage (Total 28; 14 home; 14 away) from one Championship Rugby Union team was converted into a SportsCode Elite project for post-event analysis

(SportsCode Elite V8, Sportstec Limited, Warriewood, NSW, Australia). A list of performance indicators was compiled utilising previous rugby union research and scrutinised by two elite rugby union performance analysts and two elite coaches who refined the list of performance indicators, from 40 to 31 performance indicators (minutes played prior to substitution; total tackles attempted; effectively completed tackle; ineffective completed tackle; assisted tackle; missed tackle; jackal; kick pressure; ball-in-hand; pass; into contact; ball out of tackle; recycle; lost in contact; tackled into touch; hammer; ruck clears; try; handling error; kick; penalty conceded; penalty won; turnover conceded; turnover won; line-out throw; line-out jump; lift; maul attack; maul defence; scrum engage; set piece error). The performance indicators were utilised to create a coding window in SportsCode Elite. Intra- and inter-observer reliability tests were conducted utilising a technique proposed by Hughes *et al.* (2002), to establish an error percentage (Intra – 1.37 per cent; Inter – 1.12 per cent). Following the analysis a semi-structured interview was conducted with the head coach to gain an understanding of how the information could be utilised in an applied environment. The interview lasted 19 minutes and was transcribed verbatim with grammatical alterations being conducted with the final transcript shown to the interviewee to confirm authenticity.

16.2.2 Data analysis

Performance profile data was exported to version 19 of the Statistic Package for Social Sciences (IBM, Chicago) and a Wilcoxon Signed Ranks Test was conducted with a level of statistical significance set at $p < 0.05$. The interview transcript underwent thematic content analysis to identify any unique themes.

16.3. RESULTS

Wilcoxon Signed Ranks Tests identified no statistically significant ($p > 0.05$) differences between the home and away locations for all the performance indicators. However, three main trends were identified: total tackle attempts, ball in hand occurrences and passes completed. The total number of tackle attempts each position completed, when at home in comparison to matches played away from home, was analysed (see Figure 16.1). The forwards (except Position #8) completed a higher number of tackle attempts at home compared to when playing away from home. The backs (Positions #9 to #15; except Position #14), achieved a higher number of tackle attempts when away compared to at home. Figure 16.2 shows that all playing positions, with the exception of the right second-row and full back, achieved a higher number of ball in hand occurrences when the team were playing away from home (Figure 16.3). The scrum half position and the fly half achieved the largest number of ball in hand occurrences per fixture (scrum half: home 26.5 ± 16.0; away 36.6 ± 20.6; fly half: home 17.8 ± 10.4; away 21.9 ± 13.1).

Figure 16.3 shows that all playing positions completed a greater number of passes when competing away from home (except Positions #5, #8, #12 and #15).

The tight-head prop (Position #3) completed the fewest number of passes (home 0.6 ± 1.0; away 0.7 ± 1.0), preferring to take the ball into contact (home 70 per cent; away 80 per cent).

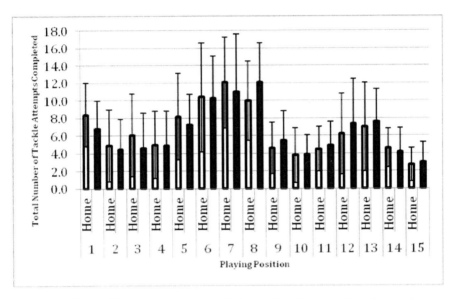

Figure 16.1 Mean tackle attempts per match per playing position when competing at home and away

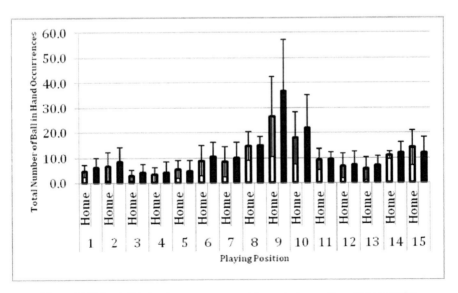

Figure 16.2 Mean ball in hand occurrence per match per playing position when competing at home and away

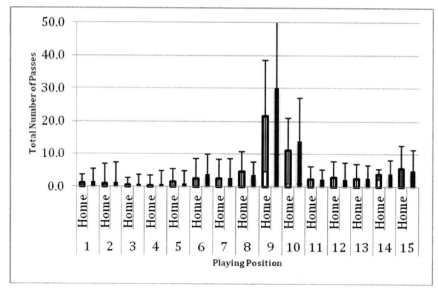

Figure 16.3 Mean passes completed per match per playing position when competing at home and away

During thematic content analysis of the coach's transcript, five key themes emerged:

- Positive use of game location positional profiles;
- Negative use of game location positional profiles;
- No use of game location positional profiles;
- Positive player performance and game location;
- Negative player performance and game location.

The coach stated that this was "the first time someone has talked to me about individual positional performances". The coach acknowledged the interesting nature of the game location positional specific profiles, however, admitted he probably would not utilise the information within his planning process. Although, the coach suggested rugby union support staff may find the data and information within the profiles useful, in particular the medical and conditioning team.

16.4. DISCUSSION

This study further developed the idea of positional profiles and their use in providing coaches with an insight into how game location affects the positional demands of each position. The findings of this research contradict those of Thomas *et al.* (2008) who identified a significant difference ($p < 0.05$) between game location and player performance, indicating the home team play an attack-dominated style of play, scoring an average of 6.6 ± 17.4 points and gain a home advantage of 73.3 per cent. Although this study does not follow the trends of previous research, three main trends were identified: the total number of tackles, ball in hand occurrences and passes.

Previous team sport research has identified that the home team would produce a greater number of attacking and defensive actions when competing. However, this study has identified that a greater number of attacking and defensive actions are completed when a team is competing away from home (see Figures 16.1, 16.2 and 16.3), with the exception of the forwards who produce a greater number of defensive actions (except Position #8) when competing at home (see Figure 16.1).

Jones *et al.* (2005) suggested that even though playing at home is associated with players demonstrating a higher level of aggression, this increased aggression may not transfer into an increased number of defensive actions. This study discovered that the backs completed fewer defensive tackles in comparison to the forwards when competing at home. Jones *et al.* (2005) suggested that players may choose to release aggression through tackle collisions and in other contact areas by generating an increased force production.

Vaz *et al.* (2010) suggested an increased number of tackles completed by the forwards may provide an increased understanding of the opposition's game plan and style of play. During the 2010/11 season, the analysed team favoured running the ball and taking the ball into contact instead of playing a kicking-dominated game plan. In addition, the team scored 70 per cent of their tries from turnover possession at contact situations or from kick receipt. Therefore, opponents may keep the ball close within the forwards to ensure minimisation of any chances for counter-attack.

The thematic content analysis highlighted the limited utilisation of performance analysis and profiling within the coach's practice. Liebermann and Franks (2008) suggested a number of key possibilities why coaches are not utilising profiling within their practice. The coach provides two reasons why he does not fully utilise performance analysis and profiling to inform his practice stating "I don't use it too much, I have been coaching for 15 plus years and I prefer to go through the video and look through it myself " and "It also takes me a long time to get my head round new ideas and processes, time which I do not have to spare."

On the other hand, the coach emphasises the importance of the game location positional specific profiles to the medical team. The coach states "They [the medical team] will be able to utilise the information gained from the profiles to design and implement game location positional specific recovery programmes" However, James *et al.* (2005) suggested that the information gained from positional profiles can assist all support staff in gaining a greater understanding of the positional specific demands ensuring that training and recovery is tailored to the individual's needs. Although this study has investigated the effect of game location on positional specific profiles and the application of these into practice, there are a number of strengths and limitations which need to be considered.

This study has provided a greater insight and understanding into the positional requirements of all 15 playing positions. Coaches and support staff are able to utilise the information to inform future practices and enable players to experience in-game demands in a controlled training environment. However, a number of limitations existed: first, a single team was utilised within this study, second, the effect of squad selection, substitutions and reductions in player numbers were not considered during this study, and finally, only one coach was interviewed to gain an understanding of how the profiles may be applied in practice.

Future examination is required within the research topic. Possible studies could aim to investigate how rugby union coaches and support staff utilise positional specific profiles within the planning and delivery of programmes; as well as the creation of positional specific performance indicators, in order to identity the key positional demands and skills utilised.

16.5. CONCLUSION

Prior to completion of this study no related research had been conducted investigating the effect of game location upon positional specific profiles within rugby union. Despite there being no significant differences between all playing positions and game location a number of interesting findings were discovered, for example, a greater number of attacking actions were completed by all positions when away from home, with the exception of the right second-row, number eight, inside centre and full back, whereas the forwards and right wing completed a greater number of defensive actions when playing at home.

The application of academic research into practice has received criticism amongst coaches and academia. Therefore, this study also interviewed an elite coach to gain a more in-depth understanding of the utilisation of performance analysis and positional specific profiles within 'real' coaching practice. The interview pinpointed that performance analysis support was not embraced within the coach's regular practice and he was sceptical of the relative merits of such assistance. This major finding highlighted that the coach preferred more traditional methods rather the use of performance analysis support in order to inform the coaching process, also suggesting that the support afforded would be more beneficial for use by the backroom staff. Therefore, this study has identified the effect of game location on positional specific profiles and provided an insight into the limited application of the profiles into practice. Clearly, it is evident that coaches still require training and assistance with the use of performance analysis and other technological advancements to highlight the benefits in enhancing and developing their practice.

16.6. REFERENCES

Hughes, M., Cooper, S. and Nevill, A., 2002, Analysis procedures for non-parametric data from performance analysis. *International Journal of Performance Analysis in Sport*, **2**(1), pp. 6–10.

James, N., Mellalieu, S. and Jones, N., 2005, The development of position specific performance indicators in professional rugby union. *Journal of Sports Sciences*, **23**, pp. 63–72.

Jones, M., Bray, S. and Oliver, S., 2005, Game location and aggression in rugby league. *Journal of Sports Sciences*, **23**(4), pp. 387–393.

Liebermann, D. and Franks, I., 2008, The use of feedback-based technologies. In *The Essentials of Performance Analysis: An Introduction,* 2nd edn, edited by Hughes, M. and Franks, I. (Abingdon, UK, Routledge), pp. 40–58.

Mellalieu, S., Trewartha, G. and Stokes, K., 2008, Science and rugby union. *Journal of Sports Sciences*, **26**(8), pp. 791–794.

Morton, H., 2006, Home advantage in southern hemisphere rugby union: National and international. *Journal of Sports Sciences*, **24**(5), pp. 495–499.

Thomas, S., Reeves, C. and Bell, A., 2008, Home advantage in the six nations rugby union tournament. *Perceptual and Motor Skills*, **106**, pp. 113–116.

Vaz, L., van Rooyen, M. and Sampaio, J., 2010, Rugby game-related statistics that discriminate between winning and losing teams in IRB and Super twelve close games. *Journal of Sports Science and Medicine*, **9**, pp. 51–55.

Part 4

Team Games

CHAPTER 17

Performance analysis of kicking and striking skills in Gaelic sports

Kevin Ball and Barry Horgan

17.1 INTRODUCTION

The Gaelic Athletic Association (GAA) sports comprise Football, Hurling and Camogie. All three sports involve goal shooting and passing the ball or sliothar which require the skilled actions of kicking/striking and hand-passing. GAA coaching resources have identified striking the ball with the hurley (stick) in Hurling and kicking in Football as two of the most important skills within each game. These are the most common methods of passing and scoring goals in both sports. Within these categories there seems to be a wide range of techniques used, with Daly (1993) noting that Football has a greater variety of kicks than any other kicking sports.

In GAA sports, few papers exist in the scientific literature examining the skills and types of execution used. The only detailed within-skill analysis in either sport compared the punt and drop kicks. McCrudden and Reilly (1993) found the punt kick to be more effective in kicking for distance but advised the choice of which kick to use should be dependent on outcome requirements. The authors also reported anthropometric factors were not linked to distance kicking. Examining game tasks more broadly, Bradley and O'Donoghue (2011) evaluated counter-attacking plays while Doggart *et al.* (1993) examined a wide range of game factors including time in play and kick profiles and quantified the effects of a rule change in Football. Locomotion patterns and activity profiles in Football matches have also been examined (e.g. McErlean *et al.*, 1998; O'Donoghue and King, 2005).

In Hurling, Gilmore (2008) quantified individual skill executions across four championship games, examining striking, gaining possession, travel methods and prevention methods. On average, 259 strikes occurred in a game with the aerial strike (hand) being the most prevalent. The author expressed surprise at the very low frequency of some of the simplest skills that were among the first to be learned. Gilmore (2008) also noted that much more detailed analyses were important future directions for this analysis to develop a baseline for skills in Hurling to guide training practices.

Within-skill analysis is a useful progression for GAA sports. This analysis involves analysing each skill execution in a game on a large number of criteria and going beyond the standard counts of kicks and strikes. This type of analysis is useful on a number of levels. First, it can identify a game-specific skill profile that can guide appropriate training procedures, as recommended by Gilmore (2008), and supports the GAA strategic vision and action plan ensuring games for learning are valid (i.e. what occurs in games is happening in games for learning). Second, this information can provide an evidence-based evaluation of a player's technical strengths and weaknesses. Ball *et al.* (2002) evaluated eight elite AF players performing set shots at goal. Using front-on and side-on video of between 10 and 40 set shot kicks for each individual, Ball *et al.* notationally analysed each performance on a large number of technical criteria (e.g. ball drop height, leg position at end of follow through). Key technical factors differed for all individuals between successful and unsuccessful kicks but these represented very individual-specific patterns. In subsequent training focussing on the technical errors with one of these players, substantial improvements were made to set shot percentage success (from 56 per cent to 78 per cent in games, Ball, 2005).

A third important use of detailed within-skill analysis is as a guide to biomechanical analyses. Typically in biomechanics the choice of skill to analyse from a particular team sport has been based on closed skills or skills that are of some importance in the sport. For example, all biomechanical research in soccer has been performed on stationary ball kicking. However, over 95 per cent of kicks performed in soccer are with a rolling ball. While these skills are appropriate to analyse, it ignores a large portion of the skills being performed in games. A complementary and potentially more valid and useful approach is to identify what skill executions are predominant in general play and analyse these performances. The use of performance analysis to identify the predominant kick executions is a sound method to select the skill execution to analyse.

The aims of this study were to evaluate kicking and striking in Hurling and Gaelic Football.

17.2 METHOD

Broadcast video footage of four Hurling matches and four Gaelic Football matches from the 2011 championship season were analysed. To gain a broad overview of skills and to attempt to avoid any team-specific bias, games were selected such that six different teams were included in the analysis. Games were also selected from quarter-finals, semi-finals and the final in each code.

Each kick or strike was evaluated on thirteen criteria under the general headings of game context, technical elements and outcome (Table 17.1). This was performed using a custom-developed Excel macro with coding form (Figure 17.1). Video recordings of each execution were played, paused and replayed as many times as required to assess each execution.

Table 17.1 Parameters and definitions

Parameter	Definition
Time	In 5 min sections
Score difference	Between the teams
Strike/kick context	General play, free, sideline, kick/puck in
Pressure	High – opponent had high influence on the execution Medium – player within 5 m and influential to hit/kick Low – player within 5 m with low influence or outside 5 m with some influence None – no influence on execution by opposition
Position from	Location on ground where the strike/kick was made. Grid setup based on ground lines for length measures. Width of ground divided into three (left, middle, right)
Position to	Location on ground where the ball/hurley was directed to
Type of hit/kick	Football – punt, hook, ground Hurling – from the hand, flick up off ground and strike without taking possession, off ground strike
Approach speed	Fast, medium, slow
Approach steps	Number of steps leading up to execution
Angle of approach	Relative to resulting ball flight
Distance	In 10 m increments approximated using ground markings. Pythagoras used when angled across the ground
Aim of strike/kick	Goal-shot, pass, clearance, centring, other
Result	Goal, point, turnover, successful pass, to a contest, out

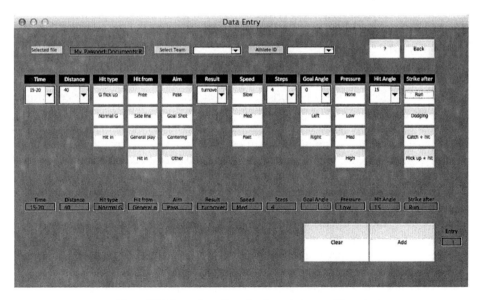

Figure 17.1 Example section of coding window used in analysis
(note – not all options included on this window)

On completion of analysis, parameter counts were totalled and percentages were calculated. Reliability was assessed by re-evaluating 50 strikes/hits the following day and comparing percentage similarity as recommended by Hughes *et al.* (2004). Reliability of the analysis was high for most parameters (Table 17.2).

Table 17.2 Reliability (percentage of cases where operator agreed on two separate occasions)

	Hurling	Football
Game context		
Game time	100%	100%
Score difference	100%	100%
Strike/kick	92%	94%
Pressure	86%	90%
Aim of strike/kick	96%	98%
Position on ground (from)	98%	96%
Position on ground (to)	96%	98%
Technical factors		
Distance	96%	98%
Type of hit/kick	100%	100%
Approach speed	88%	92%
Number of approach steps	100%	98%
Approach angle relative to ball flight	92%	90%
Result	98%	96%

17.3 RESULTS

For Hurling, on average 270 hits were performed in a game with an overall success rate of 61 per cent. Strikes comprised of 68 per cent general play, 6 per cent from the sideline, 10 per cent free hits and 17 per cent from puckouts. Eighty one per cent of strikes were performed from the hand (the sliothar or ball is released from the hand and struck while in the air), 11 per cent flicked up from the ground and struck, with the remaining 8 per cent being ground strokes. Approach speeds were spread evenly between slow (walk-jog), medium (jog-stride) and fast (stride-sprint) with three steps the most common. More than half of the strikes were under high pressure (52 per cent, an opposition player within 1 m and influencing the player with possession). Players most commonly approached the strike at zero degrees (running in the same direction as the hit, 32 per cent) and 90 degrees (21 per cent). Twenty per cent of strike distances were over 100 m (mainly puckouts) and the predominant distances of general play strikes were 50–60 m.

For Football, on average 205 kicks were performed in a game with an overall success rate of 55 per cent. Kicks comprised 74 per cent general play, 20 per cent frees and 6 per cent sideline kicks. Fifty per cent of these were hook kicks, 29 per cent punt kicks and 21 per cent were off the ground. Approach speed was most commonly moderate (41 per cent) followed by slow (33 per cent) and fast (26 per cent). Only 22 per cent of kicks were under high pressure but 60 per cent were under high or medium pressure. Of interest, similar patterns existed when examining general play and goal-shots separately. The most common approach angle was 30 degrees (35 per cent) using five steps.

17.4 DISCUSSION

Reliability of this analysis was strong for most parameters, aided by having an experienced analyser conducting the analysis. With eleven of the thirteen parameters in agreement for over 90 per cent of occasions, this reliability was similar to that reported for Bradley and O'Donoghue (2011) for counter-attacking events in Football. Level of pressure was lower in reliability as the level of influence of any opponent had to be evaluated. The initial definition of moderate pressure was an opponent within 5 m of the player. However, it became clear the term 'influence' needed to be added as there were occasions where an opponent could be within 5 m and not influencing the strike/kick. Approach speed was less reliable where a player would slow before the strike/kick after running fast. Approach angle was influenced by the last one or two steps where players would change direction suddenly or angle out in the case of kicking. Regardless, the values of reliability were still reasonably high for these parameters.

In Hurling, the most common execution elements of the strike were hitting from the hand. This was similar to the findings reported by Gilmore (2008). This strike was performed under high pressure, with an even spread of approach speeds off 4–5 steps and with angles of 0 or 90 degrees and hitting the sliothar over 50–60 m distance (for general play). The number of strikes under high pressure (52 per cent) was interesting. Further, 30 per cent were under medium pressure so pressure is an important component of the strike in Hurling. Approach speeds were evenly spread between slow, moderate and high but this analysis prompted the addition of a parameter called 'lead up', as while 30 per cent of strikes were performed with a slow approach, it was preceded by dodging motions or high intensity physical work to get clear to strike (this analysis was not performed for all games so was not included in this analysis). Gilmore (2008) recommended skills be performed in training while moving rather than stationary and this data would support this as even slow approaches required sometimes complex pre-strike movement. Strike distances were substantial with 20 per cent being over 100 m. These were predominantly from puckouts but also included clearing strikes from defence or long strikes into attack. It was also noted that many strikes were to an area rather than to a teammate.

In Football, the most common execution elements of the kick were the hook kick over 30–50 m in distance, under moderate pressure with a 4–5 step approach at moderate speed at an approach angle of 30 degrees. Of interest was the lower level of pressure evident compared to Hurling. Most kicks were performed under medium pressure (38 per cent) and only 22 per cent were under high pressure. Some influencing factors were players were able to find space to clear for the kick or execute quickly before an opponent was near. Hook kicks were the most predominant kick type used but it was noted that there were many variations of technique within these kicks. For example, different ball spin was imparted on the ball frequently (not able to be evaluated from broadcast video footage) for left-to-right, and right-to-left swing. This evaluation would be useful in future studies.

This descriptive data of the main skills in GAA have a number of uses. They can provide a guide to training specificity for GAA sports. They form a powerful tool for individual coaching in identifying performance patterns/errors for players (e.g. technical differences between good and bad kicks) as used in Australian football (e.g. Ball *et al.*, 2002). Finally they can be used to guide biomechanical analyses examining these skills, with the combined approach of game-based and lab-based technical evaluation addressing the limitations of each noted by Glazier (2010). The identification of the most common performances (e.g. kick type, approach angle/speed) is a sound scientific method of choosing the task for evaluation.

17.5 REFERENCES

Ball, K., 2005, Kick evaluation of individual players in Australia Football games. *Technical Report for Fremantle Football Club*, (Fremantle, Australia).

Ball, K., McLaughlin, P., Seagrave, C. and Marchant, D., 2002, Biomechanical aspects of set-shot accuracy in AFL football. *Journal of Science & Medicine in Sport*, **5**(4), p. 48.

Bradley, J. and O'Donoghue, P., 2011, Counterattacks in elite Gaelic football competition. *International Journal of Performance Analysis in Sport*, **11**, pp. 159–170.

Daly, P., 1993, *The Complete Coaching Guide to Hurling and Football.* (Dublin: GAA Coaching and Games Development Committee).

Doggart, L., Keane, S., Reilly, T. and Stanhope, J., 1993, A task analysis of Gaelic football. In *Science and Football II*, edited by Reilly, T., Clarys, J. and Stibbe, A. (London: E & FN Spon), pp. 186–189.

Gilmore, H., 2008, The craft of the Caman; A notational analysis of the frequency occurrence of skills used in Hurling. *International Journal of Performance Analysis in Sport*, **8**, 68–75.

Glazier, P., 2010, Game, set and match: Substantive issues and future directions in performance analysis. *Sports Medicine*, **40**, pp. 625–634.

Hughes, M., Cooper, S.M. and Nevill, A., 2004, Analysis of notational data: Reliability. In *Notational Analysis of Sport: Systems for Better Coaching and Performance in Sport*, edited by Hughes, M. and Franks, I.M. (London: Routledge), pp.189–204.

McCrudden, M. and Reilly, T., 1993, A comparison of the punt and drop-kick. In *Science and Football II*, edited by Reilly, T., Clarys, J. and Stibbe, A. (London: E & FN Spon), pp. 362–366.

McErlean, C., Murphy, M. and O'Donoghue, P., 1998, Time-motion analysis of work-rate within various positional roles of ladies' Gaelic football. *Journal of Sports Sciences*, **16**, pp. 21–22.

O'Donoghue, P. and King, S., 2005, Activity profile of men's Gaelic football. In *Science and Football V*, edited by Reilly, T., Cabri, J. and Araújo, D. (London: Routledge), pp. 205–210.

CHAPTER 18

Diversity and efficiency of the space creation dynamics in basketball teams: Age effect

Eduardo Rostaiser, Felipe Santana, Valmor Tricoli,
Dante De Rose Jr., Carlos Ugrinowitsch and Leonardo Lamas

18.1 INTRODUCTION

The dynamic of a basketball game, as in other team sports, is defined by the contest for ball possession between two teams, through individual and collective coordinated actions, in order to recover the ball or try to score, when in defence or in offence respectively (Gréhaigne and Godbout, 1995).

The skills to perform coordinated actions among players and to define proper strategies during a game depend on a long-term process that involves systematic participation in practices and in competitions. Those skills also require athletes with experience and knowledge of the game and proper teaching–learning methodologies to develop players' expertise (Ward and Williams, 2003; French and McPherson, 1999).

According to some authors the methodologies that allow someone to assess the results of different teaching–learning strategies from athlete performance are at a very initial stage of development (McGarry et al., 2002).

Lamas et al. (2011) validated a specific methodology for dynamic analysis of the occurrence of actions that should cause the rupture of defence by offensive actions. In this study, all the offensive behaviour patterns related to that objective were classified according to three aspects: a) number of players involved in the action; b) technical actions that were executed; and c) the decision context.

According to the results, seven classes of action were identified as possible behaviours that should promote the defensive rupture. Those classes of actions were denominated "Space Creation Dynamics" (SCDs):

1. *Space creation with ball dribbled (BD):* individual actions when the space to take the shot is created by the player who is dribbling, without the cooperation of teammates;
2. *Space creation with ball not dribbled (BND):* similar to BD but without a dribble, using only body displacements techniques;
3. *Perimeter isolation (PerI):* player with the ball is isolated in the perimeter, usually in the central area of the half offensive court while the other four teammates position themselves in the wings and corners of the court;

4. *Post isolation (PostI):* similar conception of *PerI* but occurring in the painted area, where centres are used to play;
5. *Space creation without ball (WB):* consists in a two players action and when one of them creates space, receives a pass from the teammate (e.g. back-door situations);
6. *On ball screen (OnBS):* one of two players positions himself in the trajectory of the defender of his teammate with the ball, interrupting the defender's line of displacement;
7. *Out of ball screen (OutBS):* similar to *OnBS* but both players involved in the screen do not have the ball.

The final purpose of an SCD is to create favourable situations for the offence to capitalise. With the increase in players' experience and with age development it is possible to hypothesise that SCDs should occur with more diversification and with higher cooperation among offensive players.

Considering that this subject was not adequately investigated before, the purpose of the present study was to evaluate the effect of competitive experience in the following performance variables: 1) diversity of the Space Creation Dynamics (SCDs); and 2) efficiency of the SCDs that resulted in score/total amount of SCDs.

18.2 METHODS

Forty six semi-final matches of all ages competing at male championships in the State of Sao Paulo, Brazil (under 12 to seniors) were analysed in this study. Table 18.1 shows the number of games that were analysed at each age group.

Table 18.1 Number of games at each age class

Age	U12	U13	U14	U5	U16	U17	U19	Senior
Games	6	6	6	5	8	5	6	4

Each game was recorded with a JVC GZ-HM 320 camera set at 5m above the floor level, just on the side of the court. The videos were viewed on a Philips DVD at a 42" TV.

The analysis of the games was conducted by a basketball expert (with an experience of at least five years in game analysis) and an assistant evaluator. Both evaluators considered three types of offensive situations: 1) set offence; 2) fast-break offence; and 3) no offence (turnovers or lost balls before the attack could find some action to create the necessary space to the scoring attempt). There were also two types of defence that were considered: 1) individual; and 2) zone.

The SCD classes used in the analysis were the same as those described by Lamas *et al.* (2011).

Researcher's reliability was tested on three occasions, one week apart using the Kappa Statistics. Minimum significance assumed was 0.75.

Data were analysed by age group according to the following variables: type of offence; type of defence; SCDs frequencies; and SCDs efficiency (i.e., SCDs that resulted in field goals made/total SCDs occurrences).

Chi Square tests were used to identify the possible significance in the association among each level of age and the variables ($p < 0.05$).

18.3 RESULTS

The results for researcher's reliability in the measures made on week 1, week 2 and week 3 were: 0.78, 0.85 and 0.85, respectively.

There was a prevalence of set offences in all age groups. The set offences were used in 82 per cent of the actions and fast breaks were used in 16 per cent of offensive actions. In 2 per cent of the offences the teams had turnovers or lost balls.

In *U12* and *U13* there was significant prevalence of zone defence (62 per cent, 57 per cent, respectively, $p < 0.05$). In *U14, U15, U16,* and *U17* there was no significant prevalence of one specific defence. However, in *U19* and *Senior* teams the individual defence was used in 64 per cent and 80 per cent of the ball possessions, respectively, which shows a prevalence of this kind of defence ($p < 0.05$).

Table 18.2 shows the results of the occurrence of SCDs against individual defence at each age group ($p < 0.05$).

Table 18.3 shows the results of the occurrences of SCDs against zone defence at each age group.

Table 18.2 Classes of Space Creation Dynamics (SCDs) among the possessions that ended in scoring opportunities, against individual defence, for each age group (values expressed in percentage)

Age group	BD	BND	PerI	PostI	WB	OnBS	OutBS
U12	51	6	4	2	15	13	9
U13	50	11	2	2	20	7	8
U14	46	9	1	6	19	13	6
U15	39	7	4	6	12	21	11
U16	33	7	3	10	11	23	13
U17	37	6	4	8	9	26	10
U19	28	5	6	5	6	32	18
Senior	27	6	8	7	11	29	12

Table 18.3 Classes of Space Creation Dynamics (SCDs) among the possessions that ended in scoring opportunities, against zone defence, for each age group (values expressed in percentage)

Age group	BD	BND	PerI	PostI	WB	OnBS	OutBS
U12	47	10	2	4	28	4	5
U13	45	9	1	6	33	4	2
U14	39	17	2	1	33	4	4
U15	47	10	1	3	28	7	4
U16	40	10	2	8	26	10	4
U17	40	11	1	7	31	7	3
U19	38	9	1	10	34	5	3
Senior	32	10	0	3	40	3	12

There was very low association for most SCD classes' efficiency among age levels and among the SCDs for each age group (differences did not achieve significance in both cases).

18.4 DISCUSSION AND CONCLUSIONS

The main result of this study is that all the age groups were similar regarding the frequencies and efficiency of SCD classes used on their offensive actions.

It seems that the type of defence (individual or zone) is the only variable that interferes on the kind of SCD with prevalence of *Space creation with ball dribble (BD)* and *On ball screen (OnBS)* when playing against individual defence and *Space creation with ball dribble (BD)* and *Space creation without ball (WB)* when playing against zone defence.

The opposition dynamics shows that the set offences are significantly more frequent than fast breaks in all age groups, just like was shown in the study made by Ortega *et al.* (2007).

The zone defence was the main defence used by the youngest players (*U12* and *U13*, $p < 0.05$) and the individual defence was the main defence used by the oldest age groups (*U19* and *Senior* players, $p < 0.05$). The same results were obtained by Okasaki *et al.* (2006) with Brazilian teams. This result points to a relevant pedagogical issue regarding the relationship between progression of strategic and tactical teaching process and the focus on short-term competitive success.

There were no defences where the most used SCDs presented higher efficiency compared to other less used SCDs. This evidence reveals another issue related to possible incoherencies between team strategies and their tactical execution by the players.

The initial hypothesis that the diversity of SCDs and the degree of cooperative interactions in offensive plays would increase with players' experience was not confirmed. The frequency homogeneity in most of the SCDs in all age levels, independence of the efficiency of those SCDs and the prevalence of *BD* against both types of defences, suggests an emphasis in individual offensive actions. The non-confirmation of the initial hypothesis induces a critical view of different aspects of the long-term process of basketball players' development.

18.5 REFERENCES

French, K.E. and McPherson, S.L., 1999, Adaptations in response selection processes used during sport competition with increasing age and expertise. *International Journal of Sport Psychology*, **30**, pp. 173–193.

Gréhaigne, J.F. and Godbout, P., 1995, Tactical knowledge in team sports: From a constructivist and cognitivist perspective. *Quest*, **47**, pp. 490–505.

Lamas, L., De Rose Jr., D., Santana, F., Rostaiser, E., Negretti, L. and Ugrinowitsch, C., 2011, Space creation dynamics in basketball offence: Validation and evaluation of elite teams. *International Journal of Performance Analysis in Sport*, **11**(1), pp. 71–84.

McGarry, T., Anderson, D.I., Wallace, S.A., Hughes, M. and Franks, I.M., 2002, Sport competition as a dynamical self-organizing system. *Journal of Sports Sciences*, **20**, pp. 771–781.

Okazaki, V.H.A., Rodacki, A.L.F., Dezan, V.H. and Sarraf, T.A., 2006, Coordenação do Arremesso de Jump no Basquetebol de Crianças e Adultos. *Revista Brasileira de Biomecânica*, **7**, pp. 15–22.

Ortega, E., Palao, J.M., Gómez, M.A., Lorenzo, A. and Cárdenas, D., 2007, Analysis of the efficacy of possessions in boys' 16-and-under basketball teams: Differences between winning and losing teams. *Perceptual and Motor Skills*, **104**, pp. 961–964.

Ward, P. and Williams, A.M., 2003, Perceptual and cognitive skill development in soccer: The multidimensional nature of expert performance. *Journal of Sport and Exercise Psychology*, **25**, pp. 93–111.

CHAPTER 19

Defensive strategy and critical match episodes in basketball game: Analysing the teams' success

António Paulo Ferreira, Anna Volossovitch,
Fernando Gomes and Sandro Didier

19.1 INTRODUCTION

In top-level basketball, the defensive strategy is prepared according to each specific opponent. This strategic match preparation intends to disrupt the opposing offensive organization and the rhythm of players' actions, taking into account the tactical advantages derived from the constraints imposed. Considering basketball as a ball possession game, the defensive phase of a match can introduce some momentary perturbations in the balance between teams and, consequently, provoke what can be called a match critical moment (Ferreira, 2006).

Several authors have discussed the existence of "game momentum" (Taylor and Demick, 1994; Burke *et al.*, 1997, 1999, 2003), "the critical game situations" (Kozar *et al.*, 1992, 1993, 1994) or even the importance of "hot hand" players (Koehler and Conley, 2003; Gula and Raab, 2004) in the basketball matches. These are different analogous expressions to designate a critical moment of the match. They suggest the existence of some occurrences during the match that introduce a momentary perturbation in the teams' balance. As a short-term consequence, these perturbations may lead to a score alteration, and depending on the match timeline, could have an important effect on the final outcome.

In basketball, as in the other sport games, defence efficacy has a great relevance for the teams' performance. For the strategic match preparation, it is very important to understand how the opposing team manipulates its defence during the match under different contextual conditions (e.g. points difference between teams or/and match quarter). Considering defensive strategy as a crucial factor for team success in a match and to better understand the strategic intentions of elite basketball teams, this study aimed to compare the defensive strategies of successful and unsuccessful top basketball teams in two different match contexts: the so-called Critical Match Episodes (CMEs) and the Normal Match Episodes (NMEs).

19.2 METHODS

The current scores of 80 matches from the Portuguese Basketball League were reconstructed, ball possession by ball possession. Each match was analysed according to the model of coach's game practical knowledge (Ferreira *et al.*, 2010). This model divides the basketball match in two different critical periods: the first three quarters and the last one. The rest time between the third and fourth quarter represents a cut reference of the game criticality. The score difference between both teams is seen as a variable that forces the game to go upward and downward among several equilibrium stages: the even stage; the alarm stage; the transition stage; and the imbalance one. Transition stage is considered as a difference between the game equilibrium and an imbalance game context.

By analogy to the dynamical systems theory, the model of coach's game practical knowledge considers the order parameters – the equilibrium match stages – as the balance attractors of the match. Game tempo and score difference are the control parameters (McGarry *et al.*, 2002) that force the match to go up and go down in the balanced scale of order parameters. A phase transition, considered as a critical game moment, occurs when the current match score switches from one equilibrium stage to another. In these cases, it is plausible to consider that the game skips to another organizational state. Using this model, a CME was considered as a transition of the match score to the equilibrium state. An NME was defined as sequence of ball possessions, in which the current score remains in the same equilibrium state.

A total of 319 CMEs and 318 NMEs were analysed. The NME were randomly selected according to a homogeneity criterion with the CME identified for each match. The number of ball possessions and the temporal framing of their occurrence were respected. A total of 2799 ball possessions from 80 basketball matches were analysed according to the referred model. As a consequence of this analysis 665 CMEs and 706 NMEs were identified. The team's success was defined by the match outcome and comparative analysis of CMEs and NMEs of winning and losing teams was carried out.

The defensive team's strategy was characterized using a multi-categorical system that included seven main categories:

1 Global strategy of the defensive transition – defines the collective organization against the offensive transition: collective conditioning, focused conditioning, no conditions observed or other conditions;
2 Outlet pass pressure – characterizes the opposition level to the first offensive pass after the ball possession is lost by the observed team: high pressure, moderate pressure, without pressure, no outlet pass or other pressure;
3 Ball pressure on the defensive transition – expresses the toughness of defensive behaviour over the ball transition from the defensive court to the offensive one: high ball pressure, moderate ball pressure, without ball pressure, no conditions to press the ball or other pressure;
4 Defensive phase – is the defensive moment where the ball possession is recovered: defensive balance, positional defence or other defensive phase;
5 Type of defence – defines the collective defensive rules related to the offence: man-to-man defence, zone defence, match-up defence, without collective organization or other type of defence;

6   Field goals opposition – means the defensive oppositions to the offensive field goal shots: active opposition, passive opposition, without opposition, opposition with foul, without shot or other type of opposition.

7   Ball recovering – characterizes how the ball possession is recovered by the defender team: opponent successful shot, defensive rebound, ball steal, block shot, offensive foul, time violations, technical violations, major fouls or other.

Three expert coaches were previously invited to the validation process of the observation instrument. Intra- and inter-observer ratings were estimated by κ-Cohen test and equalled 0.78–0.85. A Chi-Square test was performed to compare the nominal characteristics of defensive strategy of the match episodes in each type of teams' success – successful and unsuccessful teams. The p-value for significance was set at 0.05 and the adjusted standardized residuals were analysed taking into account the |1.96| boundaries.

19.3 RESULTS

The results presented in Table 19.1 showed that the differences profile between the CME and NME vary according to teams' success. Three main categories demonstrated significant differences according to final match outcome in both match episodes: *Ball pressure on the defensive transition* ($\chi^2 = 11.880$ (4, n = 1371)), *Defensive phase* ($\chi^2 = 8.690$ (2, n = 1371)) and *Type of defence* ($\chi^2 = 8.690$ (2, n = 1371)).

Table 19.1 Chi-Square values for match episodes of successful and unsuccessful teams

Main category	Successful teams χ^2	Unsuccessful teams χ^2
Global strategy on the defensive transition	5.336 (3, n = 1371)	17.187 (3, n = 1428) **
Outlet pressure	3.192 (4, n = 1371)	16.518 (4, n = 1428) **
Ball pressure on the defensive transition	11.880 (4, n = 1371) **	19.606 (4, n = 1428) **
Defensive phase	8.690 (2, n = 1371) **	11.676 (2, n = 1428) **
Type of defence	8.690 (3, n = 1371) **	16.259 (3, n = 1428) **
Field goals opposition	6.675 (5, n = 1371)	10.703 (5, n = 1428)
Ball recovering	6.181 (5, n = 1371)	46.709 (6, n = 1428) **

** significant results for p $\leq$ 0.01

Table 19.2 identifies the differences within each main category, respectively for successful and unsuccessful teams. The differences between CME and NME of successful teams were identified in *Moderate ball pressure* ($\pm$ 2.9) of the main category *Ball pressure on the defensive transition*, *Other defensive phase* ($\pm$ 2,7) of *Defensive phase* and on *Zone defence* ($\pm$ 2.3) and *Without collective organization* ($\pm$ 2.1) of *Type of defence*.

Table 19.2 Percentages (and absolute values) of nominal characteristics of critical and normal match episodes for successful teams. Bold categories indicate adjusted standardized residuals above |1.96|

Main category	Category	Critical Match Episodes	Normal Match Episodes
		%	%
Ball pressure on the defensive transition	High ball pressure	5.4 (36)	4.7 (33)
	Moderate ball pressure	**11.4 (76)**	**6.9 (49)**
	Without ball pressure	61.7 (410)	64.9 (456)
	No conditions to press the ball	14.6 (97)	18.1 (128)
	Other pressure	6.9 (46)	5.7 (40)
Defensive phase	Defensive balance	14.70 (98)	17.40 (123)
	Positional defence	78.60 (523)	79.20 (559)
	Other defensive phase	**6.60 (44)**	**3.40 (24)**
Type of defence	Man to man defence	74.30 (494)	76.10 (537)
	Zone defence	**4.40 (29)**	**2.10 (15)**
	Without collective organization	**18.00 (120)**	**19.40 (137)**
	Other type of defence	3.30 (22)	1.60 (11)

19.4 DISCUSSION

This study aimed to compare the defensive strategy of top-level basketball teams in different match episodes, mediated by teams' success. Our findings illustrate that the critical moments within a basketball match can be provoked by defensive behaviours of teams, when they try to impose their tactical goals over the opponent. Previously, Burke *et al.* (1999, 2003) identified two defensive behaviours specifically for the beginning and during *momentum* episodes – defensive stops and ball steals. However, these two individual and isolated behaviours are usually counted as basketball match statistics. According to this analysis of the top-level teams' defensive strategy, these findings allow defining three important characteristics of the CME. First, winning teams maintained a more consistent ball pressure over the defensive transition. It is suggested by the significant differences found for the categories *Ball pressure on the defensive transition* and *Moderate ball pressure*. These results are in line with the explanations for the USA basketball team's dominance at Beijing Olympic Games (2008) described by Sampaio *et al.* (2010). Authors indicated the importance of the recovered balls as indirect measure of the defensive pressure and a reason to increase the match pace. Second, the successful teams showed higher percentages of zone defence utilization in the CME comparatively to the NME. Despite the man-to-man defence that has been used by both teams as a preferential defensive system, the small percentages of zone defence utilization revealed significant differences according to the match episode type. Coaches call the structural changes during short-term match periods as an important defensive strategy to impose some offensive perturbations to the opposing teams (Ferreira *et al.*, in press); for example, the switch from a man-on-man to a zone defence or vice versa. In a short-term dimension these defensive changes could act as a positive match *momentum* for the defensive team (Stanimirovic and Hanrahan, 2004) by provoking a negative shift in the offensive performance. Third, the CME of successful teams demonstrated the presence of unconventional defensive phases and/or defensive phases without collective organization as a mark of distinction. These last characteristics show the importance of defining and understanding the existence of other defensive phases during the defensive process that are not usually described in the basketball literature.

Compared to the successful teams, the defensive profile of unsuccessful teams could not be clearly defined. The CME and NME of unsuccessful teams demonstrated a large spectrum of differences (see Table 19.1), but they revealed some contradictory results. As an example, the significant differences found in the global strategy to the defensive transition and the non-existence of ball pressure on the outlet-pass, suggest that teams try to accelerate the rhythm of ball possession through the defensive behaviour in the CME. However, in these match episodes they demonstrated a lower frequency of the defensive rebounds and the ball steals, considered as most important ball recovery defensive actions. The higher values of points missed by unsuccessful teams in the CME compared to the points missed in the NME might be interpreted as a signal of defence inconsistency that these teams tend to exhibit. Some authors usually point out defensive competence as the most important reason for the teams' match success (Stewart and Scholz, 1990; Otto, 1998; Gomez *et al.*, 2006). Although these results are related to the comparison of match episodes, it is plausible to understand this defensive inconsistency replicated to the whole match and it might be one reason to explain the unsuccessful status of these teams. To better understand the presented results, further studies should focus on the critical moments of unsuccessful teams.

Despite the unspecific profile of CME of unsuccessful teams, there are some collective behaviours that were not captured during the conventional match observation. Conversely, a CME seems to be very clear for successful teams and could be identified by the perturbation of the match rhythm. The relationship of the defensive ball pressure over transitions and the utilization of zone defences might be two important factors that allow successful teams to provoke this perturbation.

19.5 REFERENCES

Burke, K., Aoyagi, M., Joyner, A. and Burke, M., 2003, Spectators' perceptions of positive momentum while attending NCAA men's and women's basketball regular season contests: Exploring the antecedents-consequences model. *Athletic*

Insight: The Online Journal of Sport Psychology, **5**(3) (accessed on 12 February 2005 at http://www.athleticinsight.com).

Burke, K., Burke, M. and Joyner, A., 1999, Perceptions of momentum in college and high school basketball: An exploratory, case study investigation. *Journal of Sport Behavior*, **22**, pp. 303–309.

Burke, K., Edwards, C., Weigand, D. and Weinberg, R., 1997, Momentum in sport: A real or illusionary phenomenon for spectators. *International Journal of Sport Psychology*, **28**, pp. 79–96.

Ferreira, A.P., Volossovitch, A., Gomes, F. and Infante, J., 2010, Dynamics of coach's game practical knowledge in basketball, *International Journal of Sport Psychology*, **41**(4), pp. 68–69.

Ferreira, A.P., Volossovitch, A. and Sampaio, J., in press, Towards the game critical moments in basketball: A grounded theory approach. *Collegium Antropologicum*.

Ferreira, A.P., 2006, Criticality and critical moments. Basketball approaches. Unpublished doctoral thesis, (Lisbon, Portugal: Technical University of Lisbon, Faculty of Human Kinetics).

Gomez, M.A., Tsamourtzis, E. and Lorenzo, A., 2006, Defensive systems in basketball ball possessions. *International Journal of Performance Analysis in Sport*, **6**, pp. 98–107.

Gula, B. and Raab, M., 2004, "Hot hand" belief and "hot hand" behaviour: A comment on Koehler and Conley. *Journal of Sport and Exercise Psychology*, **26**, pp. 167–170.

Koehler, J. and Conley, C., 2003, The "hot hand" myth in professional basketball. *Journal of Sport and Exercise Psychology*, **25**, pp. 253–259.

Kozar, B., Vaughn, R., Whitfield, K., Lord, R. and Dye, B., 1994, Importance of free-throws at various stages of basketball games. *Perceptual and Motor Skills*, **78**, pp. 243–248.

Kozar, B., Whitfield, K. and Lord, R., 1992, Free throw shooting in critical game situations: The home-court disadvantage. *Research Quarterly of Exercise and Sport*, **March Supplement**, A-79.

Kozar, B., Whitfield, K., Lord, R. and Mechikoff, R., 1993, Timeouts before free-throws: Do the statistics support the strategy? *Perceptual and Motor Skills*, **76**, pp. 47–50.

McGarry, T., Anderson, D., Wallace, S., Hughes, M. and Franks, I., 2002, Sport competition as a dynamical self-organizing system. *Journal of Sport Sciences*, **20**, pp. 771–781.

Otto, K., 1998, Defence wins! *Scholastic Coach and Athletic Director*, **67**, pp. 24–25.

Sampaio, J., Lago, C. and Drinkwater, E., 2010, Explanations for the United States of America's dominance in basketball at the Beijing Olympic Games (2008). *Journal of Sports Sciences*, **28**, pp. 147–152

Stanimirovic, R. and Hanrahan, S., 2004, Efficacy, affect and teams: Is momentum a misnomer? *International Journal of Sport and Exercise Psychology*, **2**, pp. 43–62.

Stewart, N. and Scholz, G., 1990, *Basketball: Building the Complete Program.* (Marceline, Missouri: Walsworth Publishing Company).

Taylor, J. and Demick, A., 1994, A multidimensional model of momentum in sport. *Journal of Applied Sport Psychology*, **6**, pp. 51–70.

CHAPTER 20

Momentum in netball shooting

Catherine Roberts and Peter O'Donoghue

20.1 INTRODUCTION

Momentum has been described as "psychological power which may change interpersonal perceptions and influence physical and mental performance" (Iso-Ahola, 1980). Taylor and Demick (1994) defined momentum as a multi-dimensional construct where events can lead to positive or negative changes in cognition, physiology and behaviour which lead to changes in performance and competitive outcome. These mechanisms are believed to lead to temporal patterns in observable events within sports contests. It is hypothesised that if previous events are performed successfully, it is more likely that current events are performed successfully than if previous events had been unsuccessful. There is a perception of momentum among athletes and commentators of sport (Vergin, 2000), but scientific studies of actual sports behaviour have provided mixed evidence as to whether event outcomes are influenced by previous event outcomes within the same matches (Bar Eli *et al.*, 2006). Much of this research has been in basketball which is an indoor game with some similarities to netball. However, there are fundamental differences between the two games including differences in shooting (Barham, 1986). In netball, players can only shoot within the shooting circle and only the goal attack (GA) and goal shooter (GS) are permitted to enter the opposition's shooting circle. The shooter has 3 seconds to make a shot and opposing circle defenders are not permitted to obstruct or make contact with shooters, marking the shot from at least 3 feet away from the shooter. A further difference to basketball is that the net used in netball does not have a backboard behind it which reduces the chances of rebound opportunities where shots are missed. Shooting is an important aspect of netball because it is the scoring mechanism of the game and is one of the factors contributing to teams scoring from their possessions (O'Donoghue *et al.*, 2008). There is no published research investigating momentum effects or any other temporal aspects of netball shooting. Therefore, the purpose of the current investigation was to determine whether the outcome of shots in netball was influenced by the outcome of previously played shots. Given that shots are played from different locations, under different marking conditions and with different techniques, there are other factors that may influence the outcome of netball shots. These factors are also considered in the current investigation to see if there are any tactical differences in shooting depending on the outcome of previous shots.

20.2 METHODS

Shooting performances in 20 British National Super League matches were analysed. This included 40 team performances and 112 player performances. The outcomes of shots, number of marking defenders, whether shots were marked from the front, back or side or not and whether the shooter moved their feet during the shooting action or not were recorded. Shot location was recorded using the 9 areas identified in Figure 20.1. The two authors independently analysed one match of 139 shots agreeing on the teams performing shots ($\kappa = 1.00$), players performing shots ($\kappa = 1.00$) and outcome of shots ($\kappa = 1.00$). There was a very good strength of agreement for the number of marking defenders ($\kappa = 0.97$), whether or not the shot was marked from the front ($\kappa = 0.97$), back ($\kappa = 0.91$) and side ($\kappa = 0.88$) and whether the shooter moved their feet during the shot ($\kappa = 0.94$). The area from which the shot was taken had a good strength of inter-operator agreement ($\kappa = 0.66$) with any disagreements being between neighbouring areas of the shooting circle.

A series of chi square tests of independence were conducted on the shooting performances of each team within each of the 20 matches. Each chi square test cross-tabulated the outcome of a shot with the outcome of the previous shot. The resulting p value was not shown where there were any expected frequencies of less than 5.0. A further series of chi squares tests of independence was conducted for individual player shooting performances within matches, only revealing p values where the data satisfied the assumptions of the test. When analysing teams and individuals, a significant influence of previous shot outcome was identified by p values of less than 0.05.

Other factors that potentially influence shot outcome were considered. The percentage of shots scored was determined for different conditions within the 40 team performances. A Friedman test was used to compare the percentage of shots scored between situations where 0, 1 or 2 circle defenders were marking the shot. A p value of less than 0.05 was deemed significant. The percentage of shots scored when the shooter moved their feet and when they did not move was compared using a Wilcoxon test. A p value of less than 0.05 was deemed significant. Wilcoxon tests were also used to compare the percentage of shots that were scored between situations where the shot was marked from behind or not, marked from the front or not and marked from the side or not. These tests were deemed to be significant if p values of less than 0.017 (about 0.05/3) resulted. The percentage of shots scored was compared between the 9 areas of the shooting circle using a Friedman test with a p value of less than 0.05 being used to indicate a significant influence of shot location. The effect of distance from the goal was compared by merging the 3 inner areas together, the 3 middle areas together and the 3 outer areas together. These 3 broad areas were compared using a Friedman test with a p value of less than 0.025 indicating a significant effect. The 3 innermost areas were compared, as were the 3 middle areas and the 3 outer areas using Friedman tests with p values of under 0.008 (about 0.025/3) indicating a significant location effect.

The percentage of shots taken from the inner, middle and outer areas of the shooting circle were compared between situations where the previous shot had been scored and missed using a series of Wilcoxon tests with p values of less than 0.017 (about 0.05/3) indicating a significant influence of previous shot outcome on location of the next shot.

20.3 RESULTS

Table 20.1 shows the proportion of shots scored when the previous shot had been scored and when it had been missed for both the winning and losing team within each of the 20 matches. There was one team performance with a significant association between shot outcome and previous shot outcome ($p = 0.010$). However, the 8/30 shots scored when the previous shot had been scored was a lower proportion than the 21/36 when the previous shot had been missed.

Table 20.1 Proportion of shots scored when previous shot was scored and missed

Match	Winning team			Losing team		
	Result of previous shot		$p\ (\chi^2)$	Result of previous shot		$p\ (\chi^2)$
	Scored	Missed		Scored	Missed	
1	33/45	11/14		23/42	18/34	0.874
2	54/61	8/8		19/28	9/18	0.226
3	28/43	14/27	0.270	24/35	12/18	0.888
4	35/50	16/20	0.395	35/48	13/15	
5	38/52	14/18		21/31	11/17	0.831
6	38/51	13/14		27/43	16/23	0.582
7	23/38	15/18	0.088	8/20	12/27	0.761
8	43/59	16/18		8/19	10/18	0.413
9	8/30	21/36	0.010	8/25	17/33	0.137
10	30/42	12/15		25/40	15/19	0.206
11	35/51	16/18		22/37	14/22	0.750
12	43/59	16/22	0.989	22/35	13/24	0.504
13	38/51	14/17		18/33	15/33	0.460
14	42/53	11/12		13/25	11/24	0.666
15	45/54	9/11		24/34	10/22	0.060
16	50/61	11/16		6/20	14/24	0.060
17	37/55	18/24	0.492	20/35	15/20	0.185
18	63/73	11/12		27/34	8/14	
19	34/49	15/20	0.641	27/40	14/24	0.459
20	27/44	16/22	0.361	9/24	16/27	0.121

There were only three individual player performances out of 112 that were significant, but two of these showed the opposite to momentum (5/15 scored when the previous shot was scored and 10/13 when the previous shot was missed, $p = 0.021$; 6/16 scored when the previous shot was scored and 10/13 when the previous shot was missed, p = 0.034). The one performance where there was a greater proportion of shots scored when the previous shot had been scored (30/33) than when the previous shot had been missed (4/7) failed to satisfy the assumption of an expected frequency of at least 5.0 in each of the cells.

The number of circle defenders marking the shot had a significant influence on shot outcome (p = 0.046). The percentage of shots that was scored was 79.3 ± 31.5 per cent when both circle defenders were marking, 65.8 ± 12.8 per cent when one circle defender was marking and 66.3 ± 18.7 per cent when neither circle defender was marking the shot. Table 20.2 shows the percentage of shots scored when defenders marked the shot from the front, the back and the side or not. A significantly greater percentage of shots were scored when defenders marked from the side and from the back than when they didn't (p < 0.017).

Table 20.2 Percentage of shots scored under different marking locations

Location of marking defender	Defender at this location	Defender not at this location	p (Wilcoxon test)
Front	64.5 ± 13.0	70.7 ± 16.7	.026
Side	81.7 ± 24.6	65.1 ± 12.3	.000
Back	81.1 ± 30.2	65.7 ± 12.1	.002

The 67.2 ± 25.6 per cent of shots scored when the shooter was stationary was not significantly greater than the 62.6 ± 25.6 per cent of shots scored when she moved her feet during the shot (p > 0.05). Figure 20.1 shows the percentage of shots scored from different areas of the shooting circle. Location had a significant influence on shot outcome (p < 0.001). The percentage of shots scored was 78.5 ± 13.4 per cent from the innermost areas, 63.6 ± 13.0 per cent from the three middle areas and 53.5 ± 23.8 per cent from the three outer areas; distance from the goal was significant (p < 0.001). There was a tendency for a greater percentage of shots to be scored from the left hand sector of the shooting circle than the other areas. However, this was not significant for the inner (p = 0.016), middle (p = 0.259) or outer areas (p = 0.010).

Other factors such as marking conditions and location of shot had a significant influence on shot outcome. However, marking is an action of the defending players rather than an action of the shooter. The location of a shot was something the shooter had greater control over and so this was compared between situations where the previous shot had been scored and missed. When the previous shot was scored, players shot from the inner circle for 22.6 ± 16.1 per cent of shots, the middle circle for 62.2 ± 16.1 per cent and the outer circle for 15.2 ± 14.3 per cent of shots. Wilcoxon Signed ranks tests revealed no significant difference (0.087 ≤ p ≤ 0.820) to the percentage of shots taken from the inner (26.1 ± 24.3 per cent), middle (61.4 ± 24.9 per cent) and outer circles (12.5 ± 14.1 per cent) when the previous shot was missed.

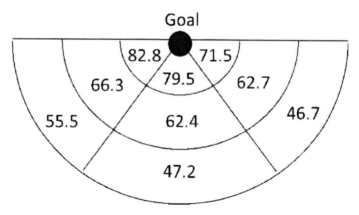

Figure 20.1 Percentage of shots scored from different areas of the shooting circle

20.4 DISCUSSION

The current investigation has not found any evidence that the outcome of shots in netball is influenced by the outcome of previous shots. There are a number of potential explanations for this finding. First, netball shooting is not a standard task within a controlled experiment. While netball is an indoor sport and the study was not affected by weather conditions like a momentum study of golf would be (Clark, 2005), there are still many factors that are outside of the control of the researchers. Some shots are played in open play while others are penalty shots where one or both circle defenders may be prohibited from marking (Navin, 2008). The ability for the shooter to step during the shot, shoot from different locations and with varying technique all mean that a particular netball shot may be a different task to previous shots within the match. Similarly, the action of the defence is not within the control of the study and leads to varying shooting conditions from shot to shot. The defensive play in netball is different to basketball, as netball is more of a man-on-man game with a smaller shooting space (Hickey and Navin, 2007, p. 29). If a shooter is perceived to be experiencing a shooting run then a defensive strategy could be implemented to prevent this from continuing.

Another explanation is that players can expect to score more shots than they miss in high level netball. The National Superleague is the highest level domestic competition in the UK and the percentage of shots scored within the current investigations was 67.1 per cent. Therefore, a missed shot may be perceived as a single event that occasionally occurs. The players may cope with missed shots by focusing on the next opportunity. The players at this level will be experienced and will have played in matches where they have missed shots before. They will have been advised by coaches of what to do in such situations and will have developed mental skills to cope with missing shots.

There may be speculation that where momentum is not observed in event sequences, it could be because players are becoming confident and attempting more difficult shots. Where more difficult shots are attempted, they could be missed, ending a sequence of scored shots. Shaw *et al.* (1992) found that repeated success leads to increased confidence over time. However, the current investigation does not provide any evidence of this; players shoot from similar areas of the shooting circle irrespective of the outcomes of previous shots.

Silva *et al.* (1988) distinguished between "micro" and "macro" approaches to analysing sports performance data when studying the concept of momentum. The current investigation has analysed individual shots. Further research could look at more macroscopic indicators of shooting performance such as shooting percentages in matches or match quarters to investigate relationships between performances.

20.5 REFERENCES

Bar-Eli, M., Avugos, S. and Raab, M., 2006, Twenty years of "hot hand" research: Review and critique. *Psychology of Sport and Exercise*, **7**(6), pp. 525–553.

Barham, P., 1986, *Netball Top Performance Techniques: A Guide to Improving Netball Performance*. (Bierton: Netball Coaching International).

Clark, D.R., 2005, Examination of hole-to-hole streakiness on the PGA tour. *Perception of Motor Skills*, **100**(1), pp. 806–814.

Hickey, J. and Navin, A., 2007, *Understanding Netball*. (Leeds, UK: Coachwise).

Iso-Ahola, E.S., 1980, "Psychological momentum": A phenomenon and an empirical (unobtrusive) validation of its influence in a competitive sport tournament. *Psychological Reports*, **46**, pp. 391–401.

Navin, A., 2008, *Netball: Skills, Technique, tactics*. (Ramsbury, UK: The Crowood Press Ltd).

O'Donoghue, P.G., Mayes, A., Edwards, K.M. and Garland, J., 2008, Performance norms for British National Super League Netball. *International Journal of Sports Science and Coaching*, **3**, pp. 501–511.

Shaw, J.M., Dzewaltowski, D.A. and McElroy, M., 1992, Self-efficacy and causal attributions as mediators of perceptions of psychological momentum. *Journal of Sport and Exercise Psychology*, **14**, pp. 134–147.

Silva, J.M., Hardy, C.J. and Crace, R., 1988, Analysis of psychological momentum on male and female tennis players revisited. *Journal of Sport and Exercise Psychology*, **10**, pp. 346–354.

Taylor, J. and Demick, A., 1994, A multidimensional model of momentum in sports. *Journal of Applied Sport Psychology*, **6**, pp. 51–70.

Vergin, C.R., 2000, Winning streaks in sports and the misperception of momentum. *Journal of Sport Behaviour*, **23**(2), pp.181–196.

Part 5

Racket Sports

CHAPTER 21

The effect of changing the scoring system on game related activity in squash

Stafford Murray, Nic James, Peter Dineen,
Mike Hughes and Goran Vučković

21. 1 INTRODUCTION

In 2000 the Professional Squash Association (PSA) introduced a reduction of 2 inches to the tin height (for professional men's squash only). This effectively increased the playing court dimensions because attacking shots to the front of the court bounce for a second time closer to the front wall meaning that the distance covered to return a shot is greater. This meant that it was easier to play winning shots (since it was harder for the opponent to return the ball) and hence it was hoped the new tin height would encourage players to be more attacking (drop shots, kills and low drives). It was thought that this would result in more exciting squash for the audience, shorter rallies and lower match durations. With the objective of reducing match durations, in 1996 the World Squash Federation changed the scoring system for professional tournaments from playing to 9 points with scoring on serve only to an alternative scoring system to 15 points, point a rally scoring system (PARS). This was further amended in 2004 so that professional matches now play up to 11 points (PARS). Shorter and more predictable match durations (PARS is more predictable that point on serve only) also make scheduling tournaments easier. Previous research in professional squash has only assessed game related activity played with the lower tin under the old scoring system to 9 points, with scoring on serve only (Vučković et al., 2009). This research showed that for elite matches the ball was in play for an average of 547s (SD = 216s) with an average of 34 (SD = 11) rallies each of duration 16.42s (SD = 4.48s). This paper will assess the extent to which the new scoring system has changed the game characteristics for professional male squash.

21.2 METHODS

21.2.1 Data collection

Matches at the 2003 World Team Championships (n = 11) and the 2010 Rowe British Grand Prix (n = 10) were recorded using a fixed overhead PAL camera (JBL UTC – A6000H, Korea) and processed using the SAGIT/Squash tracking system (Vučković et al., 2009). This is an automatic movement tracking system using a background elimination computer vision technique with operator supervision to correct any errors that might occur when players' paths cross. Game time, ball in play time, distance covered and number of rallies were calculated for each game and each player. All supplementary information (shot types and ball location) was input into SAGIT/Squash so that both movement and rally information were stored on the same timeline to ensure accuracy between measurements.

21.2.2 Reliability and data analysis

The SAGIT/Squash tracking system has been assessed for reliability (Vučković *et al.*, 2010) in terms of the software's ability to track the players' movements. The error associated with the distance covered over a one-minute period was shown to range between 1.33m and 21m depending on the nature and position of the player's movements. The errors associated with the number and times associated with rallies were analysed using intra-operator percentage error tests (Hughes *et al.*, 2002) and found to be less than 0.01 per cent. All data were exported from SAGIT/Squash to Microsoft Excel and SPSS v18 for analysis. All data were examined for normality (Shapiro-Wilk) and with some departures from normality and large differences in variance noted between groups Mann-Whitney U tests were used.

21.3 RESULTS

The new scoring system has resulted in significantly ($U = 882$, $z = 7.48$, $p < .001$, $r = 0.60$) fewer rallies (median = 20, IQR = 8) than previously found (median = 34, IQR = 15). However, the duration of rallies has not significantly reduced ($U = 2680$, $z = 0.94$, $p = .35$, $r = 0.08$) under the new scoring system (median = 14.2s, IQR = 5.0) compared to the old system (median = 15.0s, IQR = 5.4). This has resulted in the average game time (Figure 21.1) for the new scoring system (median = 533s, IQR = 351) being significantly shorter ($U = 1058$, $z = 6.83$, $p < .001$, $r = 0.55$) than for the old scoring system (median = 945s, IQR = 506).

This has also resulted in a significantly shorter ball in play time ($U = 1126$, $z = 6.58$, $p < .001$, $r = 0.53$) for the new scoring system (median = 317s, IQR = 209) than previously found (median = 511s, IQR = 292), but ball in play as a proportion of total game time did not change significantly ($U = 2404$, $z = 1.95$, $p = .05$, $r = 0.16$) for the new scoring (median = 56 per cent, IQR = 9) in comparison to the old (median = 54 per cent, IQR = 9).

In a similar pattern the distance covered by each player during a game was significantly less ($U = 943$, $z = 7.25$, $p < .001$, $r = 0.58$) for matches played under the new scoring system (median = 580m, IQR = 384) in comparison to the old (median = 1054m, IQR = 543) as was the distance covered during ball in play time (Figure 21.2) less ($U = 944$, $z = 7.25$, $p < .001$, $r = 0.58$) for the new scoring (median = 435m, IQR = 264) compared to the old (median = 752m, IQR = 408).

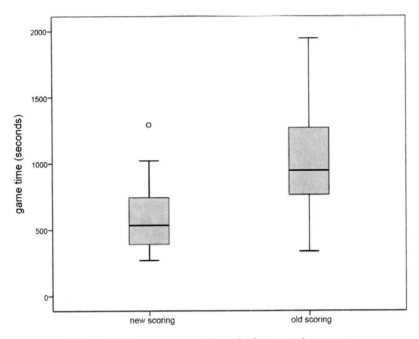

Figure 21.1 The average game time under the two scoring systems

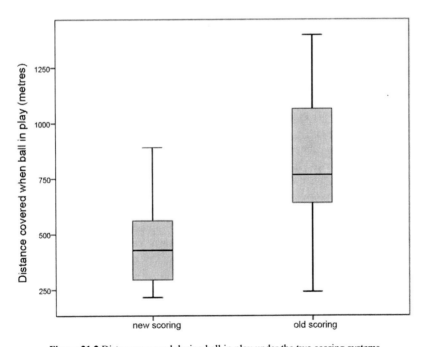

Figure 21.2 Distance covered during ball in play under the two scoring systems

Consequently the distance covered per rally has reduced ($U = 2247$, $z = 2.52$, $p < .05$, $r = 0.20$) under the new scoring system (median $= 20.2m$, IQR $= 7$) compared to the old (median $= 22.1m$, IQR $= 8$) as has each player's average speed during a rally decreased ($U = 989$, $z = 7.08$, $p < .001$, $r = 0.57$) under the new scoring system (median $= 1.35m/s$, IQR $= 0.1$) compared to the old (median $= 1.45m/s$, IQR $= 0.1$).

21.4 DISCUSSION

The Professional Squash Association's (PSA) attempt to shorten the rallies and lower the match duration by lowering the tin and adopting the new scoring system appears to have worked to some extent. This analysis has shown that game times have been reduced by about 44 per cent mainly due to an average reduction in the number of rallies by 41 per cent (due to the new scoring system). Rally durations, however, have not dramatically changed, with a reduction in time of about 5 per cent, although the players are now covering about 42 per cent less distance in total due to the lower number of rallies. The actual distance covered during each rally has significantly reduced by about 9 per cent, which suggests that some tactical changes have taken place. The reasons for this are unknown presently but scoring a point on each rally (PARS) removes the possibility of playing a different tactical plan when serving (when a point could be scored) compared to receiving serve (no point gained) for point on serve only scoring. It was generally accepted that players would play more attacking squash when hand in (serving) compared to hand out (receiving). There is no known scientific evidence to back this view up but certainly any such tactical strategy based on whether a player is serving or not has been removed with the advent of PARS.

When the distance covered per rally is put into perspective, i.e. with respect to the duration of the rally (now about 5 per cent shorter), it can be seen that players, on average, are moving about 7 per cent slower than previously. This has implications regarding the training drills and physical conditioning undertaken by players, although this paper has used average values and it is very likely that there will be differences within male professionals. For example, a match played between two players both ranked in the top 5 in the world would almost certainly be a very hard-fought match whereas a top 5 player would usually beat a player outside the top 30 relatively easily.

The finding that the players are moving 7 per cent slower is counter-intuitive to the desired outcome of making professional squash more attacking, as this implies greater speeds for the players trying to return attacking shots. Anecdotally, the consensus opinion is that there appears to be less rallying to the back of the court and more shots played to the front (this constitutes more attacking play). However, it may be the case that the lower number of rallies (one-third less) has affected the perception of spectators and coaches as to the relative frequency of different shot types. This could be akin to the classic research into basketball shooting where it was suggested that witnesses to sporting events may misperceive the pattern of events (Gilovich *et al.*, 1985). This is, of course, speculation and until research is carried out on the distribution of shots it is impossible to know what tactical changes have been implemented, if any.

21.5 CONCLUSION

Since the key objectives of the PSA were to make matches shorter, have more predictable match durations and make the elite male professional game more exciting to watch, it appears that, to some extent, this has been successful. The reduced overall match time means that over-long matches are less likely and tournament referees can schedule events more easily. It appears that shorter rallies (4 per cent), less distance covered per rally (9 per cent) and lower average velocities (7 per cent) are a consequence of the new scoring system but whether this is more exciting has not been ascertained. At present there is no research on how tactics have changed and future analyses need to assess how the game has changed in terms of the types of shot played by elite players, as this will help to identify explanations for the change in rally characteristics as well as determine if the game has indeed become more exciting to watch.

21.6 REFERENCES

Gilovich, T., Tversky, A. and Vallone, R., 1985, The hot hand in basketball: On the misperception of random sequences. *Cognitive Psychology*, **17**, pp. 295–314.

Hughes, M., Cooper, S.M. and Nevill, A., 2002, Analysis procedures for non-parametric data from performance analysis. *International Journal of Performance Analysis of Sport*, **2**(1), pp. 6–20.

Vučković, G., Perš, J., James, N. and Hughes, M., 2009, Tactical use of the T area in squash by players of differing standard. *Journal of Sports Sciences*, **27**(8), pp. 863–871.

Vučković, G., Perš, J., James, N. and Hughes, M., 2010, Measurement error associated with the SAGIT/Squash computer tracking software. *European Journal of Sports Sciences*, **10**(2), pp. 129–140.

CHAPTER 22

Consistency of key performance indicators for men's singles tennis match: Analysis from 2005 to 2011 Grand Slams

Hyongjun Choi

22.1 INTRODUCTION

Performance analysis has developed with methodological advances in the past decade. Topics in the field of performance analysis were segmented according to various stages of the analysing process. One of the fundamental steps for analysing performances is making a selection of valid performance indicators (Hughes and Bartlett, 2002) as well as selection of analysis purposes. Hughes and Bartlett (2002) have suggested a way to select performance indicators which is based on successful outcomes. The definition of a performance indicator has been discussed for real-time and lapsed-time systems (Choi, 2008).

Since the identification of performance indicators, the concept of key performance indicators (Choi et al., 2006a; 2008a; Lames and McGarry, 2007; O'Donoghue, 2008), relevant to results of performances (e.g. winning/losing, successful/unsuccessful and constructive/unconstructive), was broadly discussed as a way to identify the performance indicators in each sport. The key performance indicators that explain successful outcomes can be considered as valid.

Identifying performance indicators can involve several approaches. Statistical comparison of the performance indicators is one of these approaches. Principle component analysis (Choi et al., 2008b; O'Donoghue, 2008), multiple linear regression and artificial neural networks have also been used to identify key performance indicators. On the other hand, the confirmation of key performance indicators has been obtaining through expert group opinion (Choi et al., 2006c).

The identification of key performance indicators aids reducing data gathering and processing activity by producing an optimal set of performance indicators. Having a reduced set of key performance indicators is essential for real-time analysis (Choi, 2008). The identification of key performance indicators using statistical means, however, has not been reproduced in other studies. This means those performance indicators were only used in a specific study. Among the key performance indicators found in different data sets, there might exist consistent indicators. Those indicators can be found within many studies in sports performance. The main purpose of this study was to identify consistency of the key performance indicators within several championships in men's singles tennis at Grand Slam tournaments based on winning and losing performances (Choi et al., 2006b).

22.2 METHODS

22.2.1 Subjects

The four Grand Slam tennis competitions have been considered from 2005 to 2011 including 1,919 matches and 6,887 sets within this study. The final data used within this study were 751 matches and 687 sets that satisfied the assumptions of statistical tests used (see Table 22.1). The final data used in the study were arranged based on zero-cut where any data including a zero value for any indicator was not used for statistical comparisons.

Table 22.1 Number of data used in each championship (values in parentheses are percentages)

Championships	Matches			Sets		
	Considered subjects	Data detection	Used subjects	Considered subjects	Data detection	Used subjects
2005 WIM	125 (6.5)	45 (6.0)	80 (6.8)	445 (6.5)	397 (6.4)	48 (7.0)
2008 AUS	76 (4.0)	23 (3.1)	53 (4.5)	265 (3.8)	226 (3.6)	39 (5.7)
2008 FRA	126 (6.6)	41 (5.5)	85 (7.3)	457 (6.6)	430 (6.9)	27 (3.9)
2008 WIM	127 (6.6)	49 (6.5)	78 (6.7)	459 (6.7)	425 (6.9)	34 (4.9)
2008 US	80 (4.2)	21 (2.8)	59 (5.1)	292 (4.2)	259 (4.2)	33 (4.8)
2009 AUS	126 (6.6)	73 (9.7)	53 (4.5)	455 (6.6)	424 (6.8)	31 (4.5)
2009 FRA	127 (6.6)	56 (7.5)	71 (6.1)	450 (6.5)	418 (6.7)	32 (4.7)
2009 WIM	126 (6.6)	46 (6.1)	80 (6.8)	467 (6.8)	400 (6.5)	67 (9.8)
2009 US	81 (4.2)	31 (4.1)	50 (4.3)	276 (4.0)	237 (3.8)	39 (5.7)
2010 AUS	83 (4.3)	31 (4.1)	52 (4.5)	301 (4.4)	266 (4.3)	35 (5.1)
2010 FRA	126 (6.6)	42 (5.6)	84 (7.2)	456 (6.6)	419 (6.8)	37 (5.4)
2010 WIM	127 (6.6)	38 (5.1)	89 (7.6)	478 (6.9)	437 (7)	41 (6.0)
2010 US	127 (6.6)	68 (9.1)	59 (5.1)	455 (6.6)	422 (6.8)	33 (4.8)
2011 AUS	127 (6.6)	67 (8.9)	60 (5.1)	452 (6.6)	421 (6.8)	31 (4.5)
2011 FRA	126 (6.6)	38 (5.1)	88 (7.5)	452 (6.6)	406 (6.5)	46 (6.7)
2011 WIM	127 (6.6)	50 (6.7)	77 (6.6)	448 (6.5)	371 (6.0)	77 (11.2)
2011 US	82 (4.3)	32 (4.3)	50 (4.3)	279 (4.1)	242 (3.9)	37 (5.4)
Total	1,919	1,168	751	6,888	6200	687

22.2.2 Data collection and variables used

The data were collected from four Grand Slam tennis championships' official websites (Australian Open: http://www.australianopen.com, French Open: http://www.rolandgarros.com, Wimbledon open: http://www.wimbledon.com and US open: http://www.usopen.org). The collected data were saved into Microsoft Excel 12.0 for pre-processing and loaded into SPSS version 19.0 (SPSS, an IBM company, Amarouk, NY). The variables used in this study were the 10 indicators listed below;

- Percentage of first serves played in
- Aces
- Double faults
- Unforced errors
- Winning percentage of successful first serve
- Winning percentage of successful second serve
- Winners (included serves)
- Receiving points won
- Break point conversions
- Percentage of net approaches

In addition, the total points played was not recorded from the official statistics because winning and losing performances were already classified by match result and set result.

22.2.3 Data analysis procedure

Wilcoxon Signed Ranks tests were used to compare winning and losing performance within matches of each championship.

Table 22.2 The results of Wilcoxon Signed Ranks tests between winning and losing performance based on match data

	①	②	③	④	⑤	⑥	⑦	⑧	⑨	⑩
All data	-6.89*	-11.14*	-8.67*	-13.51*	-24.69*	-22.42*	-14.21*	-21.72*	-21.01*	-12.34*
2005 WIM	-.39	-3.00*	-.78	-3.20*	-6.29*	-5.29*	-3.00*	-6.85*	-6.43*	-3.01*
2008 AUS	-2.43*	-2.62*	-.95	-4.42*	-5.89*	-5.19*	-3.07*	-.12*	-5.48*	-5.04*
2008 FRA	-3.62*	-2.33*	-2.36*	-3.39*	-6.67*	-6.14*	-4.29*	-7.25*	-5.62*	-1.68
2008 WIM	-.71	-1.81	-2.83*	-3.67*	-6.22*	-6.54*	-2.70*	-7.52*	-4.89*	-3.39*
2008 US	-1.34	-3.59*	-1.00	-1.35	-6.19*	-4.29*	-4.04*	-6.15*	-5.06*	-2.59*
2009 AUS	-2.81*	-1.81	-2.15*	-3.75*	-5.29*	-4.17*	-2.29*	-5.87*	-3.57*	-3.03*
2009 FRA	-3.39*	-1.90	-3.20*	-3.07*	-4.92*	-5.32*	-2.58*	-6.68*	-3.97*	-3.05*
2009 WIM	-1.33	-3.24*	-3.04*	-3.92*	-5.90*	-6.93*	-4.04*	-7.23*	-4.03*	-3.94*
2009 US	-.15	-3.09*	-.75	-2.17*	-5.53*	-4.50*	-3.18*	-5.77*	-4.23*	-3.36*
2010 AUS	-.89	-3.48*	-2.29*	-1.82	-5.39*	-4.56*	-3.75*	-5.87*	-5.47*	-2.14*
2010 FRA	-.38	-3.07*	-.14	-3.20*	-6.94*	-5.73*	-4.48*	-7.58*	-5.75*	-2.96*
2010 WIM	-.58	-2.19*	-2.74*	-3.31*	-6.03*	-6.21*	-3.95*	-6.97*	-5.05*	-2.59*
2010 US	-1.07	-2.50*	-1.61	-2.48*	-5.57*	-4.28*	-3.23*	-6.30*	-3.82*	-3.78*
2011 AUS	-2.05*	-3.38*	-2.47*	-2.33*	-6.17*	-5.45*	-4.15*	-6.41*	-5.55*	-3.43*
2011 FRA	-.23	-2.64*	-1.60	-3.88*	-7.08*	-5.88*	-3.20*	-7.62*	-5.35*	-2.61*
2011 WIM	-1.81	-3.15*	-3.33*	-3.55*	-3.89*	-4.44*	-4.05*	-6.76*	-6.11*	-.31
2011 US	-2.80*	-.89	-1.82	-4.51*	-4.71*	-4.99*	-.87	-6.03*	-3.96*	-3.36*

Note: ①% of 1st serves succeed, ②Aces, ③Double faults, ④Unforced errors, ⑤Winning % of successful 1st serve, ⑥Winning % of successful 2nd serve, ⑦Winners (included serves), ⑧Receiving points won, ⑨Break points conversions, ⑩% of net approaches, $*p < .05$

22.3 RESULTS

22.3.1 Comparisons between winning and losing performances

The comparisons between winning and losing performances revealed that four indicators were consistently found to be significantly different between winning and losing performances. Table 22.2 shows the results of the Wilcoxon Signed Ranks tests.

22.3.2 Comparisons of set data between winning and losing performances

Table 22.3 shows the results of Wilcoxon Signed Ranks tests based on individual sets. Interestingly, the numbers of performance indicators which were significantly different in sets data were fewer than in match data. However, the only performance indicators found as significantly different in both methods were winning percentage of successful first serve and receiving points

Table 22.3 The results of Wilcoxon Signed Ranks tests between winning and losing performance based on set data

	①	②	③	④	⑤	⑥	⑦	⑧	⑨	⑩
All data	-5.03*	-5.72*	-4.54*	-11.25*	-17.90*	-14.94*	-11.21*	-24.52*	-7.90*	-8.46*
2005 WIM	-5.85	-2.89*	-.67	-2.30*	-3.38*	-3.87*	-2.68*	-4.87*	-.75	-1.43
2008 AUS	-3.13*	-.06	-.94	-3.28*	-3.19*	-2.30*	-1.69	-5.39*	-.02	-1.30
2008 FRA	-1.74	-.82	-.84	-1.19	-2.72*	-3.43*	-2.57*	-4.31*	-.08	-1.31
2008 WIM	-.72	-1.25	-2.09*	-1.92	-3.81*	-1.76	-1.79	-4.42*	-.72	-2.06*
2008 US	-1.85	-1.92	-.30	-1.52	-3.13*	-1.91	-2.47*	-4.55*	-.05	-.57
2009 AUS	-.26	-1.15	-.61	-2.93*	-3.50*	-2.92*	-1.98	-4.86*	-.44	-1.98
2009 FRA	-.37	-.67	-.86	-1.04	-3.11*	-2.68*	-2.66*	-4.66*	-.80	-2.29*
2009 WIM	-.33	-.21	-1.63	-2.41*	-4.20*	-3.52*	-1.36	-6.48*	-.68	-2.22*
2009 US	-.49	-2.19*	-.42	-1.70	-3.48*	-3.84*	-2.11*	-5.36*	-.07	-1.24
2010 AUS	-.53	-1.70	-.49	-1.91	-3.72*	-2.42*	-2.62*	-5.16*	-.67	-1.64
2010 FRA	-1.69	-.21	-.31	-1.22	-3.02*	-3.48*	-2.41*	-5.05*	-.44	-2.01
2010 WIM	-.20	-.83	-.69	-.11	-3.34*	-2.71*	-2.19*	-5.25*	-.08	-.62
2010 US	-1.29	-.64	-.83	-.72	-3.17*	-1.39	-2.73*	-5.02*	-1.48	-1.94
2011 AUS	-.12	-1.21	-1.97	-1.88	-4.10*	-2.39*	-1.31	-4.55*	-.70	-2.76*
2011 FRA	-.85	-1.02	-.98	-1.11	-3.62*	-2.44*	-3.21*	-4.91*	-.31	-1.33
2011 WIM	-.10	-1.46	-2.87*	-3.87*	-4.57*	-2.44*	-2.43*	-5.22*	-2.13*	-.20
2011 US	-3.47*	-.16	-1.30	-3.81*	-2.06*	-2.99*	-.63	-4.75*	-1.61	-.92

Note: ①% of 1st serves succeed, ②Aces, ③Double faults, ④Unforced errors, ⑤Winning % of successful 1st serve, ⑥Winning % of successful 2nd serve, ⑦Winners(included serves), ⑧Receiving points won, ⑨Break points conversions, ⑩% of net approaches, *p < .05

22.4 DISCUSSION

The methods used to identify key performance indicators have been discussed from various perspectives. The need for performance indicators in the field of performance analysis of sport (Hughes and Bartlett, 2002), optimal numbers of performance indicators (Choi *et al.*, 2006a), and using principle component analysis for identification of performance indicators (Choi *et al.*, 2008b; O'Donoghue, 2008) have been discussed in relation to performance indicators. However, no single agreed way to identify key performance indicators has been developed.

This study is relevant to the methodological issues in identifying key performance indicators and forms a starting point by exploring the consistency of findings in large data sets. The consistency of key performance indicators was intended to show performance similarity so that those indicators distinguishing winning and losing performances are reasonably invariant. As Choi *et al.* (2006b) mentioned, the definition of winning has to be redefined within a concept of valid identification of key performance indicators. The optimal set of key performance indicators to be used in real-time analysis systems (Choi, 2008) should be a manageable set of indicators that can be produced and used in real time based on partial match data. The identification of valid key performance indicators has to utilise many kinds of methods.

In tennis matches, there are key performance indicators involving winning shots in each rally. The key performance indicators in tennis would be consistently represented in winning performances or winners. However, the results show that there were only a couple of indicators that distinguished winning and losing performances. There were significant differences in winning percentage of successful first serves, winning percentage of successful second serves, receiving points won and break point conversion in match data. The selection of indicators also needs to consider the purposes of their use. Some indicators might be for tactical evaluation and some indicators would be for technical evaluation. The results in this study did not distinguish between these types of indicator. From a coaching perspective, individual variability of performance or tactics is often considered. To identify distinguishing indicators between winning and losing performances consistently, however, we need to able to give brief information where losing players have to enhance their performance to increase the chance of winning a set.

The numbers of indicators found to be significantly different between winning and losing performances varied between match and set data. This result was similar to previous studies by Choi *et al.* (2006b, 2008a). The previous studies also emphasised that reduction of numbers of key performance indicators is one of the ways to address limited data collection time. Thus, these reduced sets of performance indicators might be useful in real-time analysis systems as previously suggested (Choi *et al.*, 2006a; Williams, 2004). Moreover, four significant performance indicators (winning percentage of successful first serves, winning percentage of successful second serves, receiving points won and break point conversion) for matches included two significant performance indicators (winning percentage of successful first serves and receiving points won) for sets that might be consistent key performance indicators. Those performance indicators have to be considered for validity with experts' opinions or comments.

The consistency of key performance indicators not only points to optimal sets of key performance indicators. but also has implications for normative profiling (Hughes *et al.*, 2001).

22.5 CONCLUSION

The performance indicators derived from official tournament website data were considered for matches and sets. The comparison of winning and losing performances identified consistent performance indicators using Wilcoxon Signed Ranks tests. The conclusions of this study are:

1. There were greater numbers of performance indicators that significantly distinguished between winning and losing performances in match than in set data;
2. The percentage of successful first serves and break point conversions were the most consistent key performance indicators found.

22.6 REFERENCES

Choi, H., 2008, Definitions of performance indicators in real-time and lapsed-time analysis in performance analysis of sports. Unpublished PhD Thesis. (Cardiff, UK: University of Wales Institute Cardiff).

Choi, H., Reed, D., Hughes, M. and O'Donoghue, P., 2006a, The valid number of performance indicators for real-time analysis using prediction models within men singles in 2005 Wimbledon Tennis Championship. In *Performance Analysis of Sport 7*, edited by Dancs, H., Hughes, M. and O'Donoghue, P.G. (Cardiff, UK: CPA UWIC Press), pp. 220–226.

Choi, H. J., O'Donoghue, P. and Hughes, M., 2006b, A Study of team performance indicators by separated time scale using a real-time analysis technique within English national basketball league. In *Performance Analysis of Sport 7*, edited by Dancs, H., Hughes, M. and O'Donoghue, P.G. (Cardiff, UK: CPA Press, UWIC), pp. 138–141.

Choi, H.J., Kim, J.H., Kim, J.H., Hong, S.J. and Hughes, M., 2006c, A study of valid contents for an evaluation of team performance in Soccer. In *Performance Analysis of Sport VII*, edited by Dancs, H., Hughes, M. and O'Donoghue, P. (Cardiff, UK: CPA Press, UWIC), pp. 92–99.

Choi, H., O'Donoghue, P. and Hughes, M., 2008a, A comparison of whole match and individual set data in order to identify valid performance indicators for real-time feedback in men's single tennis matches. In *Science and Racket Sports IV*, edited by Lees, A., Cabello, D. and Torres, G. (London: Routledge), pp. 227–231.

Choi, H., Hughes, M. and O'Donoghue, P., 2008b, The identification of an optimal set of performance indicators for real-time analysis using principle components analysis. In *Performance Analysis of Sport VIII*, edited by Hokelmann, A. and Brummond, M. (Aachen, Germany: Shaker-Verlag), pp. 295–301.

Hughes, M. and Bartlett, R., 2002, The use of performance indicators in performance analysis. *Journal of Sports Sciences*, **20**, pp. 739–754.

Hughes, M., Evans, S. and Wells, J., 2001, Establishing normative profiles in performance analysis. *International Journal of Performance Analysis in Sport*, **1**, pp. 4–26.

Lames, M. and McGarry, T., 2007, On the search for reliable performance indicators in game sports. *International Journal of Performance Analysis in Sport*, **7**(1), pp. 62–79.

O'Donoghue, P., 2008, Principal components analysis in the selection of performance indicators in sport. *International Journal of Performance Analysis in Sport*, **8**(3), pp. 145–155.

Williams, J., 2004, The development of a real-time data capture application for rugby union. In *Performance Analysis of Sport VI*, edited by O'Donoghue, P.G and Hughes, M.D. (Cardiff, UK: CPA Press, UWIC), pp. 253–261.

CHAPTER 23

The importance of inter-shot time of ground strokes in tennis

Hiroo Takahashi, Shunsuke Murakami, Masahiko Ishihara,
Takahiro Morishige, Tetsu Kitamura,
Akira Maeda and Hidetsugu Nishizono

23.1 INTRODUCTION

Time-factors are important aspects for match analysis in tennis. O'Donoghue and Liddle (1998) analysed the length of rallies in men's and women's singles matches in Grand Slam tournaments. Richers (1995) estimated energy systems utilised by elite competitive tennis players during matches through time-motion analysis. Recently, the authors found that inter-shot times were important tactical aspects in tennis matches (Takahashi *et al.*, 2008; 2009).

Inter-shot time was defined as the difference between the time of shot by one player and the opponent. The authors clarified the tendencies of inter-shot time of ground strokes (GS) between the server and the receiver (Takahashi *et al.*, 2008) for the historical change in Wimbledon (Takahashi *et al.*, 2009). However, the analysis of each shot in the rally is needed rather than whole statistical rally analysis because players' situations in each rally are changing according to each shot.

The purpose of this study was to clarify the importance of inter-shot time as an indicator for evaluating a player's situation.

23.2 METHODS

We analysed eleven women's singles matches held in the 2010 and 2011 US Open. The total number of rallies was 1,765. Rallies of more than five shots and finished with GS were analysed in this study. Therefore, the total number of rallies included in this study was 505.

Computerised scorebook for tennis was used previously for data collection and the scorebook has been shown to record inter-shot time with high accuracy (Takahashi *et al.*, 2006). This confirmed the inter-shot time error between the data from the scorebook and the data from the recording of high-speed video. The 95 per cent limits of agreement for inter-shot time was 0.003 ± 0.05 s. It is also recommended that the scorer needed to be well trained in its operation (Takahashi *et al.*, 2007). The scorer in this study was well trained before the data collection commenced.

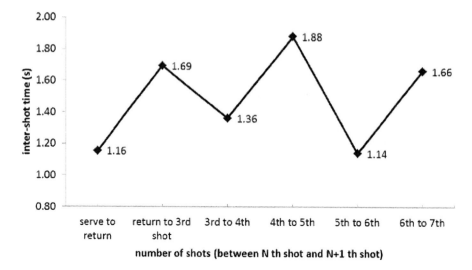

Figure 23.1 An example of a line graph of inter-shot time of GS in a rally (regular pattern)

We defined inter-shot time by server as the time interval from receiver's shot to server's shot. It means the time duration before the shot was used.

Inter-shot times of GS in each rally were plotted as line graphs (Figure 23.1). The horizontal axis showed the numbers of shots in rallies and the vertical axis showed inter-shot time of GS in each shot.

23.3 RESULTS AND DISCUSSION

23.3.1 The patterns of inter-shot time of ground strokes

It was found that the lines in the graph showed up and down regularly or irregularly. An example of regular pattern is shown in Figure 23.1 and irregular pattern in Figure 23.2. The numbers for regular or irregular rally graph patterns are shown in Table 23.1. A regular pattern was found in 199 rallies and an irregular pattern was found in 306 rallies.

It was considered that the beginning three shots were related to rally graph pattern. The first shot in the rally, Serve, was the fastest shot in the rally. Inter-shot time of serve was the shortest. The second shot in the rally, Return, is the most demanding technique in tennis (Kleinöder and Mester, 2000). Players needed to return the fastest shot safely. Therefore, inter-shot time of return was longer than other shots in the rally. The third shot in the rally, ground strokes in this study, was the next shot. It could be the first occasion for server to attack in the rally. That is why inter-shot time of third shot in the rally became shorter in this study. Such rally patterns led the regular rally graph pattern in this study.

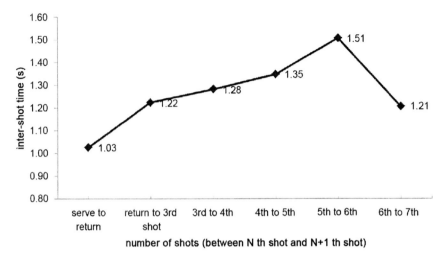

Figure 23.2 An example of a line graph of inter-shot time of GS in an irregular pattern

Table 23.1 Results of Mann-Whitney U test on inter-shot time of GS between server and receiver

Player	N	Mean	SD	p
Server	13	1.46	0.11	0.029*
Receiver	14	1.38	0.05	

*p < 0.05

We confirmed the difference of inter-shot time of GS between server and receiver. The spread of frequencies of inter-shot time of GS compared as situations was shown in Figure 23.3. There was significant difference between the server's inter-shot time of GS and receiver's according to a Mann-Whitney U test (Table 23.1). Takahashi *et al.* (2008) reported that server's inter-shot time of GS was shorter than the receiver's in men's singles matches. However, they defined the time duration after the shot as inter-shot time in that study. Those results showed that the receiver has less time to play shots prior to the receiver playing a shot.

23.3.2 Relationships between the patterns of graphs and the rallies

We also analysed the relationships between the patterns of graphs and the actual rallies. Experienced tennis coaches evaluated the actual rallies with actual videos.

It was found that players could play more aggressively when they had a longer time interval before the shot. The average inter-shot time in this study was enough time to react to the shot (Schönborn, 1999). In this study, the server had a longer time interval than the receiver. It indicated that the server had more chance

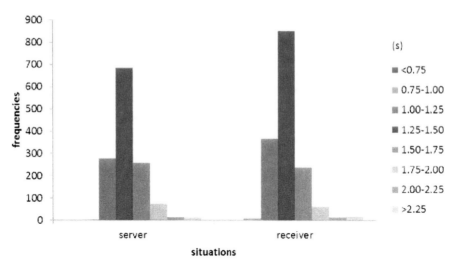

Figure 23.3 The spread of inter-shot time of GS compared as situations

to play aggressively than the receiver. This is one of the reasons why the server won more points than the receiver.

It was also found that the rallies shown as irregular patterns had the situation of changing control between the players. Coaches evaluated the rhythm of the rally type that changes to the irregular line graph pattern. For example, the rally shown in Figure 23.2 started from a second serve. The receiver played an aggressive shot at return. This is the first situation of changing control in this rally. After that, players maintained the rhythm of the rally. Eventually, the receiver attacked using a backhand stroke. This led to the server making an error. It was confirmed by coaches that the receiver took control of this rally on return.

These results suggested that we could evaluate which players controlled the rally by analysing inter-shot time of GS.

23.4 CONCLUSIONS

The importance of inter-shot time of ground strokes was confirmed in the following three aspects:

i.   The server has more time to play shots than the receiver and the receiver has to work their way into the rally.
ii. When players had a longer time interval before the shot, players could play more aggressively. That is one of the reasons why the server won more points than the receiver.
iii. We could evaluate which players controlled the rally by analysing inter-shot time of ground strokes.

23.5 ACKNOWLEDGEMENTS

This study was supported by JSPS KAKENHI 11021981 and the research fund of the National Institute of Fitness and Sports in Kanoya.

23.6 REFERENCES

Kleinöder, H. and Mester, J., 2000, Strategies for the return of 1st and 2nd serves. In *Tennis Science and Technology*, edited by Haake, S.J. and Coe, A. (Oxford: Blackwell), pp. 401–408.

O'Donoghue, P. and Liddle, D., 1998, A notational analysis of time factors of elite men's and ladies' singles tennis on clay and grass surfaces. In: *Science and Racket Sports II*, edited by Lees, A., Maynard, I., Hughes, M. and Reilly, T. (E & FN Spon: London), pp. 241–246.

Richers, T.A., 1995, Time-motion analysis of the energy systems in elite and competitive singles tennis. *Journal of Human Movement Studies*, **28**, pp. 73–86.

Schönborn, R., 1999, *Advanced Techniques for Competitive Tennis*, (Oxford: Meyer & Meyer Sport).

Takahashi, H., Wada, T., Maeda, A., Kodama, M., Nishizono, H. and Kurata, H., 2006, The relationship between court surface and tactics in tennis using a computerized scorebook. *International Journal of Performance Analysis in Sport*, **6**(2), pp. 15–25.

Takahashi, H., Wada, T., Maeda, A., Kodama, M. and Nishizono, H., 2007, The development of computerized scorebook for tennis. *Proceedings of the 6th International Symposium on Computer Science in Sport*, pp. 300–304.

Takahashi, H., Wada, T., Maeda, A., Kodama, M. and Nishizono, H., 2008, An analysis of the time duration of ground strokes in Grand Slam men's singles using the computerised scorebook for tennis. *International Journal of Performance Analysis in Sport*, **8**(3), pp. 96–103.

Takahashi, H., Wada, T., Maeda, A., Kodama, M., Nishizono, H. and Kurata, H., 2009, Time analysis of three decades of men's singles at Wimbledon. In *Science and Racket Sports IV*, edited by Lees, A., Cabello, D. and Torres, G. (Routledge: Abingdon, UK), pp. 239-246.

CHAPTER 24

Male positive affect elucidates mixed-doubles badminton tournament rank

Clare Rhoden, Julia West and Derek Peters

24.1 INTRODUCTION

Current research identifies affect as both a precursor to and a consequence of performance (Renfree *et al.*, 2012; Scott *et al.*, 2002). Pre-competition positive affect (PA) has been found to be positively correlated to wrestling (Treasure *et al.*, 1996) and climbing performance (Sanchez *et al.*, 2010) whilst pre-performance affect has been found to distinguish between faster and slower 10 km laboratory time trials (Renfree *et al.*, 2012). Walsh *et al.* (1992) reported increased levels of negative affect (NA) in failure compared to success conditions and in collegiate tennis singles, post-match NA was negatively correlated with first serve percentage (Scott *et al.*, 2002). A decrease in PA from pre- to post-competition (24 hours) was reported by male golfers who indicated their actual score was worse than their expected score (Gaudreau *et al.*, 2002).

Research findings relating to sex differences in affect are mixed. No differences in affect between males and females were discernible in both non-sport (Watson, 2000) and sport related samples (Scott *et al.*, 2002). Prior to indoor sport climbing, NA was higher for females than males; however, these differences may have been accounted for by the expertise of the females within the sample (Aşçi *et al.*, 2006). These studies investigated male and female differences *per se*; however, in team sports, what is perhaps more important is the consideration of males and females within a dyad.

The relationship within a sporting dyad is complex with many interacting factors. Research focusing on effective dyad structure, composition and process (Wickwire *et al.*, 2004) identified the ability to listen to their partner, take advice or criticism and make decisions with them, a higher level of connection and having to deal with someone else's emotions and problems, were all necessary for successful dyads; factors which have implications for the affect experienced by badminton players. Qualitative analysis of elite athlete dyads highlighted that self-efficacy stemmed from many factors, including past individual and dyad achievements, emotional factors and the intra-relationship with other-efficacy and relation-inferred self-efficacy (your estimation of how confident your partner is in you). Sources of an athlete's belief in their partner included the length of playing experience with the partner, previous partner's performance and their joint performances, third party comments and comparisons they made to previous partners and other athletes (Jackson *et al.*, 2008). Self-efficacy, other-efficacy and relation inferred self-efficacy have been shown to relate to affect (Jackson *et al.*,

2008; Treasure *et al.*, 1996), and Jackson *et al.* (2007) suggested the need to understand efficacy concepts further to ascertain if congruence between them enables sustained dyadic functioning. By inference, congruence between male and female affect profiles in a mixed-sex dyad might indicate a higher level connection between the partners and improved dyadic functioning. There may be instances where one player in the dyad exhibits a psychological profile superior to their partner and analysis of individual affect as well as total pairs affect or the discrepancy between each partner's affect could elucidate the dyad relationship further. There is, however, a paucity of research investigating affect within mixed-sex sporting dyads. This study addresses this gap directly whilst also extending empirical evidence of the relationship between affect and sports performance and sex differences in affect. The aims of this study were to examine the affect profiles of males and females both across the sample and within the dyads and to analyse the relationships between individual affect profiles and pair affect profiles with final tournament position.

24.2 METHOD

24.2.1 Participants

Eight mixed pairs of County level badminton players (males mean age = 26 ± 9 yrs, females mean age = 24 ± 6 yrs) who had played together in their doubles pair for between 1 and 5 years, consented to participate in the study. Players' length of badminton career did not differ significantly between males (16 ± 9 yrs) and females (13 ± 5 yrs, t = 0.81, p = 0.43).

24.2.2 Measures

The Positive and Negative Affect Schedule (PANAS; Watson *et al.*, 1988) was used to measure positive and negative affect via two subscales comprising 10 adjectives each (e.g. 'interested'; 'distressed'). Items on both subscales are measured using a 5 point likert scale from '*1 – not at all*' to '*5 – extremely*' giving a range from 10 to 50 for each subscale. Cronbach alphas showed acceptable internal consistency for both positive and negative affect (0.92 and 0.78 respectively).

24.2.3 Procedure

With Institutional ethics approval, players provided full written informed consent prior to data collection. Utilising a repeated measures design in a field setting, the tournament consisted of two groups with each pair playing three group matches and one final match to determine final tournament ranking. Ten minutes prior to each match, players individually rated their state affect on the PANAS.

24.2.4 Data analysis

Whole group analysis between male and female PA and NA was performed using Mann-Whitney U tests. Separating the pairs into two groups based upon their final tournament position enabled the analysis of affect profiles between good (top four ranked pairs) and poor (bottom four ranked pairs) performance groups. Within these groups Mann-Whitney U tests were performed to assess differences in male and female PA and NA. Spearman Rank correlational analysis examined relationships between tournament position and PA and NA at the i) individual (male and female) and ii) pair (pair total; pair discrepancy) levels.

24.3 RESULTS

Males reported significantly higher PA than females with PANAS scores averaged across the tournament ($p = 0.04$), but did not differ in NA (Table 24.1). Top ranked males and bottom ranked males did not differ in either PA or NA prior to any match. Top ranked females reported significantly higher pre-match NA for match 4 ($p = 0.03$, Table 24.1). For the top ranked pairs only, consistent profiles were observed across the tournament (matches 1–4) with males reporting higher levels of PA and lower levels of NA than the females. These were significant prior to match 2 ($p = 0.029$) and match 4 ($p = 0.029$, Table 24.1). Bottom ranked pairs show inconsistent affect profiles across the tournament. Prior to match 2 males exhibited lower levels of PA than females although this was non-significant (Table 24.1).

Table 24.1 PANAS median and range scores prior to each tournament match between the top and bottom ranked groups. PA – positive affect, NA – negative affect

	Match 1		Match 2		Match 3		Match 4		Tournament median	
	PA	NA	PA	NA	PA	NA	PA	NA	PA	NA
Males										
Top rank	43 33–46	13 11–21	46[a] 36–49	11 10–13	45 27–50	10 10–11	46[b] 39–48	11 10–14	45 35–48	12 10–12
Bottom rank	40 35–44	13 11–20	30 10–43	12 10–19	34 25–41	11 10–18	35 24–42	10 10–14	38 27–42	12 10–19
All males	43 33–46	13 11–21	40 10–49	11 10–19	39 25–50	10 10–18	41 24–48	10 10–14	41[c] 27–48	12 10–19
Females										
Top Rank	30 22–36	15 12–28	32[a] 20–34	17 11–21	30 23–36	18 10–22	33[b] 20–38	17[d] 13–27	33 21–36	18 12–21
Bottom Rank	35 29–39	13 11–14	35 29–41	12 10–14	34 29–37	11 10–12	26 17–40	11[d] 10–11	33 29–40	11 10–13
All females	33 22–39	14 12–28	33 20–41	14 10–21	34 23–37	12 10–22	30 17–40	12 10–27	33[c] 21–40	13 10–21

Note: [a] $p = 0.029$, $Z = -2.309$; [b] $p = 0.029$, $Z = -2.32$; [c] $p = 0.04$, $Z = -2.049$; [d] $p = 0.03$, $Z = -2.34$.

   Individual male PA was positively correlated with tournament rank in matches 2, 3 and 4 (Table 24.2). Pair total PA was positively related to tournament rank before match 4 whilst pair affect discrepancy, where the male's PA was higher than their female partners, was related to tournament rank in match 3. Individual female's NA prior to match 1 and match 4 were both correlated with final tournament rank. Similarly, the discrepancy in negative affect, where the female's score was higher than their male partner, was significantly related to tournament rank in matches 1 and 4.

Table 24.2 Correlations between pre-match affect and tournament rank (whole sample)

Affect variable	Cell contents	Match 1	Match 2	Match 3	Match 4
Males PA	rho	ns	−0.85	−0.74	−0.85
	p		0.037	0.016	0.007
Pairs discrepancy in PA	rho	ns	ns	−0.74	ns
	p			0.037	
Total pairs PA	rho	ns	ns	ns	0.79
	p				0.021
Pairs discrepancy in NA	rho	0.93	ns	ns	0.79
	p	0.001			0.02
Females NA	rho	−0.81	ns	ns	−0.72
	p	0.015			0.04

Note: ns – non significant

24.4 DISCUSSION

Male badminton players exhibited significantly higher levels of PA than females in contrast to previous findings from both Watson (2000) and Scott *et al.* (2002). Unlike the findings of Aşçi *et al.* (2006), this male–female difference was in the PA construct rather than NA. High levels of PA have been suggested to be associated with "high energy, full concentration and pleasurable engagement" (Watson *et al.*, 1988, p. 1063) and in this competitive badminton environment it suggests that the males possessed an affect profile more conducive to successful performance (Sanchez *et al.*, 2010; Treasure *et al.*, 1996).
   Analysing the findings further, however, reveals a relationship that is more complex with pre-match affect elucidating the resultant tournament rank. The male badminton players having greater PA than their female partners was evident within the top ranked pairs consistently across tournament, but this was not seen in the bottom ranked pairs. Whilst their affect profile at the start of the tournament was similar to the top ranked pairs, prior to match 2 a reversal in affect profile occurs, with the males reporting lower levels of PA than their female partners. There were, however, no differences in pre-match PA or NA between the top ranked and bottom ranked males in the sample. Thus it appears that the discrepancy between the male and female affect profile within a pair rather than the level of male PA *per*

se, is the most important factor. Crucially the match wins and high tournament positions were related to the male PA being higher than his partners.

The within dyad affect profiles differed despite identical match outcome and it is necessary to consider the reasons for this. All bottom ranked pairs were defeated in the first round match and the reductions in male PA could have been anticipated (Gaudreau *et al.*, 2002) but the mechanisms surrounding this warrant further attention. Gaudreau *et al.* (2002) found that successful coping mediated the affect-achievement relationship and as such, further research examining the utilisation of coping and its success within badminton is required.

Underpinning the effective functioning of the dyad are both individual and partner related factors, including perceived success, past achievements, interpersonal communication, self-efficacy and the intra-relationship with other-efficacy and relation-inferred self-efficacy (Jackson *et al.*, 2008) and dealing with someone else's emotions and problems (Wickwire *et al.*, 2004). These factors allude to the complexity of the dyad relationship and the mechanisms which might underpin the development of an individual's affective state. It is unknown in this study whether the fluctuating PA of the bottom ranked males is due to self-efficacy, other-efficacy or relation-inferred self-efficacy and analysing these variables and their antecedents within the badminton dyad during success and failure would be an important area of future research to support psychological diagnostics pre-intervention.

Self-efficacy, other-efficacy and relation-inferred self-efficacy have been shown to relate to affect (Jackson *et al.*, 2008; Treasure *et al.*, 1996) and congruence between them should enhance dyadic functioning (Jackson *et al.*, 2007). By implication, congruence between the affect profiles of men and women within a dyad might enhance performance. These data, however, revealed incongruence between male and female affect profiles and suggest the male PA profile appears strongly predictive of final tournament position, i.e. higher levels of PA, and lower levels of NA compared to their female partner. If these findings can be replicated in other mixed-sex sport dyads, it may confirm that a 'negative' incongruence in affect (where the male PA profile is inferior to the female PA profile) is detrimental to performance.

24.5 CONCLUSION

Higher male PA was strongly related to final tournament position. Male PA was consistently higher and NA lower than females within the top ranked pairs of the tournament. Whilst clearly highlighting within tournament variability in affect, and notable gender discrepancy even though pairs ultimately experienced identical match outcomes (win/loss), this research emphasises the importance of male PA in comparison to the females within a mixed doubles pair and its significant relationship to overall tournament position. Practical sport psychology and performance analysis outcomes for mixed doubles sports include the need to maximise male PA and incorporate coaching strategies to consider the affect profiles within pairs.

24.6 REFERENCES

Aşçi, F.H., Dermirhan, G., Koca, C. and Dinç, S.C., 2006, Precompetitive anxiety and affective states of climbers in indoor climbing competition. *Perceptual and Motor Skills*, **102**, pp. 395–405.

Gaudreau, P., Blondin, J.P. and Lapierre, A.M., 2002, Athletes coping during a competition: Relationship of coping strategies with positive affect, negative affect and performance-goal discrepancy. *Psychology of Sport and Exercise*, **3**, pp. 125–150.

Jackson, B., Beauchamp, M.R. and Knapp, P., 2007, Relational efficacy beliefs in athlete dyads: An investigation using actor-partner interdependence models. *Journal of Sport and Exercise Psychology*, **29**, pp. 170–189.

Jackson, B., Knapp, P. and Beauchamp, M.R., 2008, Origins and consequences of tripartite efficacy beliefs within elite athlete dyads. *Journal of Sport and Exercise Psychology*, **30**, pp. 512–540.

Renfree, A., West , J., Corbett, M., Rhoden, C. and St Clair Gibson, A., 2012, Complex interplay between the determinants of pacing and performance during 20km cycle time trials. *International Journal of Sports Physiology and Performance*, **7**, pp. 121–129.

Sanchez, X., Boschker, M.S.J. and Llewellyn, D.J., 2010, Pre-performance psychological states and performance in an elite climbing competition. *Scandanavian Journal of Medicine and Science in Sport,* **20**, pp. 356–363.

Scott, V.B., Stiles, K.B., Raines, D.B. and Koth, A.W., 2002, Mood, rumination and mood awareness in the athletic performance of collegiate tennis players. *North American Journal of Psychology*, **4**, pp. 457–468.

Treasure, D.C., Monson, J. and Lox, C.L., 1996, Relationship between self-efficacy, wrestling performance and affect prior to a competition. *The Sport Psychologist*, **10**, pp. 73–83.

Walsh, J., Crocker, P.R.E. and Bouffard, M., 1992, The effects of perceived competence and goal orientation on affect and task persistence in a physical activity skill. *The Australian Journal of Science and Medicine in Sport*, **24**, pp. 86–90.

Watson, D., 2000, *Mood and Temperament*, (New York: The Guilford Press).

Watson, D., Clark, L.A. and Tellegen, A., 1988, Development and validation of brief measures of positive and negative affect: The PANAS scales. *Journal of Personality and Social Psychology*, **54**, pp. 1063–1070.

Wickwire, T.L., Bloom, G.A. and Loughead, T.M., 2004, The environment, structure and interaction process of elite same-sex dyadic sports teams. *The Sport Psychologist*, **18**, pp. 381–396.

CHAPTER 25

Distribution of stroke and footwork types in top-level men's and women's table tennis

Ivan Malagoli Lanzoni,

Rocco Di Michele and Franco Merni

25.1 INTRODUCTION

The systematic analysis of technical/tactical behavior of players during actual match play is an essential practice for coaches in the majority of sports. An effective method for technical and tactical evaluation in racket sports is notational analysis (Hughes, 1998), in which relevant aspects of the actions performed by the players during match play are recorded and summarized with specific indicators. Technical and tactical skills play a crucial role as determinants of performance in table tennis. The most used technical and tactical parameters in net games are indicators of the shooting behavior, such as the distribution of shot types and of shot outcomes (Hughes and Bartlett, 2002). Another important characteristic of a shot is the footwork performed before hitting the ball, as using correct footwork allows the player to be in the most favored position for an effective ball strike (Malagoli Lanzoni *et al.*, 2007; 2010). Furthermore, it was shown that some footwork types were more associated than others with a positive outcome of the shot (Malagoli Lanzoni *et al.*, 2010).

An interesting topic from both a coaching and performance analysis perspective is that of technical and tactical differences between men's and women's matches. Otcheva and Drianovski (2002) analyzed the play style of the world's and Bulgaria's top male and female players, although the comparisons concerned only a limited number of selected stroke types. One of the most relevant finding was that the forehand topspin was used much more often by men than women. The forehand topspin being an especially aggressive stroke, it may be supposed that male players have, in general, a more offensive play style.

The purpose of this study was to analyze the distribution of stroke and footwork types, and the association of such indicators, in top-level men's (M) and women's (W) table tennis matches. It was hypothesized that male players would use a more aggressive technique with a prevalence of forehand strokes and more dynamic footwork.

25.2 METHODS

The stroke type classification was based on a general technical model associated with an internationally shared terminology (Tepper, 2003; Molodzoff, 2008), considering as stroke categories the serve, push, flick, topspin, topspin counter topspin, block, drive, lob and smash. The serve was, however, excluded from all subsequent analyses because it has no meaning to assess the serve together with other stroke types, being that stroke used to start each rally. For each shot, the forehand/backhand execution was also analyzed.

The classification of footwork included the following categories (Malagoli Lanzoni *et al.*, 2007): one step, chassé, slide, pivot, crossover and stroke without step, i.e. when the player hits the ball without executing any additional observable footwork.

In a previous study, we observed very good intra- and inter-operator reliability of stroke and footwork types as recorded using the present methods (Malagoli Lanzoni *et al.*, 2012).

Ten male and five female matches, played between 2008 and 2010, were analyzed as available from a set of matches randomly selected for previous studies. Only one match per player was considered. The 20 male players were in the top 30 position of the world ranking (from the website www.ittf.com) when the match was played, whereas the 10 female players were among the top 20 female players. Due to the homogeneity of both the samples used, we assumed that the interaction effect due to including both the players of each match did not substantially affect the outcome of the present analyses.

The mean ± SD age, height and weight, taken from the website www.ittf.com, were 26.8 ± 4.7 years, 178.2 ± 6.9 cm, and 72.4 ± 5.8 kg for males, and 25.3 ± 4.7 years, 163.3 ± 6.3 cm, and 56.0 ± 5.0 kg for females.

The selected matches were downloaded from the websites www.ittf.com and www.ettu.org. Each match was analyzed in slow motion with the software Kinovea (www.kinovea.org), at a replay speed one fifth of the actual one (0.2X).

Data collection was carried out through a dedicated Visual Basic-based application with a panel allowing a set of data to be created in the Microsoft Excel software. For quantitative variables, the mean values of M and W were compared using Student's t tests. For categorical variables, the distributions were compared using Chi-square tests. The significance was set at $p < 0.05$.

25.3 RESULTS

A total of 15 matches (M: 10, W: 5), 73 sets (M: 50, W: 23), 1354 rallies (M: 925, W: 429), and 7481 shots (M: 4790, W: 2701) were considered. The mean number of rallies per set was similar in the two genders (M: 19 ± 2, F: 19 ± 1; $p > 0.05$). Conversely, the mean number of shots per set was higher ($p < 0.05$) in W (117 ± 18) than in M (95 ± 12). The mean number of shots per rally was also higher ($p < 0.05$) in W (6.3 ± 0.9) than in M (5.2 ± 0.6).

Chi-square tests showed significant differences (p < 0.001) between M and W in the distribution of both footwork and stroke types.

Concerning the strokes, M used most of the times the topspin (32 per cent), followed by different strokes: push (20 per cent), topspin counter topspin (19 per cent), block (17 per cent), and flick (8 per cent). In W, similarly, the topspin was the most used stroke (34 per cent). However, differently from what happened in M, the defensive block was the second most used stroke (25 per cent), followed by push (15 per cent), drive (12 per cent), and topspin counter topspin (9 per cent). For both M and W, the lob (M: 3 per cent , W: ~0 per cent) and the smash (M: 1 per cent, W: ~0 per cent) were actually unused.

A more detailed analysis can be carried out considering the backhand or forehand execution of the shots. Overall, in M, the forehand and backhand executions were, respectively, 56 per cent and 44 per cent. Conversely, female players preferred backhand shots (61 per cent) to forehand shots (39 per cent). The topspin forehand was the most used stroke in M (19 per cent), followed by the topspin counter topspin forehand (16 per cent), block backhand (14 per cent), topspin backhand (13 per cent), and push forehand (13 per cent), whereas the other strokes showed an occurrence lower than 10 per cent (Table 25.1). In W, the most used stroke was the block backhand (21 per cent) followed by topspin backhand (18 per cent), topspin forehand (16 per cent), drive backhand (12 per cent), push forehand (9 per cent), topspin counter topspin forehand (8 per cent), and push backhand (6 per cent) (Table 25.2). Figure 25.1 shows the footwork distribution in M and W. The one step was the footwork preferred by males (32 per cent of cases), whereas female players executed no footwork in 43.6 per cent of cases.

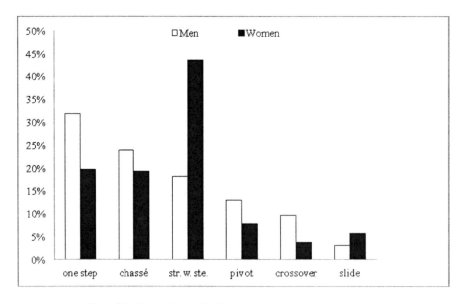

Figure 25.1 Footwork type distribution in men's and women's matches

Tables 25.1 and 25.2 display the stroke/footwork association respectively in men's and women's matches. In M, 25.5 per cent of chassé footwork was followed by a block backhand, while in 20.5 per cent of cases this footwork was used to reach the ball and execute a topspin forehand. The crossover was linked to the execution of forehand strokes in difficult conditions, namely the topspin forehand (42.3 per cent), and the topspin counter topspin forehand (35.1 per cent). The most common footwork was the one step, used especially to perform a push forehand (39.0 per cent). Concerning the pivot, it was directly linked to forehand strokes, executed from the backhand corner, namely the topspin forehand (45.6 per cent) and the topspin counter topspin forehand (42.7 per cent). The slide footwork was mostly followed by backhand strokes: block (33.1 per cent) and topspin (24.0 per cent). The stroke without step involved also backhand strokes in the majority of cases: block (36.8 per cent) and topspin (32.4 per cent).

Table 25.1 Association between strokes and footwork in men's matches

Strokes	chassé	crossover	one step	pivot	slide	str. w. ste.	overall
block backhand	25.5%	1.1%	1.0%	0.0%	33.1%	36.8%	14.3%
block forehand	4.1%	2.4%	1.1%	2.2%	9.1%	4.4%	2.9%
flick backhand	2.1%	0,0%	11.5%	0.0%	0.0%	0.3%	4.2%
flick forehand	0.5%	1.3%	10.0%	3.2%	1.7%	0.1%	3.9%
push backhand	1.0%	0.3%	20.4%	0.2%	0.0%	0.3%	6.8%
push forehand	0.3%	0.8%	39.0%	1.2%	0.0%	0.3%	12.8%
topspin backhand	15.2%	2.4%	7.3%	0,0%	24.0%	32.4%	12.9%
top c. top forehand	18.2%	35.1%	0.6%	42.7%	11.6%	11.5%	16,0%
topspin forehand	20.5%	42.3%	7.7%	45.6%	10.7%	4.7%	18.7%
other strokes	12.6%	14.3%	1.4%	4.9%	9.8%	9.2%	7.5%

Table 25.2 Association between strokes and footwork in women's matches

Strokes	chassé	crossover	one step	pivot	slide	str. w. ste.	overall
block backhand	28.7%	2.4%	0.4%	0.6%	30.8%	31.4%	21.2%
block forehand	5.0%	5.9%	0.2%	1.7%	8.5%	4.2%	3.7%
drive backhand	15.8%	2.4%	0.2%	0.0%	16.9%	18.2%	12.1%
flick backhand	0.0%	0.0%	15.4%	0.0%	0.0%	0.1%	3.1%
flick forehand	0.0%	0.0%	6.3%	0.0%	0.0%	0.1%	1.3%
push backhand	0.9%	2.4%	26.8%	0.0%	0.0%	1.8%	6.4%
push forehand	0.2%	1.2%	44.7%	1.1%	0.0%	0.1%	9.1%
topspin backhand	16.3%	1.2%	2.0%	0.0%	21.5%	30.3%	18.0%
top c. top forehand	12.8%	22.4%	0.2%	19.0%	14.6%	5.8%	8.2%
topspin forehand	18.8%	61.2%	3.6%	77.1%	6.2%	7.2%	16.2%
other strokes	1.5%	0.9%	0.2%	0.5%	1.5%	0.8%	0.7%

In W, after a chassé footwork, the most used strokes were: block backhand (28.7 per cent), topspin forehand (18.8 per cent), topspin backhand (16.3 per cent) and drive backhand (15.8 per cent). The crossover was strictly linked to forehand strokes performed in difficult situations, i.e. the topspin counter topspin (61.2 per cent) and the topspin (22.4 per cent), executed after a long displacement. As in M, the one step was the most used footwork to counter the serve. The one step was followed mostly by a push forehand (44.0 per cent) and by a push backhand (26.8 per cent). Concerning the pivot, it was strictly linked to the forehand strokes, executed from the backhand corner, namely the topspin forehand (77.1 per cent) and topspin counter topspin forehand (19.0 per cent). The slide is essentially related to backhand strokes, mainly the block (30.8 per cent) and the topspin (21.5 per cent). Finally, the stroke without step (i.e. shot executed without footwork), resulting the most used footworking technique in W, was followed mostly by a block backhand (31.4 per cent) and a topspin backhand (30.3 per cent). These combinations are the most relevant as they respectively represent 13.7 per cent and 13.2 per cent of total shots in W.

25.4 DISCUSSION

First and foremost, it is worth underlining the importance of the serve forehand and the respective response technique, often consisting of one step followed by a push forehand, as they represent two key points at the start of each rally. Indeed, it has been shown that a better serving effectiveness can strongly affect the outcome of top-level table tennis matches (Hao *et al.*, 2010).

The present results show big differences between male and female players in the use of strokes and especially of footwork during play. Overall, male players usually perform an early attack (with a topspin forehand) and continue the rally alternating a defense with a block backhand executed without a footwork, and a counter-attack, with a topspin counter topspin forehand, following a pivot or crossover footwork. The distribution of footwork types and the relationship between strokes and footwork observed in male players are similar to those reported in previous studies analyzing top-level men's matches (Malagoli Lanzoni *et al.*, 2007; 2010). The behavior of male players demonstrates an offensive and risky style of play, reflected in the use of attacking and counter-attacking shots already in the first phases of the rally, and in performing very dynamic footwork. Conversely, female players showed less dynamic footwork, often hitting the ball without any step, or performing side movements close to the table. Therefore, these observations support our hypothesis of a higher aggressiveness of male players. The stroke type distribution showed also some differences between the two categories of players, confirming the results of a previous study focused only on some selected stroke types (Otcheva and Drianovski, 2002). However, such differences observed seem less relevant than those concerning footwork types, as female players anyway adopt a rather offensive shooting style, especially with the use of backhand strokes (topspin and drive).

25.5 CONCLUSION

Notational analysis has been widely used in several racket sports, and is receiving some interest also in table tennis. Therefore, it is important to share a standard classification of the most relevant indicators in order to create a reference model for this sport. From a methodological perspective, for a complete analysis of performance, we should note that the importance of analyzing both the technical components of table tennis shots, namely the strokes and footwork, and in particular their interaction. This study has an applied interest for performance analysts, coaches and athletes, providing reference models useful to improve the technical/tactical training and the physical conditioning in the two examined categories of table tennis players. Future perspectives include the analysis of the playing style in further categories of athletes, such as junior, cadets, etc., and even in groups of players with specific play characteristics, such as left-handed athletes or defensive players.

25.6 REFERENCES

Hao, Z., Tian, Z., Hao, Y. and Song, J., 2010, Analysis on technique and tactics of Lin Ma and Hao Wang in the men's single table tennis final in the 29th Olympic Games. *International Journal of Table Tennis Sciences*, 6, pp. 74–78.
Hughes, M., 1998, The application of notational analysis to racket sports. In *Science and Racket Sports II*, edited by Reilly, T., Hughes, M.D., Lees, A. and Maynard, I. (London: E & FN Spon), pp. 211–220.
Hughes, M. and Barlett, R., 2002, The use of performance indicators in performance analysis. *Journal of Sports Sciences*, 20, pp.739–754.
Malagoli Lanzoni, I., Lobietti, R. and Merni, F., 2007, Footwork techniques used in table tennis: A qualitative analysis. In *Proceedings of the 10th ITTF Sports Science Congress*, edited by Kondric, M. and Furjan-Mandic, G. (Zagreb: University of Zagreb, Faculty of Kinesiology), pp. 401–408.
Malagoli Lanzoni, I., Lobietti, R. and Merni, F., 2010, Footwork in relationship with strokes and efficacy during the 29th Olympic Games table tennis final. *International Journal of Table Tennis Sciences*, 6, pp. 60–63.
Malagoli Lanzoni, I., Di Michele R. and Merni F., 2012, Reliability of selected performance indicators in table tennis, *International Journal of Table Tennis Sciences*, 7, pp. 62–65.
Molodzoff, P., 2008, *Advanced Coaching Manual*, Lausanne: International Table Tennis Federation.
Otcheva, G. and Drianovski, Y., 2002, Comparative analysis of the game of the finalist from the biggest international and Bulgarian table tennis competition 2000. In *Table Tennis Sciences*, edited by Yuza, N., Hiruta, S., Iimoto Y., Shibata, Y. and Harrison, J.R. (Lausanne: International Table Tennis Federation), pp. 155–166.
Tepper, G., 2003, *ITTF Level 1 Coaching Manual*, (Lausanne: International Table Tennis Federation).

CHAPTER 26

Momentum in tennis matches in Grand Slam tournaments

Peter O'Donoghue

26.1 INTRODUCTION

In physics, the momentum of an object in motion is the product of the object's mass and its velocity. An object that is already in motion requires less force to keep it moving in the same direction than a stationary object of the same mass. This has led to the term "momentum" being used in sport to represent events being influenced by preceding events. If a match is moving in a particular direction, it is likely to continue in that direction unless there is a change in momentum. The idea is that if events have been performed successfully, the player or team has momentum and this makes it more likely that subsequent events will be performed successfully than if the preceding events had not been successful. There is certainly a perception of momentum in sport with commentators frequently using the term in various sports. Tennis is no exception and commentators use the term in the majority of televised matches.

Theories have been developed based on players' perceptions of momentum including Vallerand et al.'s (1988) antecedence-consequence model, Taylor and Demick's (1994) multidimensional model and Cornelius et al.'s (1997) projected performance model. Sports science literature has used different terms for sequences of events with similar outcomes; these terms include momentum (Hughes et al., 2006), streakiness (Gould, 1989) and the "hot hand" effect (Larkey et al., 1989). The ideas of positive momentum (success breeding success) and negative momentum (failure leading to further failure) are concerned with sequences of events within sports performance. Momentum assumes that the chance of success in an event is raised if previous events have been successful. If such a force of momentum exists and is observable in actual sports performance, one would expect to see longer sequences of events of successful outcome than would be expected by chance. Consider a sports contest of 200 points between players A and B. Each point is either won by player A or by player B and we will assume each has a 0.5 chance of winning any given point. The probability of player A winning N consecutive points is 0.5^N just based on random chance. In a 200 point contest, there are $201 - N$ sequences of N points and so one would expect $(201 - N)0.5^N$ sequences of N points to have occurred by random chance. Therefore, one would expect about three sequences of six consecutive points for player A (and three for player B) within a 200 point contest through random chance. Some research in squash has concluded that momentum exists within sequences of points (Hughes et al., 2006) and perturbations (Davies et al., 2008) without comparing observed sequence lengths with what would be expected by chance. Bar Eli *et al.* (2006) surveyed research in other sports that had used appropriate statistical techniques. There is evidence for and against the existence of momentum in sports performance (Bar Eli *et al.*, 2006).

Previous notational analysis research in tennis has also provided mixed evidence as to whether sequences of points are independent of previous points (Klaassen and Magnus, 2001; O'Donoghue and Brown, 2009). Klaassen and Magnus (2001) found that winning the previous point increased the probability of winning the next point by 0.3 per cent in men's singles and 0.5 per cent in women's singles at Wimbledon (1992–5). Knight and O'Donoghue (2012) also found that players were more likely to win receiving points when they had break points than when they did not. This could suggest that good performance when receiving serve leading to break points increases the chances of breaking the opponent's serve. This can be taken as evidence in favour of the concept of momentum in tennis. However, O'Donoghue and Brown (2009) found no significant association between point outcome and previous point outcome in 26 performances of 13 men's singles matches played in 2007 Grand Slam tournaments.

Analysing momentum in terms of games in tennis is problematic due to the dominance of the serve. Therefore, the purpose of the current investigation was to analyse momentum at the set level in tennis. Previous research of four- and five-set men's singles tennis matches played at Wimbledon and the US Open found that the eventual winning player was more likely to lose sets early rather than later in a match (Jackson and Mosurski, 1997). This could be an indication of momentum in tennis performance. The data used by Jackson and Mosurski predate the 2002 introduction of surface grading and the use of Type I and Type III balls. Furthermore, women's singles matches and matches at the Australian and French Open tournaments were not included in their investigation. The current investigation examines three-set women's singles matches and four- and five-set men's singles matches played at all four Grand slam tournaments in the calendar years 2009 to 2011 inclusive.

26.2 METHODS

Completed matches from the 2009, 2010 and 2011 Grand Slam singles tournaments were included in the investigation. The criteria for inclusion also required matches to have taken three sets in women's singles and four or five sets in men's singles. Winning players always win the last set of a match and if the preceding set outcomes are independent then a chi square goodness of fit test would not find a significant difference between the distribution of matches of different set orderings and an expected uniform distribution. That is in women's singles tennis there would be just as many three-set matches where the eventual winning player lost the first set as when she lost the second set. Chi square goodness of fit tests were applied to the three-set women's singles matches, the four-set men's singles matches, the five-set men's singles matches at each individual tournament as well as overall. This analysis of men's singles matches tended to look backwards from the result of the match which does not ideally reflect the concept of momentum. Therefore, chi square goodness of fit tests were applied to men's singles matches that were in different states after the second and third sets. Any p values of less than 0.05 were deemed to be significant.

26.3 RESULTS

Table 26.1 reveals that there is evidence of momentum at the set level in men's singles with eventual winning players having lost the first set of four-set matches more than expected and eventual winning players having lost the first set or first two sets of five-set matches more than expected. In women's singles, the eventual winning player lost the first set significantly more than expected at Wimbledon.

Table 26.1 Number of completed matches of different numbers of sets in 2009, 2010 and 2011 Grand Slam singles tournaments

Gender	Sets	Aus Open	Fr Open	Wimbledon	US Open	All matches
Women 3 sets	LWW	55	61	70	61	247
	WLW	69	51	46	44	210
	χ^2_1	1.6	0.9	5.0 *	2.8	3.0
Men 4 sets	LWWW	41	40	42	36	159
	WLWW	26	47	37	35	145
	WWLW	32	17	41	28	118
	χ^2_2	3.5	14.2 ***	0.4	1.2	6.2 *
Men 5 sets	LLWWW	17	13	21	14	65
	LWLWW	12	9	10	12	43
	LWWLW	9	11	14	9	43
	WLLWW	10	11	6	12	39
	WLWLW	6	8	6	6	26
	WWLLW	12	8	17	9	46
	χ^2_5	6.2	2.0	15.0 *	4.0	18.2 **

* $p < 0.05$, ** $p < 0.01$, *** $p < 0.001$

Considering the winner of the third set in men's singles matches that were 1–1 in sets after the second set, we cannot assume an equal chance of winning the match as one player needs to win one further set before the other wins two more sets. Assuming a 0.5 chance of winning a set, the expected proportion of men's singles matches that would be won by the player with a 2–1 lead in sets is $0.5 + 0.5^2 = 0.75$. Therefore, expected frequencies of match outcomes were based on a 75:25 ratio between the player with a 2–1 lead in sets and the opponent in such matches. Overall, when a match reached 1–1 in sets, the winner of the third set went on to win the match on 373 out of 455 such matches (81.9 per cent), which was significantly greater than the expected 75 per cent of matches ($\chi^2_1 = 11.8$, p < 0.001). When a player won the first set, lost the second and then won the third, he went on to win 171 out of 214 such matches (79.9 per cent) which was not significantly greater than the expected 75 per cent of such matches ($\chi^2_1 = 2.7$, p = 0.097). However, when a player won the second and third sets having lost the first set, he won 202 out of 241 (83.8 per cent) of such matches which was significantly greater than the expected 75 per cent of such matches ($\chi^2_1 = 9.9$, p = 0.002).

26.4 DISCUSSION

Overall, the distribution of three-set matches in women's singles was not significantly different to an expected distribution of 50 per cent WLW and 50 per cent LWW. The distributions of four- and five-set men's singles matches were significantly different to the expected distributions. This agrees with the findings of Jackson and Mosurski (1997). The most frequent four-set matches were those where the eventual winner lost the first set (LWWW) and the most frequent five-set matches were where the eventual winner lost the first two sets (LLWWW). This could be an indication of shifting momentum within such matches. However, there may be many other explanations for this observation. With more matches being won by higher ranked players than lower ranked players, it could be that higher ranked players did not perform to their maximum in the first set. This could be because they under-estimated their opponent or because they wished to conceal strong elements of their game from potential opponents in future rounds of the tournament.

The only individual tournaments showing significantly different distributions to the expected uniform distributions were in the women's singles at Wimbledon, four-set men's singles at the French Open and five-set men's singles matches at Wimbledon. The shortest rallies in women's singles occur at Wimbledon (Brown and O'Donoghue, 2008) and this may help those players who come back from trailing by a set. Once the match has been levelled at 1–1 in sets, the player who won the second set may be more prepared to play a third set. Where a player had been hoping to win in two sets, losing the second set may result in a shift in momentum that may reduce motivation in the final set.

Men's singles at the French Open has the longest rallies in Grand Slam singles tennis (Brown and O'Donoghue, 2008). There were only 17 four-set matches where the losing player lost the third set. Once the player is trailing by two sets, they will require three sets to win the match in five sets. Even if they can win the match in five sets, the long rallies at the French Open may lead to fatigue and reduce their chances of winning further matches in the tournament (O'Donoghue, 2006). The two most frequent types of five-set matches at Wimbledon were the most streaky; "LLWWW" and "WWLLW". Despite the introduction of Type I and Type III balls in 2002, the serve is still more dominant at Wimbledon than at any other tournament (Brown and O'Donoghue, 2008). The fact that the opponent still needs to break serve or win a tie-breaker in the current and possibly subsequent sets may encourage players to continue competing at Wimbledon when they are trailing in sets.

There were 65 five-set men's singles matches where players won having been two sets down. This study included 118 four-set matches and 46 five-set matches where players lost the first two sets and did not come back to win. There were also three-set matches which were not included in the study where players failed to come back from being two sets behind. Investigating detailed quantitative and qualitative data from those performances where players did come back from two sets down to win in five sets is a useful area for future research.

Studies have now been done on sequences of points and sets in tennis. Further work is needed on sequences of points to adjust for the known dominance of serve in tennis. Also the observational data needs to be supported by accounts, interviews and other self-report data to contribute to theory about the mechanisms of momentum in tennis. Player rankings also need to be addressed when determining expected chances of winning matches.

26.5 REFERENCES

Bar-Eli, M., Avugos, S. and Raab, M., 2006, Twenty years of "hot hand" research: Review and critique. *Psychology of Sport and Exercise*, 7(6), pp. 525–553.

Brown, E. and O'Donoghue, P.G., 2008, Gender and surface effect on elite tennis strategy. *Coaching and Sports Science Review*, 46, pp. 9–11.

Cornelius, A., Silva III, J., Conroy, D. and Petersen, G., 1997, The projected performance model: Relating cognitive and performance antecedents of psychological momentum. *Perceptual and Motor Skills*, 84, pp. 475–85.

Davies, G., Fuller, A., Hughes, M.T., Murray, S., Hughes, M.D. and James, N., 2008, Momentum of perturbations in elite squash. In *Performance Analysis of Sport 8*, (Magdeburg, Germany: Otto-von-Guericke-Universität Magdeburg Press), pp. 77–97.

Gould, S.J., 1989, The streak of streaks. *Chance*, 2, pp. 10–16.

Hughes, M., Fenwick, B. and Murray, S., 2006, Expanding normative profiles of elite squash players using momentum of winners and errors. *International Journal of Performance Analysis Sport*, 6(1), pp. 145–154.

Jackson, D. and Mosurski, K., 1997, Heavy defeats in tennis: Psychological momentum or random effect? *Chance*, 10(2), p. 27.

Klaasen, F.J.G.M. and Magnus, J.R., 2001, Are points in tennis independent and identically distributed? Evidence from a dynamic binary panel data model. *Journal of the American Statistical Association*, 96, pp. 500–509.

Knight, G. and O'Donoghue, P.G., 2012, The probability of winning break points in Grand Slam men's singles tennis. *European Journal of Sports Science*, 12, pp. 1–7.

Larkey, P.D., Smith, R.A. and Kadane, J.B., 1989, It's OK to believe in the "hot hand". *Chance*, 2, pp. 22–30.

O'Donoghue, P.G., 2006, The advantage of playing fewer sets than the opponent in the previous two rounds of Grand Slam tennis tournaments. In *Performance Analysis of Sport 7*, edited by Dancs, H., Hughes, M. and O'Donoghue, P.G. (Cardiff, UK: CPA UWIC Press), pp. 631–635.

O'Donoghue, P.G. and Brown, E.J., 2009, Sequences of service points and the misperception of momentum in elite tennis. *International Journal of Performance Analysis in Sport*, **9**(1), pp. 113–127.

Taylor, J. and Demick, A., 1994, A multidimensional model of momentum in sport. *Journal of Applied Sport Psychology*, **6**, pp. 51–70.

Vallerand, R., Colavecchio, P. and Pelletier, L., 1988, Psychological momentum and performance inferences: A preliminary test of the antecedents-consequences psychological momentum model. *Journal of Sport and Exercise Psychology*, **10**, pp. 92–108.

Part 6

Individual Sports

CHAPTER 27

Performance analysis of show jumping strategy during British Eventing

Sophie Arundel and Lucy Holmes

27.1 INTRODUCTION

Strategy can be inferred in observational studies by considering patterns of behaviour. The selection of events performed, players involved, timing of events, the order in which events are performed and the location of those events can all indicate the strategy being adopted. The effectiveness of different strategies can be investigated by considering the success of performers adopting those strategies. The strategies of winning and losing performers within competitions can be compared. Alternatively, the strategies of performers reaching different stages of tournaments can be compared. The general aim of the current research was to investigate strategy within show jumping.

Show jumping can be conducted as an individual equestrian event or as a phase within Eventing. British Eventing is split into three elements; dressage, show jumping and cross country (Luxmoore, 2008). These three elements are split across the duration of the event; the dressage phase takes place first, establishing the initial score for the horse and rider combination (Slaughter, 2003). A horse and rider, as a combination must complete each phase. The combination that accumulates the lowest number of penalty points over the three phases is the winner (Luxmoore, 2008). Throughout the British Eventing year, points are awarded to horse and rider combinations based on the outcomes of their events solely looking at the success of the overall event. Although this information is beneficial to selection, the individual sections are also important. The different strategies involved within each segment of British Eventing have been overlooked in research (Luxmoore, 2008).

Strategy in show jumping can be inferred from the observed performance of a horse and rider combination. The path taken when completing the course and the times required for different parts of the course indicate strategic and tactical decisions that may have been taken (Hanes, 2011). Skill level is depicted by the ability of the rider to adjust the horse's stride length and the consistency of the canter strides before a fence. If the rider hurries the horse towards the fence, mistakes are more likely to occur because the preparation has been rushed (Paulson, 2012). When the horse goes slowly, it will make turns more accurately but mistakes become more evident at higher speed (Searles and Paulson, 2012).

Adjustment of speed and route within show jumping can be helpful to achieving a clear round in a relatively fast time. Gage (2005) stated that on a turn or a curving line, you can adjust the line outwards if you are reaching the fence too close and, likewise, you can take a tighter line if you are too far away from the fence. The jumps should be approached from a straight, direct approach towards the fence (Gage, 2005). Gage's assumption can be used as a means of operationalising strategy in show jumping. The number of strides within an imaginary direct straight approach to the fence indicates how soon the horse and rider turned into this direct approach path. A low number of strides in the direct approach indicates a tight turn prior to approaching the fence. A higher number of strides indicates that a longer route may have been taken from the previous fence in order to have a longer direct approach to the current fence. Cutting corners and making sharper turns can shorten the distance covered, reducing the overall time taken to complete the route (Hornsey, 2011). The speed–accuracy trade-off has been recognised in sport in general (Wrisberg, 2007). A simple variable such as number of strides within the direct approach to a fence allows an accuracy–time trade-off in show jumping to be investigated.

The effectiveness of any strategy can be evaluated using outcome indicators relating to the success of performances. A successful outcome is the completion of the show jumping course incurring zero penalties of either time or jumping faults. This is called a clear round (Hanlon, 2009). The aim of the present study was to compare the strategies of rider–horse combinations that achieve clear rounds with those that don't. Riding time between fences and the number of strides taken directly towards fences are used as indicators of strategy.

27.2 METHOD

27.2.1 Participants

Seventy-six (n=76) competitors aged 19 to 52 were recorded whilst competing on an international show-jumping course of 14 fences. The participants were in the advanced class which is restricted to qualification of previous levels and horses were restricted to those over the age of 7 years. All media rights are reserved through British Eventing and so consent was requested and granted to record and analyse the competition.

27.2.2 Data gathering

Two cameras (Sony HDR-HC9E, Sony Corporation, Tokyo, Japan) were used to film the competitors. One camera was used to film one combination fence (the triple) which has three elements, each element has a related distance of either one, two or three strides. The second camera was used to follow the competitor around the entire course of jumps. An analysis system was implemented in Sportscode (Sportstec, Warriewood, New South Wales, Australia). The approach taken to each fence was represented by the number of strides within a direct route +5° to the part of the fence the horse–rider jumped over. Figure 27.1 shows this area. Low values for strides in this area would indicate a tighter approach path than higher values for strides.

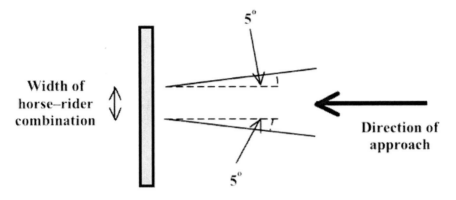

Figure 27.1 Competitors' ideal approach

Sportscode was also used to record timings for each participant. Ground time was defined as the time between the fences from when the back feet have landed on the ground after the previous fence to when the front feet leave the ground at the take-off for the current fence. Flight time was defined as the time over the fences, from when the front feet leave the ground at take-off at the fence to when the back feet touch the ground after the fence. The footage captured into Sportscode allowed the movements to be slowed down, paused and replayed to improve the accuracy of the timings and stride counts recorded.

27.2.3 Reliability

Intra-operator agreement tests were used to assess the reliability of the operator who analysed five of the competitors on two separate occasions four weeks apart. The weighted Kappa value for strides taken within a direct approach to the fences was 0.727 indicating a good strength of agreement. Mean absolute error for ground times between fences was 0.18s which was deemed sufficiently reliable for the purpose of the current investigation.

27.2.4 Data analysis

There were 27 of the competitors who achieved clear rounds and the remaining 49 did not. The number of strides taken within a direct approach had a restricted set of values (1 to 6) and 5 of the 14 ground times prior to fences failed to satisfy the Kolmogorov-Smirnov test of normality ($p < 0.05$). The ground times prior to fences and number of strides taken within a direct approach to each fence were, therefore, compared using a series of Mann-Whitney U tests to compare the 27 competitors with clear rounds with the remaining 49 competitors.

27.3 RESULTS

Table 27.1 shows the ground time that preceded each fence. Only the approach to the 14th fence showed a significantly different ground between horse-rider pairs that achieved a clear round and those that didn't ($p = 0.015$). The remaining timings are almost identical between the two groups with those achieving clear rounds starting 0.2s slower in total for the first three fences and not making this time up until the final fence when they are 0.3s ahead overall.

Table 27.1 Ground times prior to each fence (s)

Fence	Faults	Clear round (n = 27)	Non-clear round (n = 49)
1 ^	1	7.4 ± 1.0	7.3 ± 1.0
2 ^	6	8.1 ± 0.7	8.2 ± 0.8
3	4	4.5 ± 0.3	4.4 ± 0.3
4 ^	6	8.3 ± 0.5	8.3 ± 0.6
5	5	0.5 ± 0.1	0.5 ± 0.1
6 ^	6	3.5 ± 0.3	3.5 ± 0.4
7 ^	14	8.0 ± 1.3	8.0 ± 1.1
8 ^	8	4.7 ± 0.4	4.7 ± 0.4
9	5	2.6 ± 0.2	2.6 ± 0.2
10 ^	16	9.6 ± 0.6	9.7 ± 0.7
11	6	0.5 ± 0.1	0.5 ± 0.1
12	6	0.9 ± 0.1	0.9 ± 0.1
13	7	3.2 ± 0.3	3.2 ± 0.2
14	5	6.1 ± 0.4	6.5 ± 0.6

^ Fence is taken on a turn

Table 27.2 Number of competitors taking different numbers of strides (one to six) within the direct approach to fences (bold figures are group medians)

Fence	Clear round (n=27)						Not clear round (n=49)						Mann-Whitney U test
	1	2	3	4	5	6	1	2	3	4	5	6	
1	1	7	**18**	1	0	0	0	0	10	**31**	8	0	115.5***
2	1	2	7	**16**	1	0	3	12	**34**	0	0	0	246.5***
4	0	2	10	**15**	0	0	0	9	**40**	0	0	0	289.0***
6	0	1	3	**22**	1	0	1	11	**33**	4	0	0	148.0***
7	1	2	3	4	**8**	9	1	7	**25**	16	0	0	255.0***
8	0	0	1	**21**	5	0	0	0	23	**26**	0	0	310.5***
10	0	0	8	**17**	2	0	0	1	**35**	13	0	0	354.5***

*** Significant difference between competitors with clear rounds and other competitors ($p < 0.001$)

Table 27.2 shows that there were significant differences between the two groups of competitors for all seven of the fences that were taken on a turn (p < 0.001). The competitors with clear rounds had a median number of strides within a direct approach that was greater than that of the unsuccessful competitors for six of these seven fences. It was only the first fence where the competitors with clear rounds had a median of three strides compared to four strides taken by other competitors that differed from this pattern.

27.4 DISCUSSION

A strength of the current approach is that the strategy of horse and rider pairs achieving clear rounds has been compared with pairings that failed to do so. Therefore, the strategy of the unsuccessful horse–rider combinations has included fences that were cleared. There was a total of 95 observed faults over 49 unsuccessful rounds of the 14-fence course. This means that 86.2 per cent of the fences attempted by the 49 unsuccessful horse–rider combinations were successfully cleared and that the data can be taken as indicative of their strategy rather than as a consequence of technical faults. There are three main results to be discussed; (a) the similar timings between the two groups of performers, (b) the optimal strategy of the successful horse–rider combinations and (c) the individual fence strategy of the successful horse–rider combinations.

The current investigation did not find a speed–accuracy trade-off, as the timings between the two groups of performers are very similar. One explanation for the similarity in timings is that the horse–rider combinations were all of a similar high of ability, having qualified to compete in this advanced class show jumping event. Similar speeds may also be used in order to reach fences avoiding fatigue and loss of rhythm. A theory suggested by many trainers is that too fast a speed can alter the balance and rhythm of the horse, increasing the likelihood of the horse jumping 'flatly' and increasing the chance of knocking down fences (Bayley and Bowen, 2005). A further consideration is the limitation that this show jumping competition was considered in isolation from the dressage and cross-country sections of the overall equestrian event. Some horse–rider combinations may have incurred time faults during other stages requiring them to risk faults at fences during the show jumping section in order to attempt a time that would give them a higher placing in the overall equestrian event. Other horse–rider combinations could perform the show jumping course more carefully if they know opponents have already incurred time faults in other disciplines. A strong strategy is needed in all three elements of the equestrian event (Orne, 2006). A further limitation of the current investigation that may have influenced timings is the order in which horse–rider combinations compete. Competitors in the second half of the show jumping schedule may hold an advantage by being able to watch opponents, identifying where problem areas may exist in the course and revising strategy to ensure their round avoids the mistakes made by others (Copelan, 2002).

The horse–rider combinations who achieved clear rounds took more strides within the direct approach to fences 2, 4, 6, 7, 8 and 10 than those who made faults during their rounds. This suggests that the successful performers are taking a longer route with a more shallow turn into the approach to these fences, allowing a greater number of strides made directly towards the fence. This is evidence of an optimal strategy where the route is not too short with tight turns and short approaches, and not too long risking a slow overall round time. The greater number of strides made directly towards fences may improve the equality of stride length 'collecting' the horse up before take-off allowing a cleaner jump to be made (Pilliner *et al.*, 2002). Gage (2005) suggested that successful outcomes are increased when performers extend the strides made within the approach to the fence.

The unsuccessful performers had a median and mode of three strides within the direct approach to fences 2 (69.4 per cent of these 49 horse–rider combinations), 4 (81.6 per cent), 6 (67.3 per cent), 7 (51.0 per cent) and 10 (71.4 per cent), with a sizeable minority taking three strides in the direct approach to fence 8 (46.9 per cent). The 27 performers who achieved clear rounds showed much greater variability in performance, especially at fences 4, 7 and 10. This is evidence that these performers may have developed strategies for the course with different approaches being planned to different fences. For example 17 of the 27 successful performers entered the direct approach to fence 7 when they were five or six strides away from the fence.

The greater within-fence variability within this group of successful performers, especially at fences 2, 4, 7 and 10 is evidence that strategies may have been adopted that accounted for specific strengths and weaknesses of the particular horse–rider combinations. The horse's natural ability needs to be considered (Bayley and Bowen, 2005) including factors such as conformation, balance, temperament, strength, stamina, agility, partnership development, trust, confidence and responsiveness (McBane, 2006; Blanchard, 2008).

27.5 REFERENCES

Bayley, L. and Bowen, J., 2005, *The Photographic Guide to Jumping*, (Cincinnati, OH: F&W Publications Inc).

Blanchard, S., 2008, *Jump for Joy: Positive Coaching for Horse and Rider*, (Secaucus, NJ: Wiley Publishing Inc).

Copelan, S.M., 2002, Show strategies: Get ready for your championship show – or any big event – with these seven winning strategies from top trainers Steve and Andrea Archer. *Horse and Rider*, 41(8), pp 44–46.

Gage, R., 2005, Find the distance through a turn. *Practical Horseman*, 33(1), p. 66.

Hanes, T., 2011, Chasing the elusive clear round. *Horsesport*, 44(6), p. 58.

Hanlon, T.W., 2009, *The Sports Rule Book; Essential Rules, Terms and Procedures for 54 Sports, 3rd edn*, (Champaign, IL: Human Kinetics).

Hornsey, D., 2011, *Race and Track Day Driving Techniques*, (Poundbury, Dorchester, UK: Veloce Publishing Ltd).

Luxmoore, K., 2008, *Introduction to Equestrian Sports*, (Oxford, UK: Land Links Press).

McBane, S., 2006, *100 Ways to Improve Your Horse's Schooling*, (Newton Abbott, UK: David and Charles limited).

Orne, C., 2006, *Celebrity Jumping Exercises*, (Cincinnati, OH: F&W Publications Inc).

Paulson, J., 2012, How not to lose. *Horse and Rider*, **52**(2), p. 30.

Pillinar, S., Elmhurst, S. and Davies, Z. (2002), *The Horse in Motion: The Anatomy of Equine Locomotion*, (Chichester, UK: John Wiley and Sons).

Searles, D. and Paulson, J., 2012, Four-pole training. *Horse and Rider*, **51**(1), p. 2.

Slaughter, J.R., 2003, *The Woman Equestrian*, (Terra Haute, IN: Wish Publishing).

Wrisberg, C.A., 2007, *Sport Skill Instruction for Coaches*, (Champaign, IL: Human Kinetics).

CHAPTER 28

Errors in judging
Olympic boxing performance:
False negative or false positive?

Umberto Di Felice and Samuele Marcora

28.1 INTRODUCTION

In the modern era of the Olympic Games, boxing became an official sport in 1904, during the IIIrd summer Olympic Games, in St Louis, USA (www.aiba.org). Rules, weight categories and the duration of a boxing contest have changed during the last century, and in particular, there has been a change in the assessment of performance. Initially, verdicts were given by means of a scorecard that reported a subjective decision made by judges at the end of each round; in brief, judges gave an overall opinion on boxer's fighting performance (e.g., technique, tactic, strategy, style, number of hits, etc.) purely based on their expertise. A final decision of the contest's winner was then provided.

During the Games of the XXIVth Olympiad (Seoul, 1988), boxing had controversial verdicts (Alfano, 1988) such that AIBA (International Boxing Association) decided to adopt a new method for assessing boxing performance. In 1989, AIBA replaced the scorecard with the electronic scoring machine system method (SMS). By means of a combination of five judges and one automated system, the SMS was the first attempt to improve the objectivity of the verdicts, by counting the number of valid correct hits. In Beijing 2008, SMS was used for electing the contest's winner; verdicts were based on the total number of valid scoring points assigned by means of a keyboard to a correct hit by at least three out of five judges in 1 s of time (rule 11 in AIBA, 2008). Coaches were able to see immediately each assigned valid correct hit.

Despite this automated approach, SMS is prone to error because it is based on quick human observation under pressure as often shown by non-unanimous judges' decision; moreover, judges' personal biases (e.g., emotional affect toward one boxer) need to be considered (Hagemann et al., 2008; Balmer et al., 2005; Hughes and Franks, 2004).

In an attempt to propose an alternative judgement method, Coalter et al. (1998) have compared the SMS and an alternative scoring method (judge pair), with scoring based on post-contest video analysis by means of a computer analysis system, using frame-by-frame mode (boxing match analysis, BMA). Results did not support the adoption of the alternative scoring method (judge pair). Interestingly, compared to BMA, SMS failed to assign 45.6 per cent of valid scoring points by at least one out of five judges. This finding suggests that judges make considerable errors in judging boxing performance.

The purpose of the current investigation is to identify the nature of the errors that occur in judging Olympic boxing performance by means of SMS. Errors are defined as false positive or false negative. False positive is the incorrect hit that is assigned as valid scoring point. False negative is the correct hit that is not assigned to a valid scoring point. Valid scoring points were established by BMA.

28.2 METHODS

28.2.1 Sample

For the purpose of this study, we considered 10 boxing bouts ($N = 10$) performed during the XXIXth Olympiad, 2008 Beijing. These bouts are representative of all the phases of the tournament (e.g., final, semi-final, quarter-final, etc.) of five different weight categories: 51, 60, 64, 91 and +91 kg. The number (N) of bouts for each weight category is 3, 2, 1, 3 and 1, respectively. Bout duration is four rounds of 2 minutes each, with 1 minute recovery between rounds (rule 8 in AIBA, 2008). Scored points in real time using SMS, and verdicts were obtained from video footages of these bouts.

28.2.2 Boxing match analysis

One trained operator (sports scientist with past experience in competitive boxing), analysed video footages of these bouts from TV coverage (25 frame.s^{-1}). Notational analysis was performed by means of a boxing-specific performance analysis software (DFAnalysis, Umberto Di Felice, Italy), which allows quanti-qualitative analysis of technical-tactical-strategic aspects of boxing performance (www.dfanalysis.com). Video analysis modes were replay, slow motion and frame-by-frame. BMA of each bout (analysis time 11 ± 3 hours) was performed hit-by-hit for both boxers (red and blue) in order to establish valid scoring points according to AIBA (2008) guidelines (rule 11).

28.2.3 Data analysis

Four different scores were considered: SMS, false positive, false negative and BMA. SMS is the sum of hits assigned to both boxers as valid scoring points by SMS in the official verdict. False positive is the sum of incorrect hits that are scored as valid scoring points by the SMS method. False negative is the sum of correct hits that are not scored as valid scoring points by SMS. BMA is the sum of hits assigned, to both boxers, as valid scoring points by BMA method.

Data are presented as mean $\pm$ SD, unless stated otherwise. A paired 2-tailed *t*-test was used to test the difference between BMA and SMS.

28.3 RESULTS

The four scores are presented in Figure 28.1. BMA score was revealed to be significantly greater than SMS ($P < 0.01$). False positives and false negatives as percentages of SMS are 45.9 per cent and 152.3 per cent, respectively. False negative are 73.8 per cent of BMA score.

A comparison between SMS and BMA that looks at the verdict of the round and winner of the bout shows that 16/40 verdict of the round and 2/10 winners of the bouts are different in BMA when compared with SMS (Table 28.1).

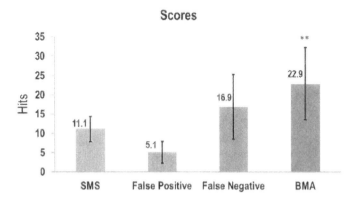

Figure 28.1 The figure shows four scores. Histograms are mean values and error bars are standard deviation. **$P < 0.01$ BMA is significantly greater than SMS

Table 28.1 Verdicts of the round and winners of the bout. Table shows the individual verdict of the round and winner of the bout, by means of the 2 methods: Scoring Machine System [a]; SMS] in comparison (vs) with Boxing Match Analysis [a]; BMA]. Verdict of the round refers to 4 rounds (1, 2, 3 and 4) of the bout. Each round gives 3 possible verdicts (R-D-B): R (Red boxer is the winner of the round), D (Draw between boxers: red corner and blue corner) and B (Blue boxer is the winner of the round). Winner of the bout indicates the boxer awarded as winner of the contest. Filled-grey box indicates that verdicts of the round and winners of the bout are different in BMA when compared with SMS. 16/40 verdicts of the round and 2/10 winners of the bout are different in BMA when compared with SMS.

a)	Scoring Machine System					vs	b)	Boxing Match Analysis				
	SMS							BMA				
	Verdict of the round (R-D-B)				Winner of the bout			Verdict of the round (R-D-B)				Winner of the bout
N	1	2	3	4			*N*	1	2	3	4	
1	B	D	B	B	B		1	R	D	B	B	B
2	B	B	B	R	B		2	B	D	B	R	B
3	R	B	D	R	B		3	D	B	R	R	B
4	B	B	B	B	B		4	B	B	B	B	B
5	B	B	R	B	B		5	R	R	R	R	R
6	B	R	B	B	B		6	B	B	B	B	B
7	R	B	D	R	R		7	R	B	R	R	R
8	B	B	B	D	B		8	D	B	B	R	B
9	R	R	D	R	R		9	R	D	B	R	B
10	B	B	B	B	B		10	B	R	B	R	R

28.4 DISCUSSION

The purpose of the current investigation was to identify the nature of the errors that occur in judging Olympic boxing performance by means of SMS defined as false positive or false negative. The most important type of error made by SMS is to miss the valid scoring points as shown by the considerable number of false negatives (16.9 ± 8.4).

28.4.1 Comparison of findings with previous research

Our results are in agreement with the Coalter *et al.* (1998) study in identifying the same kind of error: false negatives. The magnitude of false negative on the final verdict is lower in our study than Coalter *et al.* (1998); they identified 75.0 ± 35.3 scoring punches [corresponding to our valid scoring points (22.9 ± 9.3)] in their *correct solutions* analysis (corresponding to BMA), and 20.7 ± 10.3 scoring punches in the *current* approach [corresponding to SMS (11.1 ± 3.3)]. The differences between the two studies [our study vs. Coalter *et al.* (1998)] might be due to three aspects: the first is the sample size (10 vs. 6), the second is the level of performance (Olympic vs. Ulster championships), the third is the judges' skill level in detecting valid scoring points. The latter, we assume enhanced over a period of 10 years (2008 vs. 1998).

Additionally, we should consider the improvement in technical-tactical-strategic profile of boxing performance, which combined with new training methods, technologies and materials, might have further affected the discussed results.

28.4.2 Potential causes of false negatives

Potential causes of false negatives are the following:

- Rapidity of fighting action
- High hit frequencies (number of hits/s)
- Hit impact duration on target ~0.040 s
- Hit acoustic noise as result of the impact on the target
- Judges' non-optimal view due to their position around the ring
- Decrease of judges' attentive level due to mental fatigue
- Judges' focus on one boxer
- Natural (subjective) observation's biases, e.g.:
  - red colour influences the judge's decision on awarding the valid scoring point (Hagemann *et al.*, 2008),
  - emotional affect toward one athlete (Hughes and Franks, 2004),
  - influence to be a "home" or "host" boxer (Balmer *et al.*, 2005),
  - low boxer's rank position,
  - Pygmalion effect (Aronson, 2002),
  - Stigmatisation effect.

Future studies should investigate which of these factors have the most significant influence on judges' errors.

Additionally, we should not underestimate the influence of false positive and false negatives on boxers' behaviour during the match. In fact, during the Olympic Games of Beijing 2008, boxers were made aware of the scoring during the match.

28.4.3 Judges' education programmes

The need to improve judges' ability to assign valid scoring points is further emphasised by our finding that 16/40 verdicts of the round and 2/10 winners of the bout would have had a different outcome (Table 28.1). Judges' education programmes should be considered in order to reduce the magnitude of errors that occur in judging Olympic boxing performance, by enhancing the judges' valid scoring point detection skill. Judges could enhance their performance by means of computer simulation training. Specifically, by means of a video feedback, it is possible to observe patterns for which false negatives (e.g., valid scoring points that are not assigned because biased by the boxer's rank position) and false positives (e.g., valid scoring points given to incorrect hits such as those landed with the inside of the glove or to those that are accompanied by a higher acoustic noise) are characterised. The possibility to perform unlimited recalls of the events that occurred during a match offered by the frame-by-frame mode allows to develop a deeper comprehension of the characterising phases of the "valid scoring point", before, during and after its occurrence.

In conclusion, adoption of SMS in 1989 has been a step forward in the direction of a more objective assessment of boxing performance. Based on the present findings, the SMS method may be improved further by improving judges' ability to avoid false negatives. This goal may be reached by developing judges' education programmes which may include BMA as a reference.

28.4.4 Future perspectives

In the future, there might be two ways to explore, in order to enhance the judgement of Olympic boxing bouts with a more systematic and objective approach.

For the first way, BMA should replace SMS. With a technologically organised team of judges highly skilled in detecting valid scoring points by mean of BMA, the verdict will be delayed a few minutes after the end of the contest. (The time will depend on the number of judge-operators. It is hypothesised that it should be possible to provide a verdict within 20 minutes with a team of 9 judge-operators.) In this scenario, the BMA method must reduce the magnitude of errors and, hence, improve the accuracy of the verdict.

The second way would be to award more points to a single valid scoring point, which has been performed according to a higher level of fighting skill (e.g., 2 points for a valid scoring point that has been intentionally prepared to be landed in attack or different points accordingly to the types of punch: tactical, with accent and powerful). This additional qualitative evaluation of the boxing contest will lead coaches and boxers to develop punch-combinations that allow a higher score.

Further research is required to investigate whether these proposals (introduction of BMA and different points to be awarded to a single valid scoring point) obtain a higher accuracy and fairness of the verdicts, with enhanced quality of technical tactical-strategic boxing skills

28.5 ACKNOWLEDGEMENTS

I wish to thank the following persons that have made it possible to produce this final manuscript. First, the Boxing Analysis Research Team (Alberto Di Felice BSc, Mr Giuseppe Antonini, Luca Berardinelli PhD, Alessia Di Matteo MSc and Ilario Di Felice MSc) for the informatic support and team work. Second, the funders of this research project, the "Italian Boxing Federation" (Federazione Pugilistica Italiana, www.fpi.it), in particular: Chair Cav. Franco Falcinelli and Professor Massimo Scioti. Lastly, Rosella Cardigno Colonna PhD and Giovanni d'Avossa MD, for their support.

28.6 REFERENCES

Alfano, P., 1988, The Seoul Olympics: Boxing ends in controversy. *Special to the New York Times.*

Aronson, J.M., 2002, *Improving Academic Achievement: Impact of Psychological Factors on Education*, (Academic press, Elsevier Science, USA) chapter 2.

AIBA International Boxing Association, 2008, *Technical and Competition Rules.* (www.aiba.org, June 2008).

Balmer, N.J., Nevill, A.M. and Lane, A.M., 2005, Do judges enhance home advantage in European championship boxing? *Journal of Sports Sciences*, **23**(4), pp. 409–416.

Coalter, A., Ingham, B., McCrory, P., O'Donoghue, P. and Scott, M., 1998, A comparison of alternative operation schemes for the computerized scoring system for amateur boxing. *Journal of Sports Sciences*, **16**, pp. 16–17.

Hagemann, N., Strauss, B. and Leissing. J., 2008, When the referee sees red.... *Psychological Science*, **19**(8), pp. 769–771.

Hughes, M.D. and Franks, L.M., 2004, *Notational Analysis of Sport.* (New York, NY: Routledge).

CHAPTER 29

Analysing individual performance in golf using the ISOPAR method

Michael Stöckl, Peter F. Lamb and Martin Lames

29.1 INTRODUCTION

Classical performance analysis in golf usually relies on statistical performance indicators. Most of these indicators are defined by classifying shots with respect to the distance to the hole (James, 2007). Performance indicators such as driving distance, approach shot accuracy or putting average are commonly used for performance analysis in golf (James and Rees, 2008) but ignore most of the factors which make up the difficulty of a shot. They do not take into account environmental influences like the ball lie, break or slope in putting, and compare shots within certain classes which are not comparable. Furthermore, most of these performance indicators each represent more than one ability. For example, putting is a composite measure of several abilities since the starting position of the first putt is determined by the approach shot. Hence, players who are able to perform approach shots well give themselves easier putts. Moreover, the starting location of the approach shot is determined by its previous shot. Thus, putting average is a composite measure of several abilities.

The lack of performance indicators for individual shots leads us to the development of the ISOPAR method (Stöckl et al., 2011) alongside two other groups developing similar performance indicators (Broadie, 2012; Fearing et al. 2011). Whereas the approaches of Fearing et al. (2011) and Broadie (2012) are statistical and are based on distance (Broadie, 2012 also includes a classification of the ball lie), the ISOPAR method indirectly considers all factors which influence the performance of a golfer (Stöckl et al., 2012). The ISOPAR method provides a) visualisation of unique areas on a golf hole and b) a measure of performance for individual shots, *Shots Saved*. The performance indicator Shots Saved describes the quality of a shot with respect to the field's performance by the difference between the difficulty of its starting location and the difficulty of its finishing location. Additionally, Shots Saved describes the shot's contribution to the overall performance of a player.

In this study, we analysed PGA Tour ShotLink™ data measured during tournaments in 2011 using the ISOPAR method focusing on the THE PLAYERS Championship. Based on the stability findings of Scheid (1990) we studied the stability of individual players' performance with respect to different shot types.

Scheid revealed that a player's hole score or round score is not affected by his/her performance on the previous hole(s) or by holes performance in the previous round(s). Using the performance indicator Shots Saved we investigated the stability of individual players' performance for example, whether driving performance was stable throughout the four rounds of THE PLAYERS Championship. Furthermore, we analysed whether golfers with certain playing characteristics might have an advantage playing at TPC Sawgrass – the site of THE PLAYERS Championship.

29.2 METHODS

ISOPAR values and ISOPAR maps are calculated using information about shots. This information needs to contain the location from where a shot was taken and the number of remaining shots until the ball was holed from this location. In this study we used data from the PGA Tour ShotLink™ database. This database contains information on every shot taken during all PGA Tour tournaments since 2003 (except majors and match-play events). We calculated ISOPAR values and ISOPAR maps for 2,754 holes played in 153 rounds based on data of 1,009,362 measured shots from 38 PGA Tour tournaments in 2011.

The calculation of ISOPAR values and ISOPAR maps is realised in three and four steps respectively. The algorithm of the ISOPAR method was programmed with MATLAB 2011b using built-in MATLAB procedures for many of the steps. More details of the method are given in Stöckl *et al.* (2011) and Stöckl *et al.* (2012). For this reason only a summary of the different steps is provided:

1 A two-dimensional grid is assigned to the hole. In this study a mesh size of 2 inches was used.
2 At the grid nodes ISOPAR values are calculated using an exponential smoothing algorithm (Hamilton, 1994). In this study a smoothing parameter of 0.17 was used.
3 Based on the ISOPAR values from the previous step a three-dimensional, continuous ISOPAR surface is generated through a cubic spline interpolation (Fahrmeir *et al.*, 2009).
4 Using the continuous ISOPAR values so-called *iso*-lines are calculated for certain levels of performance. In this study we calculated *iso*-lines at 0.2 intervals.

Furthermore, the ISOPAR method allows a description of the quality of a player's performance using the performance indicator Shots Saved. Shots Saved describes the quality of a shot with respect to the performance of the field and the contribution of each shot to the overall performance of a player (Stöckl *et al.*, 2012). For the different analyses in this study we looked at the performance of five different shot types identified by ShotLink™: drives, long approach shots, short approach shots, around the green shots, and putts.

29.3 RESULTS AND DISCUSSION

In this section we focused our analyses on one tournament, THE PLAYERS Championship in 2011. First, we analysed an ISOPAR map of the famous island green 17th hole at TPC Sawgrass. Second, we studied individual players' performance with respect to different shot types.

29.3.1 The island green at TPC Sawgrass

We analysed an ISOPAR map of the famous island green at TPC Sawgrass (see Figure 29.1). The island green 17th is a par three, which typically plays between 130 and 140 m. The green is divided up into three different areas; there is a tier each at the right (section C in Figure 29.1) and the left of the green (section A in Figure 29.1) which are located slightly lower than the middle tier (section B in Figure 29.1). *iso*-lines represent areas of equal number of remaining shots until the ball was holed. Similar to isobar maps, from where the method gets its name, closely packed *iso*-lines represent larger change in difficulty and spread-out *iso*-lines represent less change in difficulty (Lamb *et al.*, 2011; Stöckl *et al.*, 2012).

In round four of THE PLAYERS Championship the pin was located on the lower right tier of the green (section C in Figure 29.1). The *iso*-lines are not circularly shaped around the hole which indicates that difficulty did not increase equally as distance from the hole increased. In contrast, classical performance analysis supposes difficulty being equally distributed around the hole and increasing equally as the distance to the hole increases (see Fearing *et al.*, 2011; James, 2007). Furthermore, the density of the *iso*-lines shows the change in difficulty from tier to tier. The pack of *iso*-lines $iso_{1.6}$, $iso_{1.8}$ and $iso_{2.0}$ roughly illustrates the gradient between the right tier and the middle tier. The left tier was also separated from the middle tier by an *iso*-line, the $iso_{2.2}$.

On the middle tier there are two interesting areas from which the shot difficulty differed – the area within the closed $iso_{2.0}$ (section D in Figure 29.1), from where the field took fewer than 2.0 strokes, and the area within the closed $iso_{2.2}$ (section E in Figure 29.1), from where the field took more than 2.2 strokes. From the area within the $iso_{2.0}$ players faced nearly a straight downhill putt and some of them were even able to make their putts from there. From the area within the $iso_{2.2}$ players had to deal with break and therefore find the right speed so that the ball reached the fall line leading to the hole. These putts were more difficult to play, shown by the higher ISOPAR values. Therefore, from this area within the $iso_{2.2}$ some players needed three putts to hole out.

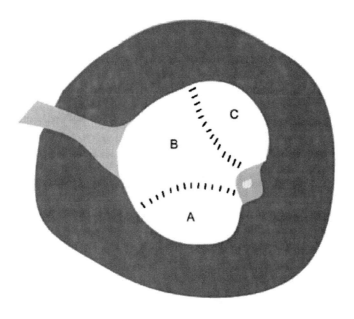

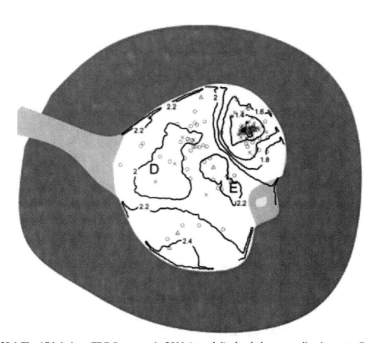

Figure 29.1 The 17th hole at TPC Sawgrass in 2011 (round 4); the dark surrounding is water. On the left panel three distinct changes in elevation (shown by hashed lines) divide the green into sections A, B and C. On the right, the *iso*-lines and ball locations (X – 1 putt, circle – 2 putt, triangle 3 putt) are superimposed on the green. D and E represent putts of different difficulty although the distance is similar

29.3.2 Analysing individual players' performance

First, we analysed whether THE PLAYERS Championship, which always takes place at TPC Sawgrass, favours certain characteristics of play. To answer this question we calculated Spearman rank correlations between players' tournament ranks and players' performance ranks in the different shot types (see Table 29.1). To be able to find out whether these findings are unique to THE PLAYERS Championship we calculated Spearman rank correlations between players' money per event ranks in 2011, which we used to represent average performance throughout the year, and players' average performance ranks for the different shot types in 2011 (see Table 29.1). The correlation coefficients for THE PLAYERS and the average of 2011 are quite similar. There are only small differences in correlations for two shot types: around the green shots ($\rho = .10$ at THE PLAYERS and $\rho = .27$ in 2011) and putting ($\rho = .34$ at THE PLAYERS and $\rho = .22$ in 2011).

Table 29.1 Spearman rank correlations between players' performance in different shot types and players' performance at THE PLAYERS Championship and players' average performance in 2011, represented by the PGA Tour's money per event ranking, respectively

	Drives	Long approach shots	Short approach shots	Around the green shots	Putts
THE PLAYERS	.57	.42	.22	.10	.34
Money per event (2011)	.61	.46	.29	.27	.22

Furthermore, the correlations in Table 29.1 reveal that the performance in the long game (drives, long approach shots) influences overall performance more than the performance in the short game (short approach shots, around the green shots, and putts). Similarly, Broadie (2008) also reported that for prototypical professional golfers, long game shots contributed more to overall performance than short game shots.

Second, we analysed players' performance at THE PLAYERS compared to their average performance in 2011 and eventually compared their performance of different rounds at THE PLAYERS. Table 29.2 shows the performance of the top three of THE PLAYERS with respect to the different shot types. Choi and Toms, who had to play a playoff to determine the winner, show different characteristics of play. Accordingly, Choi had roughly an average long game but performed well in the short game, especially putting where he saved 1.890 shots per round with respect to the average performance of the field. Toms had a very good long game where he picked up about 1.8 strokes per round by driving and long approach shots on the average of the field. Compared to their average performance in 2011 the top three performed better in nearly all shot types. Of course, this is not surprising since THE PLAYERS Championship was one of their best performances of the season.

Table 29.2 Shots Saved values per round for the different shot types of the top three at THE PLAYERS Championship including their Shots Saved values per round in 2011

Player	Tournament or year	Drives	Long approach shots	Short approach shots	Around the green	Putts
Choi	PLAYERS	0.173	−0.162	0.403	0.379	1.890
	2011	−0.078	0.200	0.111	0.233	0.139
Toms	PLAYERS	1.086	0.775	0.042	0.315	0.545
	2011	0.005	0.147	0.021	0.114	0.369
Goydos	PLAYERS	1.060	0.494	0.161	0.663	0.052
	2011	−0.407	−0.046	0.219	−0.103	−0.527

Table 29.3 shows each Choi's performance, winner of the tournament, and Donald's performance, who was ranked as the world's best golfer for several weeks in 2011, in the four rounds of THE PLAYERS. The pattern of both players' performance illustrates unstable performance from round to round in all shot types. So, players do not only perform unstably from round to round (Scheid, 1990), but also perform differently in these five different shot types from round to round.

Table 29.3 Sum of Shots Saved for the different shot types of Choi, the winner, and Donald

Player	Round	Drives	Long approach shots	Short approach shots	Around the green	Putts
Choi	1	0.012	1.148	0.259	−0.807	1.264
	2	−0.002	−0.082	0.014	−0.012	4.123
	3	0.371	−1.133	1.145	1.062	2.265
	4	0.311	−0.580	0.192	1.271	−0.093
Donald	1	0.313	−0.376	NA	−0.781	2.857
	2	0.501	1.006	0.105	0.704	0.685
	3	0.955	−0.738	0.313	0.113	−0.202
	4	−1.215	2.161	−0.039	−0.081	−1.914

29.4 CONCLUSION

In this study we have applied the ISOPAR method to performance analysis of the PGA Tour. THE PLAYERS Championship was shown to slightly favour good short game performance compared to the rest of the tournaments in 2011. Analysis of individual players revealed that the top finishers at THE PLAYERS Championship had contrasting strengths and weaknesses. This suggests that there is not a prerequisite style of play to perform well at TPC at Sawgrass.

29.5 ACKNOWLEDGEMENTS

The authors would like to thank the PGA Tour for providing access to the ShotLink™ database. We also would like to thank our colleague Malte Siegle for helpful discussions and comments.

29.6 REFERENCES

Broadie, M., 2008, Assessing golfer performance using Golfmetrics. In *Science and Golf V: Proceedings of the 2008 World Scientific Congress of Golf*, edited by Crews, D. and Lutz, R. (Mesa: Energy and Motion, Inc), pp. 253–262.
Broadie, M., 2012, Assessing golfer performance on the PGA TOUR. *Interfaces,* **42**(2), pp. 146–165.
Fahrmeir, L., Kneib, T. and Lang, S., 2009, *Regression*, (Berlin: Springer).
Fearing, D., Acimovic, J. and Graves, S., 2011, How to catch a Tiger: Understanding putting performance on the PGA Tour. *Journal of Quantitative Analysis in Sport*, **7**(1), article 5.
Hamilton, J.D., 1994, *Time Series Analysis*, (Princeton: Princeton University Press).
James, N., 2007, The statistical analysis of golf performance. *International Journal of Sports Science and Coaching*, **2**(suppl. 1), pp. 231–248.
James, N. and Rees, G.D., 2008, Approach shot accuracy as a performance indicator for US PGA Tour golf professionals. *International Journal of Sports Science and Coaching*, **3**(suppl. 1), pp. 145–160.
Lamb, P.F., Stöckl, M. and Lames, M., 2011, Performance analysis in golf using the ISOPAR method. *International Journal of Performance Analysis in Sport*, **11**(1), pp. 184–196.
Scheid, F.J., 1990, On the normality and independence of golf scores, with various applications. In *Science and Golf: Proceedings of the World Congress of Golf*, edited by Cochran, A.J. (London: E & FN Spon), pp. 147–152).
Stöckl, M., Lamb, P.F. and Lames, M., 2011, The ISOPAR method: A new approach to performance analysis in golf. *Journal of Quantitative Analysis in Sport*, **7**(1), article 10.
Stöckl, M., Lamb, P.F. and Lames, M., 2012, A model for visualizing difficulty in golf and subsequent performance rankings on the PGA Tour. *International Journal of Golf Science*, **1**(1), pp. 10–24.

CHAPTER 30

Evidence of chaos in indoor pedaling motion using non-linear methods

Juan-Carlos Quintana-Duque and Dietmar Saupe

30.1 INTRODUCTION

Quantitative studies of human motion have typically focused on properties of the average motion, and their fluctuations were considered noise. Recent publications (for example, Davids *et al.*, 2006) found evidence that the alleged noise, called motion variability, contains important information useful to characterize mature motor skills and healthy states. Motion variability is always present in healthy human beings and even Olympic athletes show motion variability despite several years of intense training of specific movements. Lack or excess of variability are now understood as a *deficiency* in motor skills.

Recently, non-linear methods for analysis of time series have been applied to quantify the amount of motion variability. In that approach, a dynamical system is presumed such that time series can be considered as noisy measurements of some function of particular solutions to the system. Dynamic invariants characterize properties of the solution space of the corresponding unknown dynamical systems.

Dynamic invariants can be calculated from trajectories in the state space of a dynamical system. Only in rare cases, when a very simple dynamical system is given explicitly, it may be possible to rigorously compute dynamic invariants. Thus, in practice only a numerical approximation is feasible. Moreover, as mentioned above, for many applications, and in particular for all practical applications in sport science, the underlying dynamical system is assumed to model a very complex system like the human body performing a certain task. In this case the dynamical system is not known explicitly. Even if it was, it would typically contain a myriad of variables defying any mathematical or even numerical analysis.

However, since the discovery by Takens (1981) of a topologically faithful reconstruction of state space of dynamical systems in a lower dimensional so-called embedding space, it became possible to estimate dynamic invariants only from the aforementioned noisy measurements of some function or projection of a trajectory in the original (unknown) state space. For example, in sport science applications one does not have access to all neural and muscular signals of the human body (i.e., the state space) or complete knowledge of their governing dynamical system to directly calculate the dynamic properties of the human motion control system, but one can record the resulting human motion using video analysis or direct motion capturing. In the case of cyclical motion of an athlete on an ergometer that we consider in this paper, we propose to measure the three-dimensional spatial position of one of the knee joints which serve as observations of the underlying complex dynamical system. The time series of one component of the coordinate position (e.g., the X-coordinate) may be enough to reconstruct the dynamic behavior of the human motion system that is to be quantified by dynamic invariants.

The dynamic invariants calculated from a time series are meaningful only when there is indeed deterministic non-linearity in the time series. However, time series data can be anything between purely random and strictly deterministic. In order to test the presence of deterministic non-linearity in a time series, it has been suggested to calculate the maximal Lyapunov exponent (this dynamic invariant will be explained in following) and to use the surrogate data methodology.

A positive maximal Lyapunov exponent is a characteristic of chaotic time series but this exponent alone cannot be used for proving strictly deterministic chaos because random data may also produce a positive maximal Lyapunov exponent. Furthermore, the surrogate data methodology is used to test a given time series for membership of a specific class of dynamical systems, comparing features of the original data and certain surrogate data which can be generated algorithmically from the original data. In order to complement the evidence of chaos, the surrogate data must keep most of the original linear characteristics of the original data while making the original chaotic characteristics random. If the result of the surrogate data test is negative and there is a positive maximal Lyapunov exponent within time series, one can conclude that the time series data come from a non-linear chaotic dynamical system.

Previous works on gait analysis (e.g., Nessler *et al.*, 2009 and Stergiou *et al.*, 2006) presented results confirming the hypothesis that gait motion data come from a deterministic chaotic system. This conclusion was reached comparing original with surrogate data created by a method operating in the frequency domain (i.e., phase randomization). However, this method is inappropriate for original data exhibiting strong cyclic components because it destroys the essential periodic original features. For such kind of cyclical motion data it is more natural to ask if there can be demonstrated determinism for durations longer than the data cycle length (Miller *et al.*, 2006). Thus, the reported evidence of deterministic chaos on gait motion data using the surrogate data obtained from randomizing the phase in the frequency domain, might be incomplete. The chaotic relation between cycles was not tested. The finding was only that the gait motion data is not random, which is obvious. In the case of gait motion (and in general for any cyclical motion), one needs to validate the hypothesis that intercycle fluctuations are deterministic chaos and not random noise.

Knowing this, we propose to analyze whether intercycle dynamics of indoor pedaling motion come from a deterministic chaotic system using the pseudo-periodic surrogate (PPS) method described in Small *et al.* (2001). The PPS method creates surrogate data from original time series data preserving the original intracycle dynamics (dynamic patterns within one period of a cyclic pattern) while changing the original intercycle dynamics (dynamic patterns between different periods across a cyclic pattern).

As far as we know, there is no previous work about evidence of chaos in pedaling motion. Here we analyzed the time series of the angle and the *X*-coordinate position of the knee joint recorded during pedaling under different constraints (low and high cadence with low and high pedal brake force). In order to find evidence of chaos within pedaling motion data, we calculated the maximal Lyapunov exponent. Additionally we used the surrogate methodology with correlation dimension as test statistic and with surrogate data created by methods based on the frequency domain and the embedding space. We found that our recorded motion data of indoor pedaling have intercycle chaotic dynamics.

30.1.1 Dynamical systems and dynamic invariants

A dynamical system consists of the dynamics taking place in a state space. The state space usually is a linear space of all possible world-states of the system in question. Each world-state represents a complete snapshot of the system at some moment in time. In the discrete-time case, the dynamics is given by a function that transforms one point in state space (world-state), representing the state of the system "now", into another point representing the state of the system one time unit "later" (i.e., a second world-state). Thus, if points in state space are denoted by vectors x_n of *m* components and the dynamics are given by a function f we have

$$x_{n+1} = f(x_n), x_n = [x_{n,1}, x_{n,2}, x_{n,3}, ..., x_{n,m}]. \tag{30.1}$$

Once an initial world-state is chosen, the dynamics determines the world-state at all future times forming a trajectory in state space.

In real-world applications, usually we do not have complete knowledge, let alone access to the *m*-dimensional state space but we have to work with one or several one-dimensional observations y_n. Takens' theorem, described in Takens (1981), guarantees that the observations y_n will be enough to reconstruct the attractor of the dynamical system in the embedding space with dimension d_e if the observations are infinite and without noise. In practice, a sequence of observations is enough to approximate the attractor when the data is sufficiently large and contains low levels of noise. The embedding is defined by equation (30.2) with the embedding dimension d_e and the embedding delay τ as parameters, where the dimension d_e of the embedding space must be larger than twice the box counting dimension of the attractor plus one. (See more details in Eckmann and Ruelle, 1985.)

$$v_n = (y_n, y_{n-\tau} ..., y_{n-(d_e-1)\tau}).$$
(30.2)

The accuracy of numerical estimation of invariants from experimental data depends on the quantity and quality of the time series data as well as on the quality of the reconstruction of the complexity of the dynamical system using an embedding space.

30.1.2 Dynamic invariants: maximal Lyapunov exponent

Lyapunov exponents describe the average expansion respectively contraction of the evolution of trajectories on an attractor of a dynamical system. The most robust and important one is the maximal Lyapunov exponent λ. This dynamic invariant is calculated from a time series using embedding points defined by equation (30.2).

Let v_{n_0} and v_{n_1} be two points in the embedding space with a sufficiently small Euclidian distance $\delta_0 = \left\| v_{n_0} - v_{n_1} \right\|$ and denote by $\delta_{\Delta n}$ the distance between the trajectories emerging from these points at some time Δn ahead, $\delta_{\Delta n} = \left\| v_{n_0+\Delta n} - v_{n_1+\Delta n} \right\|$. Then, if $\delta_{\Delta n} \approx \delta_0 e^{\lambda \Delta n}$ for a range of values Δn and in expectation for points v_{n0} on the attractor the maximal Lyapunov exponent is λ. If λ is positive, there is a strong signature of chaos in the time series data. The higher the instability and the divergence of neighboring trajectories in embedding space, the larger is the value of λ.

Numerically, the maximal Lyapunov exponent λ is calculated as the slope of the average logarithmic divergence of the neighboring trajectories in the reconstructed attractor in the embedding space. The algorithm for calculating λ is the following: A reference point v_{n_0} is chosen and its nearest neighbors $v_{n_1, n_2, ...}$ with distance to the reference point less than r are selected from the reference point's neighborhood $\mathfrak{A}$. Then, one computes the distances of all selected neighbors to the reference point following the trajectories as a function of the relative time Δn for $0 \le \Delta n \le \Delta n_{max}$. Repeating the latter for many (N) reference point's v_{n_0} and calculating the averages $S(\Delta n)$ of these results, see equation (30.3), noise in the data and fluctuations of the effective divergence will average out. If for some range of Δn the function $S(\Delta n)$ exhibits a robust linear increase, its slope is a stable and robust estimate of the maximal Lyapunov exponent. (See more details in Kantz and Schreiber, 2004.)

$$S(\Delta n) = \frac{1}{N} \sum_{n_0=1}^{N} \ln \left(\frac{1}{\left| \mathfrak{A}\left(v_{n_0}\right) \right|} \sum_{v_n \in \mathfrak{A}(v_{n_0})} \left\| v_{n_0+\Delta n} - v_{n+\Delta n} \right\| \right)$$
(30.3)

30.1.3 Dynamic invariants: correlation dimension

The correlation dimension d_c is a topological property of an invariant set (attractor) of a dynamical system. One considers the probability that two points chosen randomly from the invariant set, and according to the dynamics of the system, will be within distance ε of each other. Then one examines how this probability changes as the distance ε varies. If the probability scales as ε^{d_c} then the exponent d_c is called the correlation dimension.

The correlation dimension can be numerically computed from a long trajectory as follows: One calculates the correlation sum C(N, ε), equation (30.4), which approximates the desired probability. This sum is the relative number of pairs of embedding points (v_i, v_j) within distance less than ε of each other. By definition, equation (30.5), as the data size grows, N $\to \infty$, and for small $\varepsilon \to 0$, one expects that correlation sum scales with a power law C(N,ε) $\propto \varepsilon^{d_c}$. In practice, one inspects the function ln C(N, ε), versus ln ε for a linear region. If the linear region exists, the slope of this region is an approximation of the correlation dimension d_c.

In order to avoid the influence of temporal data correlation in the correlation sum C, one excludes those pairs of embedding points which are close, not because of the geometry of the attractor but just because they are closer than n_{min} in (discrete) time. The time window n_{min} is called the Theiler window. Furthermore, the formula in equation (30.4) is defined using the Heaviside step function Θ, which is $\Theta(x) = 0$ for $x \le 0$ and $\Theta(x) = 1$ for $x > 0$. (See more details in Kantz and Schreiber, 2004.)

$$C(N,\varepsilon) = \frac{2}{(N-n_{min})(N-n_{min}-1)} \sum_{i=1}^{N} \sum_{j=i+n_{min}}^{N} \Theta\left(\varepsilon - \|v_i - v_j\|\right) \tag{30.4}$$

$$d_c = \lim_{\varepsilon \to 0} \lim_{N \to \infty} \frac{\partial \log(C(N,\varepsilon))}{\partial \log \varepsilon} \tag{30.5}$$

However, locating the linear part, i.e., the scaling region, of the function log C(N, ε) versus log ε is often subjective. A modification for the calculation of correlation dimension proposed by Judd (1992) aims at reducing such effects by modeling the growth of correlation sum as

$$C(N,\varepsilon) \propto \varepsilon^{d_c} p(\varepsilon) \tag{30.6}$$

where p(ε) is a (e.g., quadratic) polynomial. This has an interesting benefit. For many natural objects the dimension is not the same at all length scales. If one observes a large river stone its surface at its largest length scale is very nearly two-dimensional, but at smaller length scales one can discern the details of grains which add to the complexity and increase the dimension at smaller scales. Consequently, it is natural to consider dimension d_c as a function of ε and write $d_c(\varepsilon)$ (Small *et al.*, 2001). The scale dependent correlation dimension $d_c(\varepsilon)$ and the coefficients of the polynomial can be estimated together by unconstrained non-linear optimization using correlations sums $C(N,\varepsilon')$ in a suitable chosen scaling range near ε.

30.1.4 Surrogate data

Surrogate data are new time series created from original time series data keeping some of the original linear characteristics and making the original non-linear characteristics random. The choice of method to generate surrogate data depends on the null hypothesis that one wants to test, comparing features of the original and surrogate data. The methods can be based on the original time series, on the data in the frequency domain or in the embedding space. In this paper we used the last two.

The method to create surrogate data based on embedding space called pseudo-periodic surrogate algorithm PPS, proposed in Small and Tse (2002), is used to test the null hypothesis that the original time series data, exhibiting pseudo-periodic dynamics, come from a dynamical system with an attractor whose

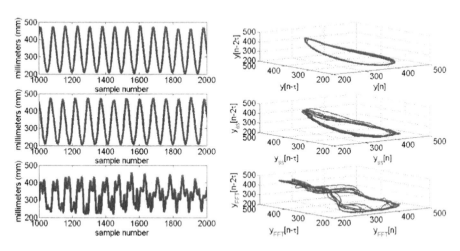

Figure 30.1 Effects of different surrogate methods on time and in embedding space. Top: Original data; middle: Surrogate data based on embedding; bottom: Surrogate data based on FFT. We plotted the time series (left) and the corresponding embedding space (right). The embedding is with dimension $d_c = 3$ and delay parameter $\tau = 15$. The surrogate method based on embedding keeps the intracycle structure of original data (see the similarity between original and surrogate time series) while destroying the intercycle structure (see the noisy attractor in embedding space). The surrogate method based on FFT destroys both the intracycle and the intercycle structure (the attractor in embedding space has a different shape).

periodic orbit is driven by uncorrelated noise. For this algorithm, the attractor of the observed dynamical system is first reconstructed from the time series data y_n using an embedding space defined by equation (30.2). After that, the embedding points of neighboring trajectories in the reconstructed attractor are used to create a new attractor with noisy trajectories. That is, one selects an initial embedded point v_i from the reconstructed attractor as start point of the surrogate trajectory. For the following point in time of the surrogate trajectory, one of the embedding neighbors z_i of v_i is randomly selected with a probability depending on the noise level parameter ρ, given by equation

$$\text{Prob}(v_i = z_i) \propto \exp(-\|z_i - v_i\|/\rho). \tag{30.7}$$

The following point in time z_{i+1} of the selected embedding point z_i is selected as the next point of the surrogate sequence being created. The last step is repeated for last selected embedding point until the number of desired points is achieved creating in this way a noisy attractor. Finally, the new surrogate time series data is constructed from the embedding points of the noisy attractor. With an appropriate choice of the embedding parameters (τ and d_e) and the noise parameter ρ, intracycle dynamics are preserved but intercycle dynamics are not (see Figure 30.1 middle). If ρ is large, then the points are simply temporally uncorrelated random points. If ρ is too small then the surrogate and original are identical. (See more details about how to select a suitable value of ρ in Small and Tse, 2002.)

The method to created surrogate data based on frequency space, proposed in Theiler *et al.* (1992), is used to test the null hypothesis that the original time series data correspond to linearly filtered noise. One generates phase-randomized surrogates from the time series data y_n by computing Fast Fourier Transforms (FFT), randomizing the phase spectra, and finally computing the inverse FFT. With this method, the power spectrum and correlation function are preserved from the original time series while the probability distribution of the values is changed and the intracycle dynamics is destroyed (see Figure 30.1 bottom).

30.2 METHODS

The pedaling motion of a healthy rider without muscle fatigue was recorded with a sampling rate of 100 Hz using a motion capture system (LUKOtronic) and a configurable cycling ergometer (Cyclus2). Four tests of 2 minutes each were made with several cadences (80 and 100 rpm) and pedal brake forces (120 and 140 newtons). The dynamic invariants were calculated from the time series data of the X-coordinate of the knee joint position and the knee joint angle (formed by three markers attached on knee, ankle, and hip joints). Raw data were used for the reconstruction of the attractor in embedding space. The calculation of the embedding parameters and the maximal Lyapunov exponent was done using the TISEAN software described in Hegger *et al.* (1999) and the surrogate data analysis was done using the ANTA software described in Small (2005).

The calculation of the embedding parameters d_e and τ was done separately for each time series. The first zero-crossing of the autocorrelation was used as embedding delay τ, and in order to choose the embedding dimension d_e, the false neighbor algorithm (FNN) was applied with the previously calculated embedding delay τ as parameter. (See Kantz and Schreiber, 2004, for a description of the used methods.)

The hypothesis, that intercycle irregularities of pedaling motion data are most likely due to deterministic chaos rather than random inputs, was analyzed using the graphical method proposed in Small and Tse (2002). This method consists of a graphical comparison between the correlation dimension values of 50 different surrogate time series and the correlation dimension value of the original time series. The contour plot in each panel in Figure 30.2 is a representation of the probability distribution function (PDF) of the scale dependent correlation dimension $d_c(\varepsilon)$ of surrogate data for distinct values of ε. Each vertical slice (i.e., for a given ε) corresponds to a single PDF calculated using the density kernel estimation algorithm (Silverman, 1986) with a Gaussian kernel. The isocline lines of the contour plot are selected automatically and uniformly. Points outside the outermost isocline correspond to correlation dimension values that are outside the range of dimensions for the surrogate data.

For the calculation of the maximal Lyapunov exponent from equation (30.3) we used a neighborhood $\mathfrak{A}(v_{n_0})$ of a size $\sigma(y_n)/100$, with $\sigma(y_n)$ as standard deviation of the discrete time series y_n. In order to get reliable results of this invariant for each time series, we calculated averages of the maximal Lyapunov exponent values obtained from embedding spaces created using embedding dimensions d_e, d_e+1, d_e+2, d_e+3, and d_e+4.

30.3 RESULTS

Table 30.1 shows the embedding parameters (embedding dimension de and embedding delay τ), and the maximal Lyapunov exponent λ calculated for all four tests. Pedal brake force is given in newtons (N), the cadence in revolutions per minute (rpm) and the power in watts (W). The maximal Lyapunov units are given in s^{-1}.

In Figure 30.2, we show the results of graphical method proposed in Small and Tse (2002) to compare correlation dimension values between original data and surrogate data. We used two different methods to create surrogate data based on frequency domain and embedding space. Additionally, in order to check whether a correlation between power and correlation dimension exists, we plot the correlation dimension for all tests in Figure 30.3.

Table 30.1 Calculated embedding dimension d_e, embedding delay τ, and maximal Lyapunov exponent λ of time series of knee joint angle and knee joint position

	140 N 100 rpm (218 W)			120 N 100 rpm (187 W)			140N 80 rpm (176 W)			120 N 80 rpm (150 W)		
	d_e	τ	λ	d_e	τ	λ	d_e	τ	λ	d_e	τ	λ
Knee angle	4	23	0.2211 ±0.0223	4	22	0.1872 ±0.0279	4	23	0.211 ±0.0393	4	33	0.32 ±0.0240
Knee X-coordinate	4	18	0.1849 ±0.0094	4	21	0.2373 ±0.0357	4	21	0.1999 ±0.0195	4	25	0.2607 ±0.0254

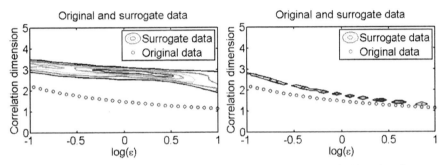

Figure 30.2 Results obtained from 50 surrogate data sets created with a method based on frequency domain (left) and on embedding space (right) for the time series data of the test 140 N 100 rpm

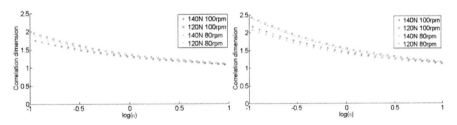

Figure 30.3 Comparison of correlation dimension values between all tests using knee joint angle data (left) and X-coordinate of knee joint position data (right). There is no evidence of a linear relation between the value of invariants and workload intensity

30.4 CONCLUSIONS AND FUTURE WORK

Evidence of deterministic chaos was found in all time series of knee motion data recorded during indoor pedaling following the methodology suggested in Small and Tse (2002). This methodology consists of the search for evidence of chaos within time series based on the calculation of the maximal Lyapunov exponent and on a test of non-linearity using surrogate data with the correlation dimension $d_c(\varepsilon)$ as test statistic.

Table 30.1 shows that the time series of all tests done with different workloads have positive maximal Lyapunov exponents λ, which is a characteristic of chaotic dynamical systems. In addition to this, analysis using surrogate data (e.g., Figure 30.2) was done in order to test two different null hypotheses: (1) the time series data correspond to linearly filtered noise (i.e., surrogate data were created based on frequency domain method) and (2) that the data come from a dynamical system with an attractor whose periodic orbit is driven by uncorrelated noise (i.e., surrogate data were based on embedding space method). For both null hypotheses, we found clear differences between the surrogate data and original data suggesting that any long-term determinism of period longer than the data cycle length exists within time series data, and that the pedaling motion comes from a deterministic chaotic system. In general, these differences were more evident for the surrogate data created using frequency method than from that using embedding space (see Figure 30.2). Evidence of chaos in other cyclic human motion such as gait data was reported in Dingwell and Casumano (2000) and in Miller *et al.* (2006), but as far as we know, there are no previous works about evidence of chaos in pedaling motion.

Furthermore, there is no evidence of a linear relation between the value of invariants and workload intensity with speed constraints (see Table 30.1 and Figure 30.3). Similar conclusions have been reported before in literature about gait data and speed constraints, for example in Buzzi and Ulrich (2004).

Our future research will focus on (1) the effects on dynamic invariants due to external (i.e., cadence and workload) and internal constraints (i.e., fatigue and muscle training), and (2) which invariants are more suitable for analysis according to the characteristics of pedaling motion.

30.5 ACKNOWLEDGMENTS

This work was supported by the DFG Research Training Group 1042 Explorative Analysis and Visualization of Large Information Spaces at the University of Konstanz.

30.6 REFERENCES

Buzzi, U.H. and Ulrich, B.D., 2004. Dynamic stability of gait cycles as a function of speed and system constraints. *Motor Control*, **8**(3), p. 241.

Davids, K., Bennett, S. and Newell, K., 2006, *Movement System Variability*, (Champaign: Human Kinetics Publishers).

Dingwell, J.B. and Cusamano, J.P., 2000. Nonlinear time series analysis of normal and pathological human walking. *Chaos*, **10**, pp. 848–863.

Hegger, R., Kantz H. and Schreiber, T., 1999, Practical implementation of nonlinear time series methods: The TISEAN package. *Chaos*, **9**, 413.

Judd, K., 1992, An improved estimator of dimension and some comments on providing confidence intervals. *Physica D: Nonlinear Phenomena*, **56**(2–3), pp. 216–228.

Kantz, H. and Schreiber, T., 2004. *Nonlinear time series analysis*, (Cambridge University Press).

Miller, D., Stergiou, N. and Kurz, M., 2006, An improved surrogate method for detecting the presence of chaos in gait. *Journal of Biomechanics*, **39**(15), pp. 2873–2876.

Nessler, J., Leone, C.D. and Gilliland, S., 2009, Nonlinear time series analysis of knee and ankle kinematics during side by side treadmill walking. *Chaos: An Interdisciplinary Journal of Nonlinear Science*, **19**(2), pp. 26104–26104.

Small, M., 2005, *Applied Nonlinear Time Series Analysis: Applications in Physics, Physiology and Finance* (London: World Scientific Pub Co Inc).

Small, M. and Tse, C., 2002, Applying the method of surrogate data to cyclic time series. *Physica D: Nonlinear Phenomena*, **164**(3–4), pp. 187–201.

Small, M., Judd, K. and Mees, A., 2001, Testing time series for nonlinearity. *Statistics and Computing*, **11**(3), pp. 257–268.

Silverman, B.W., 1986, *Density Estimation for Statistics and Data Analysis*, (Chapman & Hall, London).

Stergiou, N., Harbourne, R. and Cavanaugh, J., 2006, Optimal movement variability: A new theoretical perspective for neurologic physical therapy. *Journal of Neurologic Physical Therapy*, **30**(3), p. 120–129.

Takens, F., 1981, Detecting strange attractors in turbulence. In *Dynamical Systems and Turbulence, Lecture Notes in Mathematics, vol. 898*, edited by Rand, D.A. and Young, L-S. (Springer), pp. 366–381.

Theiler, J., Eubank, S., Longtin, A., Galdrikian, B. and Doyne-Farmer, J., 1992, Testing for nonlinearity in time series: The method of surrogate data. *Physica D: Nonlinear Phenomena*, **58**(1), pp. 77–94.

CHAPTER 31

The efficacy of judging within trampolining

Polly Johns and James Brouner

31.1 INTRODUCTION

It has been stated by Franks (2004) that 'real time' analysis is less accurate than post-analysis, which can be replayed, due to errors in memory. There has been research in many sports to investigate judging bias demonstrating that knowledge of previous performance can affect the results given (Findlay and Ste-Marie, 2004; Plessner, 1999; Rainey et al., 1989). Due to the small differences in elite performance, any level of open feedback can lead to the potential for social conformity and bias within the judging system which can result in the difference between winning and losing for an athlete (Vanden Auweele et al., 2004; Boen et al., 2006; Scheer et al., 1983). Therefore, an objective observation of performance is crucial to quantify performance and gain a true outcome of competition. Objective analysis has also been shown to aid both coaches and athletes on how to improve performance (Franks, 2004).

Trampolining is a recreational sport that developed into a competitive international elite sport due to the increase in technology and complexity of skills (Kunze et al., 2009). A panel of five Form judges and two Tariff judges analyse routines at competitions marking a score out of ten. The Form judges assess the aesthetics of a routine and the Tariff judges mark the difficulty, the Federation Internationale de Gymnastique (FIG) certifies all judges in the United Kingdom. The 'form' of a routine increases with the consistency in height of bouncing, fluidity of routine, execution of skills and limited travel across the bed (Kunze et al., 2009). A routine consists of 10 skills, each skill carrying a single point weighting, a maximum of 0.5 can be deducted from the mark of each skill. The highest and lowest score given from the Form judges is discarded with a total score being generated with addition of the difficulty score given by the Tariff judges. The panel of judges simultaneously displays scores after the completion of the routine to the Chair of Judges, competitors, coach and audience. A ranking order of competitors is then generated from the sum of both routines, compulsory and voluntary, including difficulty (Kunze et al., 2009).

In order to enhance the notation of sporting performance, human limitations need to be decreased by reducing subjective analysis. To improve the accuracy and reliability of judging, many sports have integrated the use of computer analysis to enhance correct outcomes of performance (Liebermann and Franks, 2004). For example, within the sport of amateur boxing the integration of new computerised notational techniques has eliminated judging bias (Coalter et al., 1998).

The aim of this study was to compare the accuracy of objective computerised post-event notational analysis with the current subjective hand notational system in place within trampolining. Errors in subjective hand notation, as discussed, can be due to many different factors including human which can contribute to the limitations of the current hand notational system. By altering this to a computerised system it is hypothesised to result in an improvement of accuracy and reliability of the results, making the scores given from the judging system more valid.

31.2 METHODS

31.2.1 Participants

The 13 athletes who participated in the study were over the age of 18 and British Artistic Gymnastic Association (BAGA) affiliated trampolinists of a high standard. The five judges, all qualified trampoline judges certified by BAGA with a ranging level of experience, were examined within the study. Full informed consent was gained from all participants; however, information was withheld from the judges so as not to give any influence or bias of their results. The title of the study was altered, explaining to the judges that it was about creating a new system, not analysing the current system and their results. A debriefing was given after the data was collected to give the participants the right to withdraw after the true study has been revealed.

31.2.2 Design

The method of this study used post-performance statistical analysis compared to in-event judge's hand notational analysis of performance. The design of this study was observational as the researcher went to a competition and observed the behaviours and actions of the judges and the competitors in their natural environment (Thomas *et al.*, 2010).

31.2.3 Procedure

The lead researcher, a qualified BAGA certified judge with 6 years of experience, observed the South West Closed Trampoline Competition and recorded each participant competing two routines. Two digital video cameras (JVC Digital Video Camera GZ – MG20, Japan) were used, one on a sagittal plane of the performance (where the judges viewed the routine) and another camera on the frontal plane of the performance. The marks from the five Form judges and the ranking of competitors were collected after completion of the event.

Key performance indicators (KPIs) were used to analyse each aspect of each routine. The KPIs that were used to analyse each skill during the routines have been developed using the FIG code of points (Kunze *et al.*, 2009) and from the

British Gymnastics Trampolining Coaching Manuals (British Gymnastics, 2009a, b, c and d). Due to the complexity of trampolining each skill has been broken down into three phases: take-off, flight and landing. If the move involves a body landing, an additional flight and landing phase will be necessary for the performer to return to their feet for example, seat landing to feet.

All routines were analysed post-event via a video statistical package (GameBreaker Plus, SportsTec, Warriewood, NSW Australia). Recordings from both the sagittal and frontal planes were utilised to achieve maximum objectivity of each skill. A score was then generated for each skill/routine using the KPIs and FIG guidelines, which was considered as the 'true' mark for the routine. This was completed for both the compulsory and voluntary routine of all 14 competitors. The results from the two notational systems were compared to discover if the judges' scores correlated with the 'true score' generated via computer analysis, testing for accuracy.

31.2.4 Statistical analysis

The ranking order of athletes was performed to discover whether the results given in each form of analysis would still have given the same ranking order from 1st to 14th place. Statistical analysis was performed to compare the marks awarded by the judges and the mark given from objective video analysis to see if the results were significantly different between the two systems. The data collected was non-parametric due to the nature of the results not meeting the assumptions of parametric tests (Thomas *et al.*, 2010). The results needed a statistical direct comparison between the two results, as they were related samples. Therefore, the data was analysed using a Wilcoxon matched-pairs signed-ranks test to assess if the difference in scores of the same subjects is significant (Thomas *et al.*, 2010).

31.2.5 Reliability

The intra-operator reliability of the objective analysis is key in gaining a true function from resulting outputs. By calculating an individual's accuracy and consistency of analysis, results displayed can be said to be of sound definition and a true reflection of performance (Hughes *et al.*, 2004).

Intra-operator reliability was tested within the post-performance analysis to examine whether the researcher's score generated was consistent each time a routine was assessed. This was generated by using a Kappa value (McGinn *et al.*, 2004) and percentage error (Hughes *et al.*, 2004). The intra-reliability was conducted by repeating the marking of a routine, not included in the study data set, once and repeated after a week time period so the analyst could not recall marks from memory (Hughes *et al.*, 2004).

The Kappa statistic measures observer variability by examining measurement agreement and the measurement agreement expected by chance. The results expressed the degree of agreement achieved (McGinn *et al.*, 2004).

31.3 RESULTS

Results from the reliability checks performed on the post-event analysis demonstrate an excellent level of reliability. Percentage error score showed a 0.1 per cent difference between tests with a Kappa score resulting in an 'almost perfect' outcome.

Table 31.1 Final results awarded by the judges, calculated score by the judges and post-analysis result
(∧ indicates an increase in placement, ∨ denotes a decrease in placement)

Competitor	Awarded score	Calculated score	Post-analysis score
1	16.2	16.1 ∨	16.8 ∧
2	15.0	15.0	15.1 ∧
3	9.9	9.9	10.0 ∧
4	14.8	14.8	14.5 ∨
5	15.9	16.0 ∧	16.5 ∧
6	15.4	15.3 ∨	15.5 ∧
7	14.3	14.2 ∨	14.5 ∧
8	16.6	16.4 ∨	16.0 ∨
9	12.3	12.3	11.7 ∨
10	13.9	14.1 ∧	13.5 ∨
11	12.1	12.3 ∧	12.6 ∧
12	16.1	16.0 ∨	15.8 ∨
13	16.8	16.8	17.1 ∧

Table 31.2 Rankings of competitors after final scores were generated by judges compared to post-analysis (numbers in superscript indicate movement in ranking)

Ranking	Official rank	True calculated rank	Post-analysis rank
1	13	13	13
2	8	8	1 [+1]
3	1	1	5 [+2]
4	12	12 & 5 [+1]	8 [-2]
5	5		12 [-1]
6	6	6	6
7	2	2	2
8	4	4	4 & 7 [+1]
9	7	7	
10	10	10	10
11	9	9 & 11 [+1]	11 [+1]
12	11		9 [-1]
13	3	3	3

31.4 DISCUSSION

All competitors were given different scores in event as opposed to the objective post-event analysis, with a maximum range of 0.5 marks, which is a large difference. At the Beijing 2008 Olympics 0.5 was the difference between 2nd and 4th place (Trampoline Women's Final Results, 2008). When studying Table 31.1, a clear difference in total results can be seen. None of the competitors were awarded the same result when analysed by the post-performance computerised objective method compared to the real-time subjective hand notational method of the judges. However, the results from Table 31.1 were not found to be significant, demonstrating no difference between methods of judging. (P=0.925). The results shown in Table 31.1 clearly show the range in values given, with the largest being 0.6 marks. When observing Table 31.2, the rankings awarded to the competitors differed in all but four competitors. Within the rankings, 1st, 6th, 7th and 10th places were the only rankings that remained the same; all other positions were awarded differently. This therefore highlights the change in competitors being awarded medals. First place was still awarded to the same athlete; however, the amount by which they won was largely different when comparing methods, a total difference of 0.6 marks. Competitor 5 went from 5th to 3rd place, therefore changing their results and awarding them bronze medal. Consequently, competitor 1 moved from 3rd to 2nd also improving their final score and ranking. However, the rankings were also found not to be significant (P=1), showing that although the results are different the power of the results does not show statistical significance. However, with such drastic changes to the final places of the competition being shown, the results have a meaningful difference and warrant further investigation.

When examining the judges' raw data/marking of raw data sheets it can be seen that the deductions given to the competitors do not correlate with the results given. These discrepancies could be due to either poor arithmetic skills when calculating the results, bias or social conformity to other judges. Social conformity has been identified and has tried to be eliminated in such sports as gymnastics, rope skipping and synchronised swimming (Scheer *et al.*, 1983; Boen *et al.*, 2006; Vanden Auweele *et al.*, 2004). The judges have been found to change their scores to gain social acceptance when seen by the other judges. This may account for why there is a change in the calculated score and the score given. However, this could also be due to poor arithmetic of the judges as they are under pressure to calculate the score as quickly as possible. Mistakes were made by all the judges therefore not just the ability of one judge can be responsible for the errors.

Currently, to become a judge of trampolining you must attend a day course set by British Gymnastics followed by an exam (Kunze *et al.*, 2009). The criteria to qualify for this course are low. Therefore, only a small amount of background knowledge of the sport is required and a minimum age of 15 (Kunze *et al.*, 2009). The demand for judges within the sport is high due to every club having to enter judges at competitions; therefore many parents attend the courses. There is no consideration of experience or knowledge of trampolining when evaluating applicants to attend the course. If the candidate passes the exam they will be deemed as a valid judge, this is not in support the expertise theory of Starkes and Ander Ericsson (2003)

The expertise of the judges has been shown to be of importance within sport using different knowledge to gain insight into the performance (Starkes and Ander Ericsson, 2003). Declarative knowledge entails the understanding of the rules of the sport and procedural knowledge requires the technique of the performance to be analysed (Thomas and Thomas, 1994). A study researching behaviours of gymnastic judges showed that the expert judges paid 10.9 per cent more attention to the routines than that of novice judges (Ste-Marie, 2000). This demonstrates that experience and training may have an impact of the quality and accuracy of the scores being generated (Cooper *et al.,* 2007).

The post-performance objective computerised method could be adopted and used for the training of judges. It shows the true value and a high level of reliability, which may aid the education of newly trained judges to help them become more accurate. Similarly within the studies by Catteeuw *et al.* (2010) and Coalter *et al.* (1998) the rules of judging within trampolining could be altered to improve the accuracy of the judging. All routines are recorded, allowing re-analysis to be made. Currently if there is a range greater than 0.5 within the judging panel there is no system in place to question that accuracy apart from the coach's appeals (British Gymnastics, 2011). However, when the error discrepancy exceeds this 5 per cent, the routine could be remarked in order to increase the accuracy of the judges' scores given to the competitors. With the introduction of this new rule, consistency of accuracy may be seen and an increased level of focus may be displayed within the judging panel to ensure proficiency so that the scores are correct.

31.5 CONCLUSION

The aid of using computerised support has been shown to aid many sports (Harding and James, 2010; Harding *et al.,* 2008a; 2008b; Cassel *et al.,* 2005; Coalter *et al.,* 1998) and could also be achieved within trampolining. The introduction of using technical equipment such as iPads may eliminate the arithmetic errors that occur within the judging panel. If the judges typed their marks in to a computerised device, the score could automatically be calculated for them to aid their accuracy and decrease human error.

The final results suggest that the current system is adequate enough to generate accurate results. However, with the consistent human error displayed amongst all judges and the post-event analysis awarding different final marks to all competitors the judging process in trampolining must be considered. It appears not to be crucial to change the scoring system within trampolining; however the accuracy of judging could be enhanced using computerised technology as adopted by other sports (Harding and James, 2010; Harding *et al.,* 2008a; 2008b; Cassel *et al.,* 2005; Coalter *et al.,* 1998).

31.6 REFERENCES

Boen, F., Vanden Auweele, Y., Claes, E., Feys, J. and De Cuyper, B., 2006, The impact of open feedback on conformity among judges in rope skipping. *Psychology of Sport and Exercise*, 7, pp. 577–590.

British Gymnastics (2009a, b, c, d) *UKCC 1/2/3/4 Coaching Manual –Trampolining.*

British Gymnastics (2011) *Trampoline National Competition Structure*, GB.

Cassel, R., Collet, C. and Gherbi, R., 2005, Real-time acrobatic gesture analysis. *Gesture in Human-Computer Interaction and Simulation, Lecture Notes in Computer Science Volume* 3881, pp. 88–99

Catteeuw, P., Gilis, B., Garcia-Aranda, J.M., Tresaco, F.,Wagemans, J. and Helsen, E., 2010, Offside decision making in the 2002 and 2006 FIFA World Cups. *Journal of Sports Sciences*, **28**(10), pp. 1027–1032

Coalter, A., Ingham, B., McCrory, P., O'Donoghue, P. and Scott, M., 1998, A comparison of alternative operation schemas for the computerised scoring system for amateur boxing. *Journal of Sports Science*, **16**, pp. 16–17.

Cooper, S.M., Hughes, M.D., O'Donoghue, P.G. and Nevill, A.M., 2007, A simple statistical method for assessing the reliability of data entered into sport performance analysis systems. *International Journal of Performance Analysis in Sport*, 7(1), pp. 87–109.

Findlay, L.C. and Ste-Marie, D.M., 2004, A reputation bias in figure skating judging. *Journal of Sport and Exercise Psychology*, **26**, pp. 154–166.

Franks, I.M., 2004, The need for feedback. In *Notational Analysis of Sport: Systems for Better Coaching and Performance in Sport, 2nd edn*, edited by Hughes, M. and Franks, I.M. (London: Routledge), pp.8–16.

Harding, J.W. and James, D.A., 2010, Performance assessment innovations for elite snowboarding. *Procedia Engineering*, **2**, pp. 2919–2924.

Harding, J.W., Toohey, K., Martin, D.T., Hahn, A.G. and James, D.A., 2008a, Technology and half-pipe snowboard competition insight from elite-level judges. *The Engineering of Sport*, 7, pp. 467–476.

Harding, J.W., Mackintosh, C.G., Hahn, A.G. and James, D.A., 2008b, Classification of aerial acrobatics in elite half-pipe snowboarding using body mounted inertial sensors. *The Engineering of Sport*, 7, pp. 447–456

Hughes, M., Cooper, S-M. and Nevill, A., 2004, Analysis of notation data: reliability, In *Notational Analysis of Sport: Systems for Better Coaching and Performance in Sport, 2nd edn,* edited by Hughes, M. and Franks, I.M. (London: Routledge), pp. 189–204.

Kunze, H., Makarov, N., Shuyska, T., Lambert, C., Andersson, U., Zeman, V. and Beeton, J., 2009, *Fédération Internationale de Gymnastique Code of Points: Trampolining.* Retrieved 26 November 2011 from http://www.fig-gymnastics.com/vsite/vtrial/page/home/0,11065,5187-187975-205197-45048-285446-custom-item,00.html

Liebermann, D.G. and Franks. I.M., 2004, The use of feedback technologies. In *Notational Analysis of Sport: Systems for Better Coaching and Performance in Sport, 2nd edn*, edited by Hughes, M. and Franks, I.M. (London: Routledge), pp. 40–58.

McGinn, T., Wyer, P.C., Newman, T.B., Keitz, S., Leipzig, R. and Guyatt, G., 2004, Tips for learners of evidence-based medicine: 3. Measures of observer variability (kappa statistic). *Canadian Medical Association Journal,* **171**(11) pp. 1369–1373.

Plessner, H., 1999, Expectation biases in gymnastics judging. *Journal of Sport and Exercise Psychology*, **21**, pp. 131–144.

Rainey, D.W., Larsen, J.D. and Stephenson, A., 1989, The effects of a pitcher's reputation on umpires' calls of balls and strikes. *Journal of Sport Behaviour*, **12**, pp. 139–150.

Scheer, J.K., Ansorge, C.J. and Howard, J., 1983, Judging bias by viewing contrived videotapes: A function of selected psychological variables. *Journal of Sports Psychology*, **5**, pp. 427–437.

Starkes, J.L. and Anders Ericsson, K., 2003, *Expertise Performance in Sports: Advances in Research in Sports Expertise*, (Champaign, IL: Human Kinetics).

Ste-Marie, D.M., 2000, Expertise in women's gymnastic judging: An observational approach. *Perceptual and Motor Skills*, **90**, pp. 543–546.

Thomas, J., Nelson, J. and Silverman, S., 2010, *Research Methods in Physical Activity, 6th edn*, (Champaign, IL: Human Kinetics).

Thomas, K.T. and Thomas, J.R., 1994, Developing expertise in sport: The relation of knowledge and performance. *International Journal of Sports Psychology*, **25**, pp. 295–312.

Trampoline Women's Final Results (2008, 18 August) Retrieved 17th April 2012, from http://www.gymnasticsresults.com/2008/olympics2008traw.html.

Vanden Auweele, Y., Boen, F., Geest, A.D. and Feys, J., 2004, Judging bias in sychronised swimming: Open feedback leads to non-performance-based conformity. *Journal of Sport and Exercise Psychology*, **26**, pp. 561–571.

CHAPTER 32

Characterisation of the current level of performance in individual competitions in Rhythmic Gymnastics

Tina Breitkreutz and Anita Hökelmann

32.1 INTRODUCTION

Rhythmic Gymnastics is an Olympic sport which belongs to the group of acyclic technical-compositional sports with the main purpose 'to perform the movement of the own body with involvement of apparatus and perhaps partners according to the norms' (Kirchner and Stöber, 1994). According to the former IOC President Juan Antonio Samaranch it is the 'most charming and feminine sport of the world' (Welkow-Jusek and Labner, 2011). Individual and group competitions are characterised by 'numerous, difficult movement structures and choreography compositions including the apparatus rope, hoop, ball, clubs, and ribbon' (Schwabowski *et al.*, 1992). Body movement elements can be grouped in pivots, jumps, flexibilities and balances. Rhythmic Gymnastics links high athletic performance with body control, concentration, sense for space and time, aesthetic, grace, creativity, and artistic skills on a very high level. Therefore, it combines culture of movement, art and sport, which makes it a very complex athletic performance (Figure 32.1).

According to Kwitniewska *et al.* (2009), 'the fast tempo of movement and the large number of sporting actions, make evaluating the performance a complex and difficult task'. Especially, the evaluation of qualitative factors (grace, expressivity, creativity, composition between music and movements) is highly influenced by subjective bias. Thus choreography analyses are mainly focussed on quantifiable

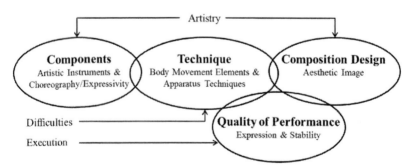

Figure 32.1 Structure and complexity of performance in Rhythmic Gymnastics

parameters such as the number of body and apparatus techniques, and space utilisation. However, those analyses may help to rank performances, to create databases and performance profiles of individual athletes. Additionally, it facilitates to describe the current performance level and development trends in this complex sport.

32.2 AIM

The aim of this study is to use choreography analyses to clarify the most influencing indicators of performances in Rhythmic Gymnastics, to determine the current performance level and the trends of development. This knowledge is required for an active training and competition control. The following research questions are discussed:

1. What kinds of pivots were performed and how many revolutions were demonstrated?
2. What type of jumps were performed according to the flight phase (translator or rotatory)?
3. Are there body movement elements which are performed most frequently with one specific apparatus?
4. Is there a link between specific apparatus techniques and body movement elements?
5. Which zones of the gymnastic mat are used most frequently?

32.3 METHODS

The finals of the Berlin Masters individual competition were recorded with a 25Hz camera. A total of 32 routines with the different apparatus (ball, hoop, ribbon, clubs [8 each]) were than analysed post-event utilising the software Utilius vs. (CCC-Software, Markkleeberg, Germany). The research issue was the number of body movement elements and apparatus techniques and where these elements were demonstrated on the competition floor. With regards to the zones of the gymnastics mat it was decided to separate the floor area into nine zones (Figure 32.2). The arrow shows the main direction of the choreographies. Therefore, zones 1–3 are located directly in front of the jury. Reliability was tested applying the Cohen's Kappa test (Table 32.1).

Table 32.1 Intra- and Inter-Reliability Testing

Discipline	Intra-operator reliability	Inter-operator reliability
Ball	0.91	0.98
Ribbon	0.79	0.69
Hoop	0.90	0.91
Clubs	1.00	0.77

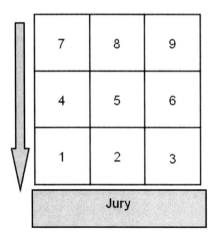

Figure 32.2 Zones of the gymnastics mat/floor area

32.4 RESULTS

32.4.1 Pivots

Pivots are highly important elements in Rhythmic Gymnastics choreographies. These body movement elements contribute the creative aspect of choreography due to numerous possibilities to initiate (relevé, piqué, lifting) and perform pivots (with diverse behaviour of the swing and stance leg as well as trunk and arm positions). Original and inventive routines including technically correct basic body and apparatus elements are more likely to be evaluated with the highest scores. Thus, it is important to analyse pivots in more detail in order to derive both the current performance level and the trends of performance development.

In total 115 pivots were demonstrated during all examined routines. Pivots with free leg in split were performed the most frequently (27), followed by pivots with free leg in horizontal position (25) and fouetté turns (18). The most common number of revolutions was two to three full rotations. However, pivots of 1440° were also observed in the most successful routines (Table 32.2). It was also observed that the highest number of pivots and also the highest number of pivots with multiple revolutions (up to four full rotations) were demonstrated with the clubs (Table 32.2). Additionally, it became clear that gymnasts prefer the relevé initiation followed by an equilateral pivot (Table 32.2).

32.4.2 Jumps

Jumps are body movement elements which are not supported by the ground for the whole time of demonstration. After a one-legged or two-legged take-off the main phase – flight phase – follows. The flight phase can be translatory or rotatory. The

Table 32.2 Number of revolutions, initiations, and direction of the performed turns

Apparatus	Number of revolutions						Initiation of pivot (%)			Direction of turn (%)	
	1	2	3	4	>4	Total	Relevé	Piqué	Lift	Equilateral	Inequilateral
Ball	2	5	5	2	3	17	89	3	8	86	14
Ribbon	6	15	7	2	5	35	93	5	2	86	14
Hoop	7	8	5	4	4	28	84	8	8	89	11
Clubs	7	6	10	6	6	35	87	8	5	85	15
Total	22	34	27	14	18	115					

Table 32.3 Flight phase behaviour of jumps

Apparatus	Flight phase behaviour in jumps			
	Translatory	Rotatory	Vertical	Total
Ball	13	23	0	36
Ribbon	12	23	0	35
Hoop	15	4	5	24
Clubs	19	1	3	23
Total	59	51	8	118

flight phase behaviour has an influence on difficulty and creativity of the movement and therefore, on the success of the performance.

In 32 final routines 118 jumps were observed. The highest number of jumps were performed in ball and ribbon routines. Jumps in these routines were mainly of translatory nature while jumps with rotations during their flight phase were more frequently performed in choreographies with hoop and clubs (Table 32.3).

32.4.3 Flexibilities and balances

Flexibilities may be performed on every part of the body and the body position is not required to be fixed at any point of the movement. In comparison balances need to be demonstrated on one foot (in relevé) or on one knee. The body position needs to be fixed at some point of the movement. All body movement elements are required in all apparatus disciplines.

Flexibilities are most frequent in ball routines. A large number of balances was observed in the club finals.

32.4.4 Body movement elements

In the apparatus discipline hoop all four groups of body movement elements were demonstrated with a similar frequency whereas the utilisation of the body movement elements with ball and ribbon were very inhomogeneous.

The body movement group of jumps are performed in all four apparatus disciplines with a frequency of more than 20per cent and thus are the most frequently demonstrated element (Figure 32.3).

32.4.5 Apparatus techniques

Apparatus techniques are specific for each apparatus discipline and body movement elements.

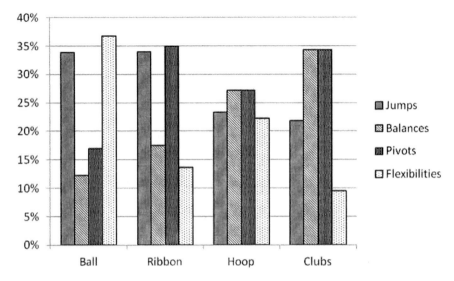

Figure 32.3 Percentage of flexibilities and balances in the four apparatus finals

It was observed that the apparatus technique 'throwing and catching' was linked with jumps in all four apparatus finals. Specific techniques like 'roll on body' (ball) or 'bounce with hand' (ball) were performed during balances most frequently. In ribbon finals this observation was made according to pivots and 'spirals'. In routines with clubs pivots were mainly linked to 'handling'. Another strong link was observed between balances and 'twisting' the hoop (Figure 32.4).

32.4.6 Space utilisation

Space utilisation is very important from a stage psychological and compositional point of view. According to the Code de Pointage (Federation International de Gymnastique, 2009) the entire gymnastics floor needs to be utilised consistently in a routine. However, the analysis shows that the centre of the gymnastics mat is used most frequently in all examined routines, especially in ball choreographies. For hoop, ribbon and clubs disciplines a better space utilisation with regards to the distribution of body and apparatus elements on the floor was observed. However, routines with clubs tend to be performed in the rear part of the mat (Figure 32.5).

Additionally, it was observed that jumps were initiated in the centre and directed to any other zone of the gymnastics floor.

32.5 DISCUSSION AND CONCLUSIONS

The analysis of the Berlin Masters 2011 has an important contribution to the description of the performance structure in Rhythmic Gymnastics. The results are

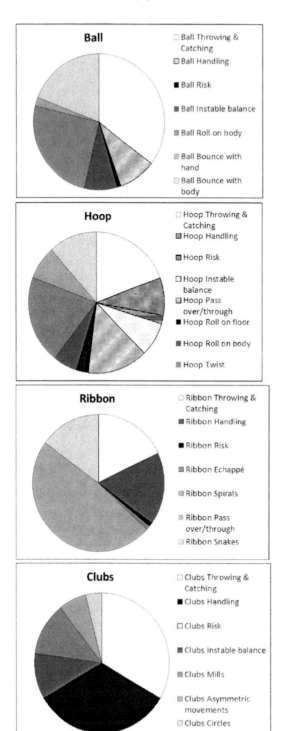

Figure 32.4 Specific apparatus techniques with regards to apparatus discipline and body movement elements

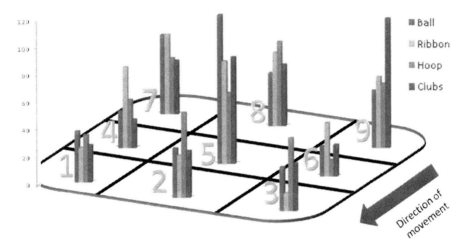

Figure 32.5 Number of body movement elements per zone on gymnastics mat in all four apparatus disciplines

in context with the requirements of the Code de Pointage and/or can be described by biomechanical laws. For example the highest number of pivots was observed with clubs and ribbon. It can be assumed that these apparatus operate as an elongation/increase of the gyrating mass (arms) and thus, have a positive influence to the generation of the angular momentum. However, turns with two or three revolutions were performed most frequently but there is a tendency to perform a higher number of rotations especially for the more successful gymnasts. The initiation by relevé is beneficial to the transfer of the angular momentum due to the quick and powerful extension of the previously bent supporting leg (Imura *et al.*, 2010). Additionally, it became clear that turns in the direction of the pivot leg are preferred. This is due to the preference of the relevé initiation which facilitates equilateral turns more than inequilateral ones. It can be concluded that specific apparatus seem to facilitate turns and thus support the trend of performance to increase the number of revolutions and execute pivots in difficult body positions.

With regards to the analysis of the jumps the following conclusion can be drawn: jumps with rotatory flight phases provide a greater variety of movements and thus contribute to the originality of the choreography. However, jumps with rotatory flight phases are more difficult compared to translatory flight phases. Therefore, easy jumps are mostly linked with complicated and specific apparatus techniques. With respect to a possible improvement of the performance in individual competitions it can be recommended that gymnasts should perform a higher number of jumps with rotatory flight phases – especially in the disciplines clubs and hoop. With respect to the specific apparatus techniques, gymnasts should demonstrate more risky elements in their choreographies to improve the overall performance. Risks are eye-catching and, if performed successfully, improve the final score and outcome of the competition (Schwabowski *et al.*, 1992). Jumps and flexibilities are most frequently linked to the discipline of ball, jumps and balances are mainly demonstrated in ribbon routines, balances and pivots can mainly be observed in choreographies with clubs, and body movement elements are balanced in the discipline of hoop.

In conclusion, it can be stated that the observations are compliant to the requirements of the Code de Pointage and gymnasts try to fulfil those in order to reach high scores by demonstrating highly complicated movements and combinations of different movement and apparatus techniques.

According to the Code de Pointage the gymnasts have to use the gymnastics mat evenly. However, based on the analysis it became clear that the centre and the rear part of the gymnastics floor were utilised most frequently in order to demonstrate body movement and apparatus difficulties. Only a few elements were demonstrated directly in the front of the jury desk. These observations can be explained based on stage psychology (Humphrey, 1986). Elements which are performed in the centre of the mat gain the most attention from the spectators and the jury. Difficulties demonstrated in the rear part of the floor appear to be mysterious and offer an aesthetic perspective. According to Humphrey (1986) the front part of the gymnastic mat is more beneficial for the demonstration of elements of expression as gestures, facial expressions, and comedy.

However, it also must be stated that some errors may have been between neighbouring areas in the reliability test. A weighted version of the kappa should be applied for further studies. Furthermore, more detailed information for determination of the current performance level and performance development in Rhythmic Gymnastics require additional choreography analyses of top level athletes in individual competition. Based on this it is possible to create a database and execute a longitudinal study of trends and developments in Rhythmic Gymnastics.

32.6 REFERENCES

Federation International de Gymnastique, 2009, *Code of Points – Rhythmic Gymnastics, 2009–2012*. Downloaded 25 February 2011 at http://www.fig-gymnastics.com/vsite/vnavsite/page/directory/0,10853,5187-188050-205272-nav-list,00.html.

Humphrey, D., 1986, *Die Kunst, Tänze zu machen. Choreographie des Modernen Tanzes*. (Berlin: Henschel).

Imura, A., Iino, Y., Kojima, T., 2010, Kinematic and kinetic analysis of the fouetté turn in classical ballet. *Journal of Applied Biomechanics*, **26**, pp. 484–492.

Kirchner, G. and Stöber, K., 1994, Ordnung in der Vielfalt – taxanomische Ansätze und Anforderungsprofile. In *Sportmotorik. Grundlagen, Anwendung und Grenzgebiete*, edited by Hirtz, P., Kirchner, G. and Pöhlmann, R. (Kassel: Universität-Gesamthochschule), pp. 335–355.

Kwitniewska, A., Dornoskoi, M. and Hökelmann, A., 2009, Quantitative and qualitative analysis of international standing in group competitions in the sport of rhythmic gymnastics. *Baltic Journal of Health and Physical Activity*, **1**(2), pp. 118–125.

Schwabowski, R., Brzank, R. and Nicklas, I., 1992, *Rhythmische Sportgymnastik. Leistung – Technik – Methodik.* (Aache: Meyer und Meyer Verlag).
Welkow-Jusek, G. and Labner, R., 2011, *Rhythmische Gymnastik in Österreich. Plattform für Expertinnen und Insider.* Downloaded 2 March 2011 at http://www.oeft.at/rg/basis-info.htm.

CHAPTER 33

A preliminary investigation into the effects of jumping saddle design on rider posture

Cassie White and Lauren Birkbeck

33.1 INTRODUCTION

Competitive athletes strive to improve performance, often incorporating the use of equipment perceived to give them a competitive edge (Hughes, 2008). In equestrian sports, the use of 'close contact' saddles has increased dramatically over the past decade, due to the perception that the saddle design permits closer connection between horse and rider. The primary aim of the saddle is to stabilise the rider so that posture may be maintained and the aids used to control and direct the horse effectively applied. Whether the saddle design assists in this has not been scientifically proven. The aim of this study was to analyse rider posture in two types of saddle commonly used in jumping over the past 20 years; a modern 'close contact' saddle and a 'traditional style' two flap jump saddle.

33.1.1 Rider posture

Riding is mainly a postural sport (Panni and Tulli, 1994). Rider posture plays a significant role in the oneness of horse and rider (Kang *et al.*, 2010) and rider safety (Peham *et al.*, 2004). Postural control, required to maintain stability and a good position, is dependent on skill, experience, training and discipline (Lovett *et al.*, 2004).

Trunk, hip and knee angles in the walk and trot have been shown to vary significantly ($P<0.05$) in both mean and variance between advanced and novice riders (Schils *et al.*, 1993; Kang *et al.*, 2010) and advanced riders also showed greater ability to allow for and harmonise with the movements of the horse (Peham *et al.*, 2001; Lovett *et al.*, 2004). No differences in rider posture according to gender have been reported.

33.1.2 The saddle

The key role of the saddle is to stabilise the rider. Modern saddle designs aim to provide maximum comfort, security and control, whilst positioning the rider as close to the horse's centre of mass as possible (Edwards, 2007). The saddle provides a key line of communication between horse and rider via the seat, vital for application of the aids and control of the horse (Powers and Harrison, 2004). This is a two-way communication, as the saddle can be expected to follow the movement of the horse's back, specifically the mid thoracic region (Byström *et al.*, 2009), and thus different saddles have characteristic motion patterns (Galloux *et al.*, 1994).

Stability of the rider is achieved by a central dip in the seat to encourage the rider to sit in the deepest part, knee and leg rolls and blocks to assist and secure the correct leg position. Stirrup bars are recessed to avoid unnecessary bulk and the saddle waist is narrowed to allow closer contact of the thighs (Edwards, 2007). The shape of the saddle seat is known to influence the position of the rider (Belton, 1997), and potentially centre of mass (Panni and Tulli, 1994). Jump saddles typically differ from their dressage counterparts in panel cut (forward as opposed to straight), seat depth (shallower), and stirrup bar placement (further forwards as stirrup length is shorter). This allows the leg to be maintained in the most stable position, with the ankle beneath the hip (Edwards, 2007). There are also forward positioned knee rolls to enable the correct position and support the extra weight taken through the knee (Belton, 1997; Edwards, 2007).

Manufacturers of close contact saddle designs aim to aid balance via the reduction of bulk between horse and rider (Devoucoux, 2011). Typically this is achieved by using smaller, flatter panels, a single saddle flap and extended girth straps, so that buckle bulk is taken away from the thigh. Newer models use knee and hind leg blocks to offer security (Edwards, 2007). What is not documented, however, is whether these changes in saddle design have an effect on rider posture.

33.2 METHOD

33.2.1 Participants

The participants in this study were nine experienced riders (eight female and one male), mean height 1.69m (± 0.08m), mean weight 59.42kg (± 7.42kg). All riders were competitive at British Eventing affiliated level.

Each participant was asked to wear their own tight fitting clothes, and normal riding equipment. Circular, self-adhesive markers of 3.5cm diameter were placed on the left side of each rider at selected anatomical landmarks, in accordance with Lovett *et al.* (2004), Schils *et al.* (1993) and Terada *et al.* (2006) (Figure 33.1).

33.2.2 Saddles

Participants rode in two saddles, on a Ride Master Pro 2006 equestrian simulator. Saddle A is a single flap 'close contact' design cross country saddle. Knee blocks and rolls support the knee, and hind blocks also feature. Saddle B was a traditional style jump saddle design, consisting of forward cut panels with two leather flaps between the rider's leg and the horse. It featured knee rolls but no excess blocking. Both saddles had an 18.5" seat and the same 55cm (eighteen holes) stirrup leathers and stirrup irons were used for each saddle and participant.

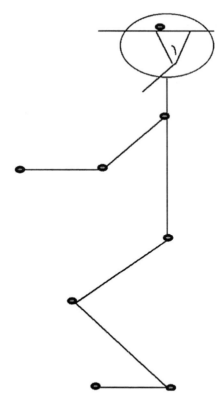

Figure 33.1 Anatomical marker locations: hat (above ear, behind harness), shoulder (glenohumeral joint centre), elbow (lateral epicondyle of the humerus), bony prominence of the wrist, hip (greater trochanter of the femur), knee (lateral side on the centre of the flat portion of the condyles of the femur) heel and toe of boot

33.2.3 Study design

Participants were split into two groups, in a cross-over designed experiment. Once mounted, stirrups were adjusted to a comfortable length for cross country (forward seat canter and jumping) riding. Subjects were given five minutes to become accustomed to and comfortable on the riding simulator. All riders were filmed using an HD Casio EXILIM EX-FH100 (240Hz).

Participants were recorded in all gaits for 30 seconds, at speeds predetermined by the external controller. The rider then dismounted, and stirrup leather length was recorded.

Raw footage was edited in Dartfish ProSuite® Video Analysis Software to comprise of 2 seconds of halt and 10 seconds of walk, sitting trot, seated canter and forward seat canter. Seated and forward seat canter were chosen as the most applicable to analysis from an eventing and jumping perspective, as cross country riding and jumping typically takes place from these positions. Halt was used as a control.

33.2.4 Data analysis

The same experienced observer was utilised throughout the trial and for each participant, all measurements were taken thrice and averaged. Absolute angles for ankle, knee and hip were calculated for each gait, and stirrup length was also measured. Data were tested for normality of distribution using the Kolmogorov-Smirnov test. Differences in variables between saddles were tested using Related Samples Wilcoxon Signed Ranks Test. A P-value of <0.05 was considered statistically significant in all statistical comparisons. PSAW Statistics 19 was used throughout.

33.3 RESULTS

33.3.1 Stirrup length

Stirrup bar placement was measured and no significant difference was found between the two saddles. Therefore, individual preferred stirrup length were analysed and participants were found to ride with significantly longer stirrups (t = –3.124, P = 0.035) in the close contact saddle (mean = 50.66 cm ± 1.91 S.E.) than the traditional saddle (mean = 46.10 cm ± 1.17).

33.3.2 Rider posture

Absolute angles for hip, knee and ankle were analysed for each gait, and no significant differences were identified for any angle at halt. There were no significant differences in ankle or hip measurements in walk, sitting trot and seated canter (P>0.05). Significant differences were, however, found for the knee in walk, trot and seated canter (see Table 33.1).

Table 33.1 Median absolute angles for the knee in each saddle and gait

Gait	Median absolute angle of knee (°)		P Value
	Close contact saddle	Traditional style saddle	
Walk	36.2	31.7	<0.001
Sitting trot	34.8	31.4	<0.001
Seated canter	27.3	25.9	0.008

In forward seat canter, there were no significant differences in knee or ankle angle (P > 0.05). However, a significant difference was found in the absolute hip angle (Z = –2.50, P = 0.012). The close contact saddle was found to have a median absolute angle of 128.1° compared to the traditional style saddle (median 133.3°).

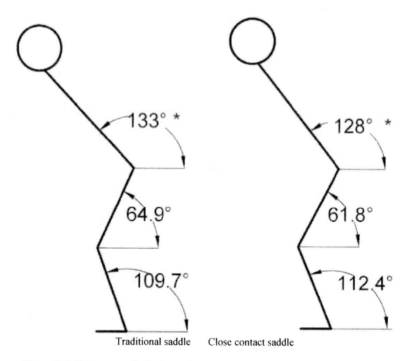

Traditional saddle   Close contact saddle

Figure 33.2 Rider posture in the forward seat canter (showing median absolute angles).
* denotes significant change in angle

A summary of overall changes seen between saddles in the forward seat canter is illustrated by Figure 33.2.

33.4 DISCUSSION

This study measured the stirrup length and absolute angles of experienced participants riding in two differing saddle designs. Whilst it is accepted that the general saddle design influences the rider (Belton, 1997), there is a paucity of information about the overall effect of different saddle designs on rider posture.

Experimental results revealed significant differences ($P < 0.05$) in stirrup length between the two saddles, with all participants selecting to ride longer in the close contact saddle. As participants were able to select their own stirrup length, it is fair to suggest that a change in saddle design has effected this change in rider position. Whether this has an impact on rider balance or harmony with the horse is unclear at the moment but worthy of further research.

Absolute knee angle was significantly different between the two saddles during walk, sitting trot and seated canter, with a more open knee seen in the close contact saddle throughout. This result may relate to the aforementioned longer stirrup length adopted by participants.

In the forward seat canter, no significant difference was found in absolute knee angle; however, a significant difference in hip angle was recorded. This suggests participants rode with greater flexion through the hips in the traditional style saddle compared to the close contact saddle; in which they adopted a more vertical alignment between the hip and ankle.

33.5 CONCLUSION

Riding is mainly a postural sport, the control of which has been shown to be dependent on skill, experience, training and discipline (Lovett *et al.*, 2004). Rider posture is important for control, communication and harmony with the horse. This study has shown rider posture to vary significantly between two types of jump saddle, including a difference in preferred stirrup length. Knowledge of factors influencing rider posture may serve to improve performance and horse–rider relationship. Whether a change in weight distribution and centre of mass occurs when riding in different styles of saddle is an important area for further research, as it presents opportunities to enhance both performance and safety.

33.6 REFERENCES

Belton, C., 1997, *The Principles of Riding, The Official Instruction Handbook of the German National Equestrian Federation Book 1*, (UK: Kenilworth Press).

Byström, A., Rhodin, M., von Peinen, K., Weishaupt, M.A. and Roepstorff, L., 2009, Basic kinematics of the saddle and rider in high-level dressage horses trotting on a treadmill. *Equine Veterinary Journal.* **41**(3), pp. 280–284

Devoucoux , 2011, Saddles: Chiberta (CHI) [online]. Available at: http://www.devoucoux.com/devoucoux_fr/contenu/uk/boutique_uk/fiche_prod.php ?fam=selle&prod=CHI (accessed 17 March 2011).

Edwards, E.H., 2007, *Saddlery: The Complete Guide*, (London: JA Allen)

Galloux, P., Richard, N., Dronka, T., Leard, M., Perrot, A., Jouffroy, J.L. and Cholet, A., 1994, Analysis of equine gait using three-dimensional accelerometers fixed on the saddle. *Equine Veterinary Journal Supplement.* **17**, pp. 44–47.

Hughes, M., 2008, *The Essentials of Performance Analysis*, (Oxford: Routledge).

Kang, O-D., Ryu, Y-C., Ryew, C-C., Oh, W-Y, Lee, C-E. and Kang, M-S., 2010, Comparative analyses of rider position according to skill levels during walk and trot in Jeju horse. *Human Movement Science*, **29**, pp. 956–963.

Lovett, T., Hodson-Tole, E. and Nankervis, K., 2004, A preliminary investigation of rider position during walk, trot and canter. *Equine and Comparative Exercise Physiology*, **2**, pp. 71–76.

Panni, A.S. and Tulli, A., 1994, Analysis of the movements involved in horse riding. *Journal of Sports Traumatology and Related Research*, **16**, pp. 196–205.

Peham, C., Licka, T., Kapaun, M. and Scheidl, M., 2001, A new method to quantify harmony of the horse-rider system in dressage. *Sports Engineering*, **4**, pp. 95–101.

Peham, C., Licka, T., Schobesberger, H. and Meschan, E., 2004, Influence of the rider on the variability of the equine gait. *Human Movement Science*, **23**, pp. 663–671.

Powers, P.N.R. and Harrison, A.J., 2004, Influences of a rider on the rotation of the horse-rider system during jumping. *Equine and Comparative Exercise Physiology*, **1**(1), pp. 33–40.

Schils, S.J., Greer, N.L., Stoner, L.J. and Kobluk, C.N., 1993, Kinematic analysis of the equestrian: Walk, posting trot and sitting trot. *Human Movement Science*, **12**, pp. 693–712.

Terada, K., Clayton, H.M. and Kato, K., 2006, Stabilization of wrist position during horseback riding at trot. *Equine and Comparative Exercise Physiology*, **3**, pp. 179–184.

CHAPTER 34

The effects of rider specific Pilates on rider position from a lateral view: A six week study

Eleanor Boden, Hayley Randle and Charlotte Bridgen

34.1 INTRODUCTION

Maintaining a balanced position on a horse is the basis for achieving the best performance whilst engaging in equestrian activity. The relationship between horse and rider is understood to be complex (Blokhuis *et al.*, 2008; Visser *et al.,* 2003). The performance of a rider can be affected by many variables including their balance and aspects of the horse–rider interaction. Other variables can also affect rider position including the horse's temperament, conformation and the speed at which the horse is travelling (Meyners, 2004; Blokhuis *et al.*, 2008).

34.1.1 Correct rider position

The correct rider position has been described by different authors and there is wide agreement that correct rider position results in having an effective seat (Zetterqvist, 2000; von Dietz, 2005; Blokhuis *et al.*, 2008). This is particularly important because the riders' seat is the area in direct contact with the saddle through which the horse receives signals (from the rider).

The correct position is understood to be difficult to learn, teach and maintain. If the rider is in the correct position it should be possible to draw an imaginary line between the ear, shoulder, hip and heel (ESHH) so that the stirrup leather suspended from the saddle remains perpendicular to the ground. The riders legs should be able to remain long suspended from the hip, sustained by a semi-flexed knee and a semi-flexed ankle (Meyners, 2004; Ceroni *et al.*, 2007).

Only once a sustainable rider position has been established, is it possible to convey clear messages to the horse. Studies carried out to quantify the influence of the rider on ridden horses have highlighted that an incorrect riding position may restrict the movement of the horse or in severe cases compromise the welfare and well-being (de Cocq and Back, 2004). Being able to achieve consistency with a horse is a challenge for many horse riders, particularly those who are beginners; this is not surprising as the sport of horse riding is not similar to any other athletic endeavours.

34.1.2 Pilates for horse riders

Pilates was primarily developed in order to assist immobilised wounded soldiers regain condition through carrying out a range of exercises. The importance of conditioning the core abdominal muscles and subsequently stabilising the torso was accepted and its efficacy in maintaining a more correct rider position has been widely reported (Latey, 2001; Sekendiz *et al.,* 2007).

Current Pilates practices allow parallels to be drawn with weight training regimes, both improving strength and endurance during lengths of physical exercise. Pilates has also been suggested to improve static and postural balance in dance students (Fitt *et al.,* 1993; Sekendiz *et al.,* 2007). Within the equine industry, British Dressage (BD) has suggested that Pilates will support and enable individual riders to self-assess and address personal imbalances whilst enhancing strength, muscle tone and flexibility (Donati *et al.,* 2007) in order to achieve consistency in rider position.

34.1.3 The effects of gait (pace)

Each gait of the horse comprises a different sequence of foot falls, therefore each gait must be treated and measured as an individual entity (Clayton, 1989). In order to understand the components responsible for maintaining a consistent rider position it is important to understand the way the horse's gait acts upon the rider. The most common gaits used during dressage competition are walk, 'working' trot and 'working' canter.

A 'working' gait has been described by Peham *et al.* (2001) as the most natural version of the pace; between 'extended' where the strides are opened and the overall frame of the horse becomes elongated; and 'collected' where the horse becomes a lot rounder over the back. Walk is a regular, four-time beat; trot is a diagonal, two-time gait with a moment of complete suspension between strides. Canter is made up of a three-time stride motion with a moment of suspension. Lagarde *et al.* (2005) and Peham *et al.* (2001) have found that experienced riders are more consistent with the movement of the horse as a result of the horses back moving in distinctly different ways dependent on the gait.

34.1.4 Aim

The aim of this study was to investigate if a six week course of Pilates can affect the deviation from the riders' ESHH alignment whilst mounted.

34.2 METHODS

A total of 120 trials (10 riders × four gaits × three strides) × three replicates were carried out and analysed for deviation from the ESHH alignment. The differences in rider position before, at half way (+3 weeks) and after (+6 weeks) were assessed using an ANOVA to determine the effect of gait, stride, time (week) and marker placement. The significance level was set to 0.05 (Table 34.1).

Table 34.1 ANOVA for deviation from the ESHH alignment

Variable	Degrees of freedom	F-ratio	P value
Week of Pilates	2	35.81	< 0.001
Gait	3	31.49	< 0.001
Rider	9	37.11	< 0.001
Marker position	2	4.20	< 0.05
Stride	2	24.72	< 0.001

34.2.1 Ethics and pilot study

This study was carried out with approval of the University of Central Lancashire's Ethics Committee as well as full informed consent from all the candidates who took part.

The pilot study was executed using one horse and one rider which were not taking part in the proposed study. The purpose of the pilot study was to divulge any possible problems that may have arisen during the data collection, hindering the reliability of the results. The only amendment made to the methodology prior to the data collection was the use of high visibility markers to compensate for the potential lack of natural light during the data collection sessions.

34.2.2 Basis of rider selection

Ten (n = 10) female riders with an age range of 32 ± 13.8 years participated in the study. Due to the financial implications of the study, the candidates were all volunteers. Riders self-reported level of riding experience and were considered 'advanced'.

The internationally recognised British Horse Society (BHS) qualifications were used as an indicator of ability as well as the level of affiliated British Dressage (BD) that the riders were competing at. Following Symmes and Ellis (2009), all candidates had no previous injuries and were allowed to withdraw at any stage during the six week trial period. Each rider rode their own, personally owned/trained horse during each data collection in correctly fitting, familiar equipment.

34.2.3 Rider requirements

The candidates were required to wear dark jodhpurs and a dark, well-fitting long sleeved top to facilitate the visibility of the markers as well as reduce any marker displacement as much as possible. During the three data collection sessions all riders were requested to wear familiar riding boots, hat and gloves which would encourage the rider to represent a true reflection of their normal riding position whilst being filmed (Symmes and Ellis, 2009; Lovett *et al.*, 2004).

High visibility covered markers (50mm) were placed on anatomical landmarks vertically on the riders' person located on the top of the riding hat (marker A), shoulder (marker B), hip (marker C, greater trochanter of the femur) and heel (marker D) (Figure 34.1) using a method adapted from Lagarde *et al.* (2007).

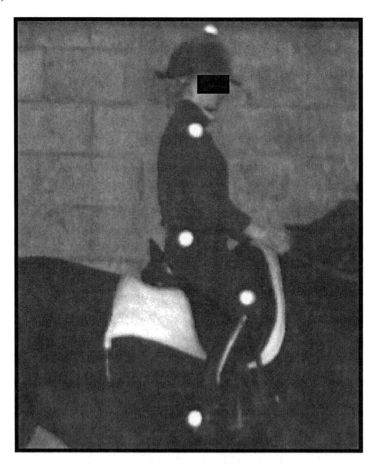

Figure 34.1 Marker placements during data collection

34.2.4 Pilates course

The Pilates course in which the riders were enlisted was a BD organised course designed to promote the key benefits of Pilates to horse riders. All six sessions over the six week trial period were conducted by a certified Pilates instructor in a fully mirrored gymnasium.

34.2.5 Data collection

The data collection was carried out in an International Arena which measured 60 metres by 40 metres on fully prepared, sand and rubber fibre mixed surface. A track was defined using dressage boards set out with 5 metres in between down the centre line, to avoid any laterality preferences of horse or rider.

After all riders had carried out a predefined 10 minute warm-up routine, each rider was required to ride down the trackway in walk, working trot, working canter left and working canter right. This sequence was repeated three times per subject.

Data validation was ensured using a 1 metre cube in each frame to enable calibration of measurements during data analysis. The data collection sessions were carried out before any Pilates sessions had taken place, after three weeks, and after the full six weeks has been completed.

34.2.6 Data analysis

Using Quintic™ Sports Biomechanics Software, measurements were collected using the hip marker to dictate the ideal alignment of the ear, shoulder, hip and heel (ESHH). The deviations of each marker, away from the ESHH alignment, were recorded (cm) in each gait for all candidates when the off forelimb was in stance phase of the stride cycle (straight, whilst in contact with the surface).

34.2.7 Statistical analysis

The raw data derived from each data collection session for each individual were analysed using a General Linear Model of Analysis of Variance (ANOVA).

34.3 RESULTS

34.3.1 Influence of gait on deviation from ESHH alignment

The gait significantly affected the deviation from the ESHH alignment ($F_{3,316} = 31.49$; $p < 0.01$). The largest variation in deviation was seen between the walk (2.9 cm ± 4.7 cm) and trot (5.5 cm ± 6.0 cm). Interestingly the direction of canter showed a difference in ESHH alignment, canter left (CL) 2.4 cm ± 6.4 cm in comparison to canter right (CR) 4.5 cm ± 5.5 cm.

34.3.2 Influence of time, post starting the Pilates treatment, on deviation

The week of data collection, subsequently number of Pilates sessions completed, showed a significant difference ($F_{2,316} = 35.81$; $p < 0.001$). Prior to the Pilates training the mean ± SD for ESHH deviation was 5.0 cm ± 7.0 cm in comparison to the half way (+3 weeks) measurements of 3.9 cm ± 5.5 cm. Upon completion a further significant decrease in ESHH deviation was seen of 3.0 cm ± 4.1 cm (Figure 34.2).

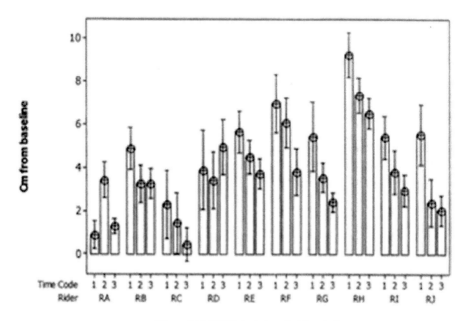

Figure 34.2 ESHH deviation of trial period

34.3.3 Influence of marker placement

The individual markers showed significant differences ($F_{2,316} = 4.20$; $p < 0.001$). The difference between marker placements highlighted the varied movements required of the body during horse riding. The marker which displayed the largest amount of deviation was the head marker, followed by the heel marker and shoulder marker respectively.

34.4 DISCUSSION

In this study it was hypothesised that a six week course of rider specific Pilates will affect rider position from a lateral view. The results of this study suggest that using

Pilates in addition to regular riding can significantly improve rider position as well as highlighting other factors which may potentially be responsible for influencing rider position.

34.4.1 Influence of rider specific Pilates course on rider position from a lateral view

The six week Pilates course has been shown to have reduced the deviation of the ESHH alignment in 8 of the 10 candidates. These findings suggest that the use of floor based, core strengthening, Pilates had the desired effect on rider position. Figure 34.2 indicates that 5 of the 10 candidates made more improvements during the first three weeks of Pilates. These initial improvements could have been influenced by the amount of horse riding carried out alongside the Pilates course which in turn would encourage immediate use of the acquired knowledge (Johnson *et al.*, 2007). Rider C (RC) and Rider G (RG) showed the greatest reduction in deviation from the ESHH alignment after the third week. The high level of competition that is already achieved suggests that these two riders already have the ability to focus on control, centring and core strength. Sekendiz *et al.* (2007) suggested that it would be expected in this instance to develop improvements later on due to requiring more established exercises to further promote core muscle strength and endurance.

34.4.2 Influence of gait and rider skill

Horse gait influences both rider position and deviation from the ESHH alignment although this may have been predictable due to the difference in stride motions (Peham *et al.*, 2004).

The gait has been shown to have a higher mean deviation from the ESHH alignment supporting the finding of Symmes and Ellis (2009) which also suggested that riders held their shoulder further forward in trot than any of the other gaits.

The difference in deviation from the ESHH alignment between CL and CR was unexpected as it is assumed that riders would be as balanced in the gait due to the familiar stride motion regardless of the direction of travel; which highlights the influence of the horse on rider position. All riders generally displayed a reduction in deviation whilst demonstrating CL.

Interestingly, past research by Warren-Smith *et al.* (2007) and Kraft *et al.* (2007) has illustrated that the rider will apply stronger force to the horse's mouth via the hands, whilst turning left than when turning right, which could subsequently have an effect on rider position.

The walk, as expected, exhibited the lowest deviation from the ESHH alignment and this finding supports Peham *et al.*'s (2004) description of the walk as not being transparent enough to enable postural imbalances as a result of it being symmetrical, four-time beat and the slowest gait.

34.5. CONCLUSION

Riding in a consistently efficient manner due to continuation and preservation of the ear, shoulder, hip and heel alignment is affected by factors such as rider skill and gait.

A six week course of rider specific Pilates has been demonstrated to be effective in achieving reduced deviation from the ear, shoulder, hip and heel alignment whilst riding in walk, trot, canter left and canter right.

34.6 REFERENCES

Blokhuis, M., Aronsson, A., Hartmann, E., van Reenan, C. and Keeling, L., 2008, Assessing the rider's seat and the horse's behaviour: Difficulties and perspectives. *Journal of Applied Animal Welfare Science.* **11**, pp. 191–203.

Ceroni, D., De Rosa, V., De Coulon, G. and Kaelin, A., 2007, The importance of proper shoe gear and safety stirrups in the prevention of equestrian foot injuries. *The Journal of Foot and Ankle Surgery*, 46(1), pp. 32–39.

Clayton, H.M., 1989. Locomotion. In: *Equine Sport Medicine*, edited by Jones, W.E. (Philadelphia: Lea and Fiebiger), pp. 149–187.

de Cocq, P. and Back, W., 2004, Effects of girth, saddle and weight on movements of the horse. *Equine Veterinary Journal*, 37 (3) p. 231.

de Cocq, P., Mariken, A., Clayton, H., Bobbert, M., Muller, M. and Van Leeuwen, J., 2010, Vertical forces on the horse's back in sitting and rising trot. *Journal of Biomechanics*, **43**, pp. 627–631.

Donati, M., Camomilla, V., Vannozzi, G. and Cappozzo, A., 2007, Enhanced anatomical calibration in human movement analysis. *Gait and Posture*, **26**, pp. 179–185.

Fitt, S., Sturman, J. and McCain-Smith, S., 1993, Effects of Pilates based conditioning on strength, alignment and range of motion in university ballet and modern dance majors. *Kinesiology and Medicine for Dance*, 16(1), pp. 36–61.

Johnson, E., Larsen, A., Ozawa, H., Wilson, C., and Kennedy., K., 2007, The effects of Pilates-based exercise on dynamic balance in healthy adults. *Bodywork and Movement Therapies*, 3(4) pp. 238–242.

Kraft, C., Urban, N., Wallney, T., Scharfadt, A., Jager, M. and Pennekamp, P., 2007, Influence of riding discipline and riding intensity on the incidence of back pain in competitive horseback riders. *Sportverletz and Sportschaden*, **21**, pp. 29–33.

Lagarde, J., Peham, C., Licka, T. and Kelso, J., 2005, Co-ordination dynamics of the horse and rider system. *Journal of Motor Behaviour*, 37(6), pp. 418–424.

Latey, P., 2001, The Pilates Method: History and Philosophy. *Bodywork and Movement Therapies*, pp. 275–282

Lovett, T., Hodson-Tole, E. and Nakervis, K., 2004, A preliminary investigation of rider position during walk, trot and canter. *Equine Comparative Exercise Physiology*, 2(2), pp. 71–76.

Meyners, E., 2004, *Effective Teaching and Riding.* (Missoula, MT: Goals Unlimited Press).

Peham, C., Licka, T., Schobesberger, H. and Meschan, E., 2001, Influence of the rider on the variability of the equine gait. *Human Movement Science*, **23**, pp. 663–671.

Sekendiz, B., Altun, O., Korkusuz, F. and Akins, S., 2007, Effects of Pilates exercises on trunk strength, endurance and flexibility in sedentary adult females. *Journal of Bodywork and Movement*, **11**, pp. 318–326.

Symmes, D. and Ellis, R., 2009, A preliminary study into rider asymmetry within equitation. *Veterinary Journal*, **181**(1), pp. 34–37.

Visser, E., Van Reenen, C., Rundgren, M., Zetterqvist, M., Morgan, K. and Blokhuis, H., 2003, Responses of horses in behavioural tests correlate with temperament assessed by riders. *Equine Veterinary Journal*, **35**, pp. 176–183.

von Dietze, S., 2005, *Balance and Movement: How to Achieve the Perfect Seat*. (Pomfret, VT: Trafalgar Square Books).

Warren-Smith, A., Curtis, R., Greetham, L. and McGreevy, P., 2007, Rein contact between horse and handler during specific equitation movements. *Applied Animal Behaviour Science*, **108**, pp. 157–169.

Zetterqvist, M., 2000, Didactics in horse jumping. *Proceedings of the 51st Annual Meeting, European Association of Animal Production*, (The Hague, The Netherlands), p. 360.

Part 7

Systems

CHAPTER 35

Use of barcode scanning for notational analysis

Donald Buchanan, David Cook and John Seeley

35.1 INTRODUCTION

Improvements in sports performance are information dependent. However, for many major sports, match play is dynamic in space and time, there are numbers of participating players and competition unfolds over approximately hour-long periods. These features make sports notation challenging. Notational techniques overcome the limitations imposed by the information-processing capacity of the human brain, memory encoding and individual bias (Franks and Miller, 1986; Franks, 2004; Breedlove *et al.*, 2010). Written accounts of notation present the variety of approaches to acquiring data, from pencil and paper methods to computer-based video processing (Reep and Benjamin, 1968; Liebermann and Franks, 2004; Carling *et al.*, 2005).

The notation method reported in this paper was developed when one of the authors was working with a non-league football club. Matches were recorded using video but there was still a need for timelines of match events – set-pieces, attempts on goal and so forth. Some of the information sought by management (on passing sequences, for example) required more detailed notation. This aspiring junior club was no different from many others: resources were limited. Even if they had been inclined to purchase one of the pieces of sophisticated software used for modern notation, they would not have had the staff to operate it. The barcode scanning method reported here was developed with this type of club in mind but is flexible enough to be used for a wide variety of notational purposes, both for real-time coding and in working from video.

35.2 THE METHOD

We have been using small, highly portable barcode scanners to make time-coded recordings of events in competitive sport, mainly football and taekwondo. In the case of football, recordings were made both in real-time and from video footage; for taekwondo, recordings were made solely from video. Competition records were tabulated, analysed and prepared for presentation using Excel software. The method operates in the following way:

1   The sport events to be recorded are coded as short, abbreviated strings of characters.

2   The event codes are arranged on a **coding sheet** as a set of text boxes in a standard font.
3   The text boxes are reformatted to barcodes using a barcode font.
4   The coding sheet is printed.
5   Barcodes are scanned as the action of live competition or the video moves forward. The event records are stored in the scanner along with the date and time of their occurrence. The times of events are recorded to the nearest second.
6   After completion of scanning, the barcode readings are downloaded as a text file to a personal computer.
7   The text file is opened within Excel and a time series of events is then compiled. Commonly, the codes are represented in standard English.
8   Additional analysis and reporting is carried out within Excel or using additional software.

We have used inexpensive Opticon barcode scanners (OPN-2001, 6.2 cm × 3.2 cm × 1.6 cm, supplied along with software by Kelgray Products, West Sussex, UK) and barcode font IDAutomation HC39M, obtained free from the IDAutomation website (www.idautomation.com). Codes for match events have normally been arranged to be made up of a standard number of characters since this makes it easier to decode the events using Excel. PowerPoint or other graphics software was used to draw up the coding sheet. Individual codes were incorporated onto the sheet as text boxes. !HCOA!, for example, might represent a corner (CO) taken by the home side (H) from the left-hand corner of the pitch (A). The leading and trailing exclamation marks are converted to asterisks when the normal text font is converted to a barcode font and signify the start and end of the barcode (Figure 35.1).

Figure 35.1 Transition from text to barcode

The code for a match event is generated in the form of a text box and begins and ends with an exclamation mark (left). Reformatting to a barcode font forms the final barcode (right).

To make scanning both easier and faster the positioning of a text box on the coding sheet matches the position of the event on the pitch. As the action and the scanning proceed the scanner moves over the coding sheet in the same manner as the ball moves over the pitch. The coding sheet is therefore arranged for spatially congruent scanning responses (Magill, 2010). Our routinely used coding sheet for football has about 130 barcodes and therefore looks somewhat forbidding (Figure 35.2). This number of codes reflects the variety of football events, the use of two codes for most events (one for each team) and our division of the pitch into 12 sections. We have two pitch representations on the sheet: one for common events such as passes and the second for less common events such as goals and free kicks (Figure 35.2). It has been convenient to use a standard sheet and to aggregate events in the match report according to need. Naturally, many reports could make do with far fewer barcodes. More details on barcodes are reported below under Supporting Investigations.

Coding sheets were normally drawn up using the graphical features of PowerPoint. The figure shows a coding sheet in which the spatial distribution of events is of primary interest. The pitch is divided into 12 sections and reproduced schematically twice over – on the left for frequent match events (completed passes, throw-ins etc) and on the right for infrequent events (free kicks, shots on- and off-target, goals etc). There are normally two barcodes, one for each team. The bottom sections of home team barcodes are covered here with a semi-transparent blue rectangle.

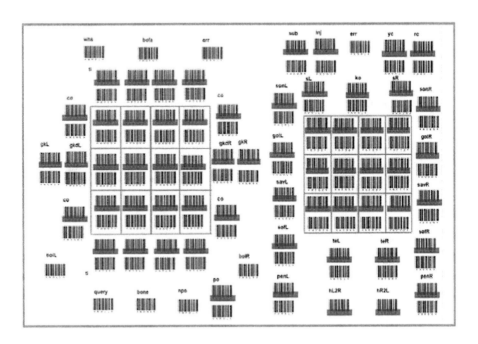

Figure 35.2 Coding sheet for football

The scanner links to a personal computer via a USB connection. This is the means of charging the device. We have routinely scanned approximately 1,000 events for each football match, which is well within the storage capacity of the scanner (ca. 3,000 scans) and its battery life (ca. 10,000 scans). Recorded scans are downloaded to a computer using simple software, which controls operation of the scanner, acquisition/deletion of scanned codes and time settings. A graph of events for a single football match is shown in Figure 35.3 and illustrates both the number and variety of events recorded. This was prepared for sports science purposes. Reports to clubs consist of a timeline of main events (goals, shots, corners and so forth) and aggregate statistics by (decoded) event type, which are readily calculated using Excel functions.

35.3 SUPPORTING INVESTIGATIONS

Sometimes, in initial testing of the scanner, it failed to record a barcode (as registered by the instrument failing to generate a confirmatory "beep"). This raised concerns about its reliability for sports purposes and we therefore undertook an extensive series of tests that related to barcode size, colour and print quality and the distance and orientation of the axis of the scanner head relative to the barcode.

Barcodes were inkjet printed in a range of font sizes from 8 to 32 point in black, blue, dark blue, dark purple, green and light blue colours. As font size decreased there were increasing numbers of failed scans. A 12-point font size was selected as a standard for testing since this was sufficiently large to be scanned with good reliability yet sufficiently small to allow fair numbers of barcodes to be printed on the A3 coding sheet. (Laser printing of barcodes does reduce usable font size.) The scanner was normally held approximately 5 cm from the code with the long axis of the scanner head parallel to the long axis of the barcode.

In testing, the conjoint responses of the operator and scanner were recorded using a combination of Best Metronome and Audacity 1.3.12 software (both available as free downloads from the Internet). The metronome software delivered both a visual and an auditory stimulus. On the **visual** metronome command the operator scanned the barcode under test whilst recording both the metronome tick and the scanner beep using Audacity software. The time interval between metronome tick and scanner beep were measured from the Audacity intensity–time trace for recorded sounds. The scanner tests therefore mimicked the sports situations of interest. For each test situation 230 separate trials were made, arranged in a manner that minimised any anticipation by the operator.

Response times for the variously coloured barcodes (mean ± standard deviation) ranged between 0.42 ± 0.08 s (dark blue) and 0.57 ± 0.18 s (dark purple). Whilst there were statistically significant differences in response times for the different colours (data not given) there were **no functionally significant differences** for this colour set. Since there were differences – albeit small – in response times for different colours, the original idea of printing barcodes in inks corresponding to team colours was abandoned. A see-through coloured rectangle was printed over the base section of one player's/team's barcodes, as seen in

Figure 35.2. In this way, rapid, accurate selection of the appropriate code could be made but the actual scans were invariably of a black barcode.

Scanner responses to red barcodes were rather different. Six different shades of red were used for the barcodes in this test. For five of the sets, responses ranged between 0.64 ± 0.40 s and 1.09 ± 0.77 s with increases in both the average response time and the variability in responses. Failed scans ranged between 2 per cent and 50 per cent and averaged at 27 per cent for the five sets. For a sixth set and a particular shade of red the scanner completely failed to respond. We concluded that red should not be used for barcodes but have found red to be a useful, non-interfering colour in marking up grids on coding forms. (Other, darker lines do interfere with scanning.)

The scanner failed to record 0.8 per cent of scans over the 3,320 tests of colour, distance and orientation (red barcodes not included). The failure rate appeared to increase somewhat for oblique orientations and light-coloured barcodes. One per cent could therefore be taken as an upper limit on scan failure rate under normal scanning conditions.

The influence of distance between scanner and barcode was tested using black barcodes over the range 3 to 7 cm, being the likely extreme range of distances for real-time scanning of sports events. Scanning distance was controlled by a measured piece of string attached to the scanner. There was a slight (statistically significant) increase in response time with distance: 0.43 ± 0.08 s for 5 cm; 0.45 ± 0.13 s for 7 cm. Clearly this effect is unimportant in terms of usage.

Increasing the angle between the scanner long axis and the long axis of the barcode also increased response times. Angles were measured by attaching the scanner to a NokiaTM N900 phone that was running the Angle meter SW application. For standard black barcodes and a 5 cm scanning distance observed values were: 0.43 ± 0.08 s (0 degrees); 0.49 ± 0.14 s (40 degrees); 0.52 ± 0.17 s (angle just less than diagonal to the barcode). Functionally, the orientation of the scanner has negligible influence on scanning operations. Overall the scanner operated in a highly reliable manner, variations in response times all lying within the 1 s time increment that is recorded by the scanner.

Limited testing of the repeatability of event scanning was carried out using video footage of football matches. Over four 45-minute periods, 98 per cent of events were recorded on a scan–rescan basis as occurring within a period of 2 seconds. Of the remaining 2 per cent, 1.4 per cent of those disagreements involved assignment of the same event to adjacent sections of the football pitch.

35.4 MATCH EVENTS

We routinely use the standard recording conditions that were derived from our investigations of the scanner. Figure 35.3 shows a timeline of events for a non-league football match. For judgements of difficult events (shots on-/off-target, for example) a scan–rescan approach was adopted. For taekwondo notation, for which this method has also been employed, repeated scanning was used with a defined set of events being notated for each viewing of the video footage.

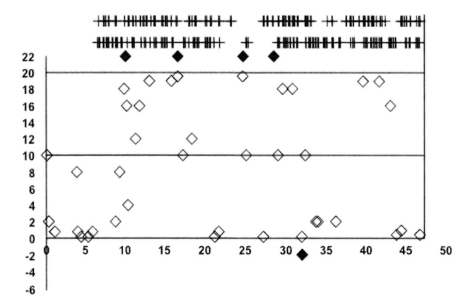

Figure 35.3 Match events in football

Figure 35.3 shows a timeline of match events for one half of a football match. Match time in minutes is on the horizontal axis. Away team goals are represented by a vertical axis value of 22 and the home team goal by a value of −2. Completed passes are recorded on the top two lines from 7 minutes in. Other symbols represent corners, goal kicks, goalkeeper distributions, kick-offs, shots on goal and throw-ins. Approximately 1,000 events were recorded in real-time over a match.

35.5 DISCUSSION

Our initial scepticism over the reliability of scanning was perhaps the result of working with smaller, poorly printed barcodes. It proved to be entirely unfounded. Both careful testing and use of scanning in practice has established the high reliability of the method.

The notation work for football has focused on the distribution of match events about the pitch (Carling *et al.*, 2005). This is evident in the spatial arrangement of barcodes in Figure 35.3. Since this barcode scanning method is readily adaptable, an alternative focus on player actions could be arranged. Real-time scanning of match events is readily achievable after quite modest practice with the method (Magill, 2010) and, for football matches, we were routinely recording events at 3–5 second intervals. Our coding sheet included a query code that signified judgements that required confirmation from subsequent viewing of video footage (Franks and Miller, 1986). Estimation of shots as being on- or off-target is another situation that required use of video. One might view the scanning method as involving a single scan for the many readily judged match events and double scan for a small minority of judgements. The arrangement of scanning was quite different for taekwondo, for which many judgements are difficult and much of match play involves rapid event sequences. Scanning of taekwondo involved repeated scanning of the entire match with the operator focusing on only a limited number of events for each run. The match report is a summation of the separate scanning replays. Since taekwondo matches commonly occupy less than 10 minutes in total, the re-scanning approach is not particularly arduous, though it does require careful "clapperboard" synchronisation to mark the start of each round of a fight.

Many commercial notation products such as the SportsCode suite seamlessly integrate video streams and sports event marking. Whilst the barcode scanning method is a low-cost option and is relatively straightforward to operate, it does not provide convenient integration of data and video (SportsCode Gamebreaker Manual, 2012). However, given the direct access to raw data and the options for graph plotting using Excel or other packages, the barcode method can provide convenient opportunities to represent event timelines and various measures of match flow. As recorded in relation to barcode use for both football and taekwondo, the method is adaptable in operation. We conclude that barcode scanning is a useful addition to the range of tools available for sports notation.

35.6 REFRENCES

Breedlove, S.M., Watson, N.V. and Rosenzweig, M.R., 2010, *Biological Psychology, 6th edn*, (Sunderland, MA: Sinauer Associates).

Carling, C., Williams, A.M. and Reilly, T., 2005, *Handbook of Soccer Match Analysis*, (London and New York: Routledge).

de Coq, P. and Back, W., 2004, Effects of girth, saddle and weight on movements of the horse. *Equine Veterinary Journal*, 37 (3) p. 231.

Franks, I.M., 2004, The need for feedback, In *Notational Analysis of Sport, 2nd edn*, edited by Hughes, M. and Franks, I.M. (London and New York: Routledge), pp. 8–16.

Franks, I.M. and Miller, G., 1986, Eyewitness testimony in sport. *Journal of Sport Behaviour*, **9**, pp. 39–45.

Liebermann, D.G. and Franks, I.M., 2004, The use of feedback-based technologies, In *Notational analysis of Sport, 2nd edn*, edited by Hughes, M. and Franks, I.M. (London and New York: Routledge), pp. 40–58.

Magill, R.A., 2010, *Motor Learning and Control, 9th edn*, (New York: McGraw-Hill).

Reep, C. and Benjamin, B., 1968, Skill and chance in association football. *Journal of the Royal Statistical Society A*, **131**, pp. 581–585.

SportsCode Gamebreaker Manual, 2012 (Warriewood, Australia: Sportstec).

CHAPTER 36

Using spatial metrics to characterize behaviour in small-sided games

António Lopes, Sofia Fonseca, Roland Leser, Arnold Baca
and Ana Paulo

36.1 INTRODUCTION

In team sports, each player seeks to coordinate with his/her team players in order to achieve a common goal (McGarry *et al.*, 2002). Thus, a team can be studied as a multi-agent action system (Saltzman and Kelso, 1987) when described by the interactions of its components – e.g., team-players. This interpersonal coordination is specific to task constraints (Araújo *et al.*, 2004) and self-organized structures, like offensive and defensive patterns that describe the system's/team's behaviour, that can emerge from these complex interpersonal interactions of performers (McGarry *et al.*, 2002; McGarry and Franks, 2007). Individual and collective playing behaviour in team sports can be subsumed under the term "tactics". Teodorescu (1984) defined tactics from a traditional viewpoint as a group of collective and individual norms and behaviours aiming for a successful performance from an active and conscious contribution during the game. On the other hand, Jäger *et al.* (2007) outline that tactical behaviour includes both individual and team tactics in certain game situations and it usually refers to the athletes' actions. They emphasize that the position of every athlete of a team on the playing court is strongly influenced by the tactical concept of that team, adding that configurations of a team vary from one moment to another and they may thus be considered as a time dependent process. From this relation, spatial patterns emerge representing the players' behaviour. According to Garganta (2009), tactical features in team sports strongly depend on the strengths of the opponent, the cooperation within a team and the capability of technical skills in order to act efficiently in specific playing conditions. Thus, a team's playing behaviour is constrained not only by its opponent, but also by its components (players) and by their individual action capabilities. This information is extremely pertinent when creating a representative task design, that is, with constraints similar to those present in competition settings (Davids *et al.*, 2006). For instance, some examples of relevant constraints, in association football, are the active role of opponents (Vilar *et al.*, 2012) and the distance to goal (Headrick *et al.*, 2012), which players typically use to organize their actions during performance.

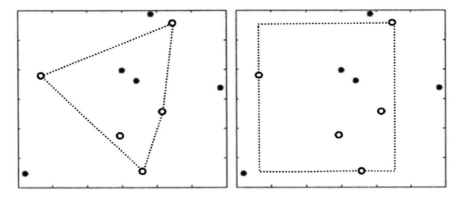

Figure 36.1 Examples of the convex hull (left) and bounding rectangle (right) for one of the two teams (white dots). The dots represent the position of the players of each team (black dots and white dots) in a given moment

In soccer and indoor soccer training, small-sided games (SSGs) are often used as they are "an optimal task to optimize training time by fulfilling the broad range of fitness requirements without compromising skill performance and decision-making" (Aguiar *et al.*, 2012). Actually, SSGs are one of the most addressed topics in contemporary soccer research (Hill-Haas *et al.*, 2009).

McGarry (2009) mentioned a couple of issues that scientific sport performance analysis should focus on in order to improve their outcomes in future. From these aspects the author stressed a) "increased attention should be paid to further developing an understanding of the associations between sports behaviours and sports outcomes"; b) "the interactions between opposing players and/or teams is key for interpreting game behaviour"; c) "the context in which the sports behaviours are produced offer important information for game analysis"; and d) "the behaviours of players both with and without possession of the sports article must be considered for a complete assessment of game performance" (p. 128).

A proper method of assessing tactical team performance in game sports is the observation of spatial organization (Garganta, 2009). An important parameter for analysing spatial patterns is the space covered by a whole team according to various spatial metrics (Bartlett *et al.*, 2012; Frencken *et al.*, 2011; Seabra and Luis, 2006). Examples of these metrics are the convex hull (CH) – the smallest convex set that contains all the players of a team, and the bounding rectangle (BR) – the smallest rectangle that contains all the players of a team (Bourbousson *et al.*, 2010; McGarry, 2009), as illustrated in Figure 36.1.

The area of the geometric forms mentioned above is often considered to be a characteristic of the tactical team behaviour (McGarry, 2009; Bourbousson *et al.*, 2010). However, that area is calculated for each team considering solely the position of all players of a team, which encloses two problems: i) configurations are only based on the players' location ignoring where they are on the field (sports related boundaries are ignored); ii) the possibility of having overlapped shapes is also ignored, which means that it may happen to have players from

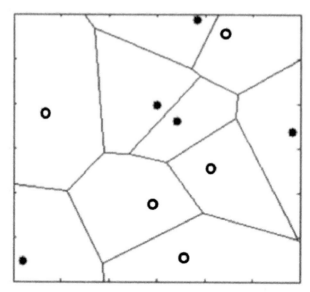

Figure 36.2 Example of the Generalized Voronoi Diagram generated for the set of coordinates of the players from two teams

both teams inside a common area, which is relevant information regarding the tactics of both teams. In order to deal with these limitations, Generalized Voronoi Diagrams (GVDs) can be used as an additional analysis parameter (Fonseca *et al.*, 2012a). This spatial construction defines specific regions on the playing field associated with each player, and hence each team, according to the field boundaries as well as to the position of all players (Figure 36.2).

Taki *et al.* (1996) and Fujimura and Sugihara (2005) have considered this construct to introduce their concept of players' dominant regions, which was defined as the region that a player can arrive earlier than all the others (Taki *et al.*, 1996). Given this, the area covered by a team can be derived by the sum of the area of the Voronoi cells of the respective players (Fonseca *et al.*, 2012a), which overcome the limitations previously mentioned.

The purpose of this work is to study team tactical behaviour in a small-sided indoor soccer game based on the players' spatial configurations. For this, different spatial constructions were investigated in order to identify the best candidate to describe such behaviour.

36.2 METHODS

36.2.1 Sample and procedure

The players and ball trajectories were collected from an indoor small-sided amateur soccer game in a 5 vs. 5 situation, with four trials with a total duration of

30 minutes, in a 33 m × 18 m field. To track players and ball positional data across each trial duration, Ubisense Location System (Leser *et al.*, 2011) was used. The area of each spatial metric defined above (CH, BR and GVD) was calculated for each team across the duration of each trial, which varied between 401 and 490 seconds, using routines implemented in Matlab® R2008a software (The MathWorks Inc, USA). The resulting time series data were considered for analysis.

36.2.2 Data analysis

In order to quantify the regularity of the spatial behaviour of each team, the normalized measure of approximate entropy (Fonseca *et al.*, 2012b), $ApEn_{RatioRandom}$ (ApEnRR) was calculated for each metric's time series. ApEnRR is the ratio between the ApEn value of a series and the mean ApEn of 100 random series of the same size. In order to assess the degree of predictability of the observed behaviour, the 95 per cent confidence interval for random behaviour was determined according to formulae given by the same authors. Also, the Pearson correlation coefficient was considered to evaluate the inter-team spatial relationship, as it is hypothesized that the teams' spatial organization presents a strong and negative correlation (Frencken *et al.*, 2011).

36.3 RESULTS

36.3.1 ApEn

The 95 per cent confidence interval for random behaviour was [0.94; 1.06], considering n = 450. For all spatial metrics, the obtained value of ApEnRR (Table 36.1) is below the lower reference limit (i.e., 0.94), which indicates that the observed spatial behaviour deviates from a random behaviour, being more regular.

Table 36.1 Normalized ApEn calculated for each spatial metric, trial and team from players' positional data (n is the duration of the trial in seconds)

Metric	Team	Trial 1 (n = 490)	Trial 2 (n = 465)	Trial 3 (n = 434)	Trial 4 (n = 401)
BR Area	A	0.801	0.780	0.761	0.760
	B	0.641	0.724	0.778	0.766
CH Area	A	0.761	0.794	0.721	0.760
	B	0.652	0.751	0.826	0.695
VD Area	A	0.697	0.717	0.790	0.708
	B	0.698	0.721	0.794	0.708

Table 36.2 Pearson correlation coefficient values, for each trial and spatial metric

Trial	BR area	CH area	GVD area
1	0.06	−0.03	−1.00
2	0.00	0.05	−1.00
3	0.00	−0.01	−1.00
4	−0.21	−0.13	−1.00

36.3.2 Pearson Coefficient

As shown in Table 36.2, both BR and CH areas measured for the two teams present low values of correlation, as it was found in previous work from Frencken *et al.* (2011), which indicates that the expected inverse relation of the team areas is not captured by these two spatial metrics. On the other hand, the GVD of the two teams present a perfect negative linear correlation (Table 36.2), indicating that this spatial metric is a strong candidate to describe the spatial interaction behaviour observed in invasive team sports.

In order to assess the ability of each spatial metric to describe the tactical behaviour of each team, a sequence of a shooting attempt from team B was extracted from the game, which evolves sequentially as described next:

1 Team B starts the sequence near its goal;
2 Team A forms a first pressure line;
3 Team B passes the ball to the goalkeeper while trying to create space;
4 Team B progresses in the field;
5 Team A forms a second pressure line in the midfield while team B protects and keeps the ball in possession;
6 Team B invades the opponents midfield with the ball;
7 Team A closes the space near the goal;
8 Team B shoots at goal and misses the target.

Figure 36.3 presents each of the three spatial metrics during this sequence, where the periods 1–3, 4–6 and 7–8 are highlighted with shading. Note that the period 4–6 (III) corresponds to a transition of the attacking team (B) to the opponent's midfield which appears to be well captured by the GVD areas. In addition, in the periods 7–8, the GVD area better captures the increase of team B's area (attacking team) and the decrease of team A's (defending team).

36.4 DISCUSSION

The current work aimed to study team tactical behaviour in a small-sided indoor soccer game, considering the players' spatial configuration. The intent was to identify the best candidate from three different spatial constructions: BR, CH and GVD.

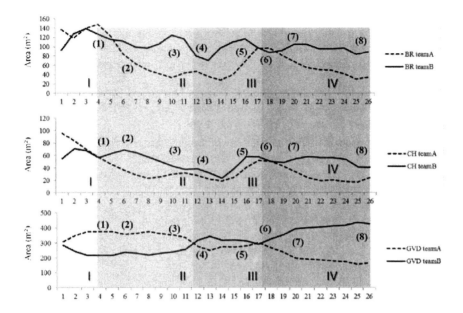

Figure 36.3 Each of the three spatial metrics during a shooting attempt sequence from team B

Data showed that teams changed their behaviours through the match. The different spatial metrics provided similar, but different, information about how teams used space by means of tactics.

The analysis of these measures has shown that the dispersion of the teams in the field tends to follow a dynamical teams' counter-phase (Yue *et al.*, 2008). In other words the area or dominant region of a team tends to contract when the opposite team area expands (Frencken *et al.*, 2011), and this was best reported by the GVD. This kind of pattern collective behaviour seems to be associated with the ball possession changes and/or disputes between teams' in play, following the results of Bourbousson *et al.* (2010), when they used similar spatial metrics (stretch index). In the example presented in Figure 36.3, the GVD appears to be the best candidate to show where/when the ball disputes happened between team (4–6, III).

The team dominant region seems to be affected by the ball position and possession, thus resulting in more or less regularity of the players' position (Taki *et al.*, 1996), which can be measured with normalized ApEn, giving the chance to assess the degree of complexity of the game within the agents' interaction.

One can argue that the regularity found in the different measures of spatial behaviour used in this work, might be related to the teams' and players' levels (novice and amateurs) in this specific task, since the spatial distribution of the player in the performed task might be dependent on the continuous set of organismic, environmental and task-related constraints offered by the system (Glazier *et al.*, 2003) throughout the game. Further research is needed to verify the current findings, due to the limited generality of this work, but still it has allowed us to identify some key events that emerge from collective patterns.

Although these spatial metrics can be considered to characterize teams' collective behaviour, more questions have arisen along this work, in particular, a number of relevant methodological and applied questions concerning the use of spatial metrics to characterize team tactical behaviour, still remain unclear and unanswered:

- Which geometrical forms should be considered to study team tactical behaviour?
- Can the identified limitations for convex hull and bounding rectangle be addressed in a different manner? (e.g., considering the overlapped region);
- Should the teams' surface areas be weighted by a specific variable? (e.g., distance from ball, distance from field boundaries, players' skills, motion direction);
- And finally, can these spatial metrics be applied to all team sports and/or game moments, or need they to be adapted with rules to specific games and "phases", in order to describe teams' tactical behaviour and compare to the principles that regulate them?

36.5 ACKNOWLEDGEMENTS

The first author gratefully acknowledges the support of the Spanish Government project Observación de la interacción en deporte y actividad física: Avances técnicos y metodológicos en registros automatizados cualitativos-cuantitativos (Secretaría de Estado de Investigación, Desarrollo e Innovación del Ministerio de Economía y Competitividad) during the period 2012–2015 (Grant DEP2012–32124).

The fifth author is being supported by a grant of the Portuguese Foundation for Science and Technology (SFRH/BD/68692/2010).

36.6 REFERENCES

Aguiar, M., Botelho, G., Lago, C., Maças, V. and Sampaio, J., 2012, A review on the effects of soccer small-sided games. *Journal of Human Kinetics*, **33**, pp. 103–113.
Araújo, D., Davids, K., Bennett, S.J., Button, C. and Chapman, G., 2004, Emergence of sport skills under constraints. In *Skill Acquisition in Sport: Research, Theory and Practice*, edited by Williams, A.M. and Hodges, N.J. (London and New York: Routledge), pp. 409–433.
Bartlett, R., Button, C., Robins, M. and Dutt-Mazumder, A., 2012, Analysing team coordination patterns from player movement trajectories in soccer: Methodological considerations. *International Journal of Performance Analysis in Sport*, 12, pp. 398–424.

Bourbousson, J., Sèvee, C. and McGarry, T., 2010, Space-time coordination dynamics in basketball: Part 2. The interaction between the two teams. *Journal of Sports Sciences*, **28**, pp. 349–358.

Davids, K., Button, C., Araújo, D., Renshaw, I. and Hristovski, R., 2006, Movement models from sports provide representative task constraints for studying adaptive behavior in human movement systems. *International Society for Adaptive Behavior*, **14**(1), pp. 73–95.

Fonseca, S., Milho, J., Travassos, B. and Araújo, D., 2012a, Spatial dynamics of team sports exposed by Voronoi diagrams. *Human Movement Science,* **31**(6), pp.1652–1659.

Fonseca, S., Milho, J., Passos, P., Araújo, D. and Davids, K., 2012b, Approximate entropy normalized measures for analyzing social neurobiological systems. *Journal of Motor Behavior*, **April**, pp. 37–41. doi:10.1080/00222895.2012. 668233.

Frencken, W., Lemmink, K., Delleman, N. and Visscher, C., 2011, Oscillations of centroid position and surface area of soccer teams in small-sided games. *European Journal of Sport Science*, **11**(4), pp. 215–223. doi:10.1080/17461391. 2010.499967.

Fujimura, A. and Sugihara, K., 2005, Geometric analysis and quantitative evaluation of sport teamwork. *Systems and Computers in Japan*, **36**(6), pp. 49–58. doi:10.1002/scj.20254

Garganta, J., 2009, Trends of tactical performance analysis in team sports: Bridging the gap between research, training and competition. *Revista Portuguesa de Ciências do Desporto*, **9**(1), pp. 81–89.

Glazier, P.S., Davids, K. and Bartlett, R.M., 2003, Dynamical systems theory: A relevant framework from performance-oriented sports biomechanics research. *Sportscience*, **7**, pp. 85–92.

Headrick, J., Davids, K., Renshaw, I., Araújo, D., Passos, P. and Fernandes, O., 2012, Proximity-to-goal as a constraint on patterns of behaviour in attacker-defender dyads in team games. *Journal of Sports Sciences*, **30**(3), pp. 247–253. doi:10.1080/02640414.2011.640706.

Hill-Haas, S.V., Rowsell, G.J., Dawson, B.T. and Coutts, A.J., 2009, Acute physiological responses and time-motion characteristics of two small-sided training regimes in youth soccer players. *Journal of Strength and Conditioning Research*, **23**(1), pp. 111–115. doi:10.1519/JSC.0b013e31818efc1a.

Jäger, J.M., Perl, J. and Schöllhorn, W.I., 2007, Analysis of players' configurations by means of artificial neural networks. *International Journal of Performance Analysis in Sport*, **7**(3), pp. 90–105.

Leser, R., Baca, A. and Ogris, G., 2011, Local positioning systems in (game) sports. *Sensors*, **11**, 9778–9797. doi:10.3390/s111009778.

McGarry, T., 2009, Applied and theoretical perspectives of performance analysis in sport: Scientific issues and challenges. *International Journal of Performance Analysis in Sport*, **9**(1), pp. 128–140.

McGarry, T. and Franks, I.M., 2007, System approach to games and competitive playing: Reply to Lebed, 2006. *European Journal of Sport Science*, **7**(1), pp. 47–53. doi:10.1080/17461390701216831.

McGarry, T., Anderson, D.I., Wallace, S.A., Hughes, M.D. and Franks, I.M., 2002, Sport competition as a dynamical self-organizing system. *Journal of Sports Sciences*, **20**(10), pp. 771–781.

Saltzman, E. and Kelso, J.A.S., 1987, Skilled actions: A task-dynamic approach, *Psychological Review*, **94**(1), pp. 84–106.

Seabra, F. and Luis, D., 2006, Space definition for match analysis in soccer. *International Journal of Performance Analysis in Sport*, **6**(2), pp. 97–113.

Taki, T. and Hasegawa, J., 2000, Quantitative measurement of teamwork in ball games using dominant region. *International Archives of Photogrammetry and Remote Sensing*, **XXXIII** (Supplement B5), pp. 125–131.

Taki, T., Hasegawa, J. and Fukumura, T., 1996, Development of motion analysis system for quantitative evaluation of teamwork in soccer games. In *International Conference on Image Processing, Proceedings*, Vol III.

Teodorescu, L., 1984, *Problemas de teoria e metodologia nos jogos desportivos*, (Lisboa: Livros Horizonte).

Vilar, L., Araújo, D., Davids, K. and Renshaw, I., 2012, The need for 'representative task design' in evaluating efficacy of skills tests in sport: A comment on Russell, Benton and Kingsley (2010). *Journal of Sports Sciences*, 30, pp.1727–1730.

Yue, Z., Broich, H., Seifriz, F. and Mester, J., 2008, Mathematical analysis of a soccer game. Part I: Individual and collective behaviours. *Studies in Applied Mathematics*, 2008, **121**, pp. 223–243.

CHAPTER 37

Application of three time motion analysis systems in semi-professional soccer match play

Jason Cook

37.1 INTRODUCTION

Time motion analysis systems have been utilised in elite level soccer to quantify the demands of match play via distances covered, running intensity and activity patterns (Di Salvo *et al.*, 2007). However, investigations specific to semi-professional soccer are limited, with a lack of infrastructure for semi-automated tracking systems which have been utilised in studies investigating positional work rate demands at an elite level (Di Salvo *et al.*, 2007).

Global positioning systems (GPS) have been validated in regards to analysing the physiological demands of intermittent activity (Coutts and Duffield, 2010; Portas *et al.*, 2010); however, obtaining permission to utilise the methodology in soccer match play is challenging. The application and the interchangeable usage of semi-automatic and GPS monitoring systems have been investigated by Harley *et al.* (2011) and Randers *et al.* (2010) in elite subject groups, with findings suggesting that conclusions regarding player work rate should not be formed when employing systems interchangeably.

Alternative methodologies utilised within previous literature which overcome the constraints of regulations regarding GPS usage include video analysis (Bloomfield *et al.*, 2007) and computer based tracking (Edgecomb and Norton, 2006; Burgess *et al.*, 2012). Post *et al.* (2010) suggest that video analysis is an accurate and repeatable methodology when estimating distances travelled during match play. However, limitations of video analysis methodologies include the lack of real-time analysis and the time consuming nature of the analysis process, as well as the subjective observation of player movement which may be exposed to observational errors in the analysis process (Edgecomb and Norton, 2006).

Computer based tracking software has been utilised in time motion analysis investigations within Australian Rules football (Edgecomb and Norton, 2006; Burgess *et al.*, 2012) and involves observation by an allocated tracker to mechanically track the speed and movement pattern of the player being analysed. The accuracy of the system is therefore dependent on the observational skills of the 'tracker' and subjective observations of player movement and speeds (Burgess *et al.*, 2012). The reliance upon subjective observations could lead to errors during the data collection; however, as with video analysis it does not compromise regulations as experienced with GPS systems.

The quantification of match play demands can facilitate the development of specific training loads which assist in player development and match play preparation (Di Salvo *et al.*, 2007; Burgess *et al.*, 2012). Current practice allows the monitoring of training loads via GPS monitors; however, with constraints associated with the use of GPS monitors in competitive match play, alternative methodologies such as video analysis or computer based tracking systems are implemented at semi-professional level. The area is of specific interest if the systems are to be used interchangeably to monitor training and match play demands throughout a season. Therefore the purpose of this study was to investigate the application of three time motion analysis systems in monitoring the movement demands of semi-professional soccer match play, assessing the concurrent level of data collected by three contrasting methodologies

37.2 METHODS

Five male semi-professional soccer players were recruited for the study (age 24 ± 0.4 years; body mass 77.2 ± 1.4 kg; stature 1.78 ± 0.06 m). All participants were recruited for the study based on playing position (midfield) and were all regular starters in their respective teams. All participants gave informed consent to participate in the study, which had received local ethical clearance. All participants were examined in six competitive match play situations via three time motion analysis systems. To account for the small sample size data collected were analysed according to the half of match play in which it occurred. Participant activity profiles were assessed during match play via global positioning systems (GPS) (SPI Pro 5Hz, GPSports, Canberra, Australia), computer based tracking software (Trak Performance v 3.2, Sportstec, Warriewood, NSW, Australia) and video based analysis (SportsCode Pro v 8.0, Sportstec, Warriewood, NSW, Australia). Five categories of intensity were considered during the study 0–11 km.hour^{-1} (standing, walking, jogging); 11–14 km.hour^{-1} (low speed running); 14–19 km.hour^{-1} (moderate speed running); 19–23 km.hour^{-1} (high speed running); >23 km.hour^{-1} (sprinting).

37.2.1 Global positioning system

Each participant was fitted with a GPS athlete tracking device via a sleeveless garment which was equipped with a pocket to house the device. The monitor was located above the mid-point of the shoulder blades and worn for the duration of match play. Data were extracted from each receiver post match via team AMS software.

37.2.2 Computer based tracking

Video recordings were collected using five digital cameras (Sony HDR-FX1000 Handycam, Sony, UK). All cameras were positioned level with the half way line at an elevation of approximately 10 m. Each camera tracked the movement of one participant throughout match play. Sufficient zoom and a radius of approximately 5 m around the tracked participant were maintained at all times during match play. Computer based tracking software was used retrospectively in accordance with the captured video to track the participants' movement on a scaled image of the playing area provided by the software throughout the duration of match play. Prior to commencement of data collection, repeated video analysis to track a participant undertaking a football specific track test (adapted from Portas *et al.,* 2010) was used and the tracker required to demonstrate an intra-observer technical error in distance covered in each speed zone of less than 5 per cent before data collection could commence (Burgess *et al.* 2012).

37.2.3 Video analysis

Initially each participant performed a 10 m locomotor test via electronic timing gates (IRD T175 system, Brower, USA) in each of the predefined categories of intensity used in the study. Each participant started locomotor activity 3 m prior to the starting timing gate and repeated the test 5 times per speed zone. Individual participant mean times for each category of intensity were calculated and used in the equation (distance = speed × time) to predict the distances travelled in each category of intensity post video analysis. The match play video recordings were analysed using a specific template including the five categories of intensity via video computer playback software. Time motion analysis using video analysis was based on the prediction of distance in each speed zone using the speed from the 10 m locomotor test and the total time recorded in each category of intensity during match play. Initially intra-observer technical error was assessed using a football specific track test (adapted from Portas, *et al.,* 2010) with a technical error of 5 per cent deemed acceptable measured against the distance of the football track test. As suggested by Duthie *et al.* (2003), 15 minute segments of each game included in the study were analysed twice to test for intra-observer reliability in each speed zone. A 5 per cent level of error in regards to distance covered in each speed zone was deemed acceptable in the study.

37.2.4 Statistical analysis

Statistical Package for Social Sciences (SPSS v 19, an IBM company, Armonk, New York, USA) was used to quantify the level of agreement between two different time motion analysis systems measuring the same parameter (distance covered). Levels of agreement between the time motion analysis systems were measured using Bland and Altman's (1986) 95 per cent limits of agreement. All results are presented as systematic bias ± random error.

37.3 RESULTS

Greater levels of agreement were recorded between the GPS and video analysis methodology in all speed zones than the GPS compared to the computer based tracking methodology, with greater systematic bias and random error evident throughout all speed zones between GPS and computer based tracking software. Greater levels of random error were found at higher speed zone intensities when comparing GPS to computer based and video analysis methodologies. Video analysis reported lower distances at intensities >19 km.hour^{-1} than those recorded by GPS. Lowest systematic bias and random error values were found at the standing, walking, jogging speed zone intensity (0–11 km.hour^{-1}) when comparing GPS with video analysis, suggesting the greatest level of agreement between the two systems at this intensity. Comparisons in total distance covered during match play elicited greater systematic bias than random error in both methodological comparisons, with the computer based tracking and video analysis reporting greater total distances than those recorded by GPS (Table 37.1).

Table 37.1 Comparison of GPS with computer based tracking and video analysis systems in regards to the mean difference and the range of mean differences between each of the systems when measuring distance travelled during match play (m) (systematic bias ± random error)

GPS compared with	Total distance	0–11 km.hour^{-1}	11–14 km.hour^{-1}	14–19 km.hour^{-1}	19–23 km.hour^{-1}	>23 km.hour^{-1}
Computer tracking	251.70 ± 80.94	41.81 ± 22.10	50.65 ± 19.21	46.92 ± 40.63	40.43 ± 54.08	47.85 ± 60.80
Video analysis	191.23 ± 41.70	15.38 ± 10.46	42.89 ± 15.35	33.92 ± 21.21	−24.06 ± 29.14	−10.07 ± 26.07

37.4 DISCUSSION

The present study investigated the application of three time motion analysis systems in semi-professional soccer match play with a focus on the concurrent nature of the data collected by the GPS compared to computer based tracking and video analysis. GPS technology has recently been validated in regards to the analysis of intermittent activity (Coutts and Duffield, 2010; Portas *et al.*, 2010) and is utilised in training load monitoring at various levels of competition. However, the restrictions of usage within match play means the use of alternative methodologies if longitudinal monitoring of match play is required to accompany the monitoring of training load via GPS.

In regards to the results of this study greater levels of agreement were found between GPS and video analysis than GPS and computer based tracking systems in relation to total distance covered. In regards to the computer based tracking methodology Edgecomb and Norton (2006) found greater distances to be recorded by computer based tracking software than GPS technology; however, these findings were from a methodology lacking in sport specific movement patterns. The inclusion of football specific movements in this current study may have contributed to the lower level of agreement found between the two systems.

Focusing on high intensity speed zones (>19 km.hour^{-1}) the video analysis methodology recorded lower distances covered than GPS, a finding concurrent with those of Randers *et al.* (2010), with previous investigations focusing upon the application of GPS suggesting that error in sampling increases with increasing velocities (Portas *et al.*, 2007). Computer based tracking recorded a greater distance covered at intensities >19 km.hour^{-1} than GPS with high levels of random error evident. Potential suggestions for low levels of agreement and greater random error could be the 'tracker's' ability, even after initial reliability tests were employed, to track the analysed player using the computer based tracking software and were exposed to difficulties subjectively identifying sprinting activity. With high levels of random error recorded at high intensity activity interchangeable use of GPS with either computer based or video analysis based methodologies should be approached with caution.

Lower levels of random error were recorded when comparing GPS with computer based and video methodologies at lower speed zone intensities (<19 km.hour^{-1}), suggesting measurement of distance in these speed zones by the three methodologies to be more agreeable than at higher intensities. Systematic bias measurements between the GPS and video analysis were lower than those recorded between the GPS and computer tracking software. However, with lower random error measurements the systems may be used interchangeably if the systematic bias is taken into consideration. Randers *et al.* (2010) found video analysis to record greater distances at lower intensities than GPS, a finding concurrent with the present study. Post *et al.* (2010) suggest that GPS loses accuracy when recording fine locomotor movements, including sideways and backwards movements, which may have contributed to the lower distance recorded by GPS compared to computer based tracking and video analysis during the current study.

In conclusion although the systems did not experience high levels of agreement the low levels of random error at low speed zone intensities and total distance covered indicate that applied practitioners are potentially able to use the GPS and video analysis or computer based tracking systems interchangeably if appropriate adjustments to the data collected are applied. Further research is required to investigate the data collected by the three contrasting methodologies, potentially using a football specific track test to assess the agreement of the systems in comparison to a defined measured distance.

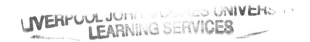

37.5 REFERENCES

Bland, M. and Altman, D.G., 1986, Statistical methods for assessing measurement error (reliability) in variables relevant to sports medicine. *Lancet*, **I**, pp. 307–310.

Bloomfield, J., Polman, R. and O'Donoghue, P., 2007, Physical demands of different playing positions in FA Premier League soccer. *Journal of Sports Science and Medicine*, **6**, pp. 63–70.

Burgess, D., Naughton, G. and Norton, K., 2012, Quantifying the gap between under 18 and senior AFL football: 2003 and 2009. *International Journal of Sports Physiology and Performance*, **7**, pp. 53–58.

Coutts, A.J. and Duffield, R., 2010, Validity and reliability of GPS devices for measuring movement demands of team sport. *Journal of Science and Medicine in Sport*, **13**(1), pp. 133–135.

Di Salvo, V., Baron, R., Tschan, H., Calderon Montero, F.J., Bachl, N. and Pigozzi, F., 2007, Performance characteristics according to playing position in elite soccer. *International Journal of Sports Medicine*, **28**(3), pp. 222–227.

Duthie, G., Pyne, D. and Hooper, S., 2003, The reliability of video based time motion analysis. *Journal of Human Movement Studies*, **44**, pp. 259–272.

Edgecomb, S.J. and Norton, K.I., 2006, Comparison of global positioning and computer-based tracking systems for measuring player movement distance during Australian football. *Journal of Science and Medicine in Sport*, **9**, pp. 25–32.

Harley, J.A., Lovell, R.J., Barnes, C.A., Portas, M.D. and Weston, M., 2011, The interchangeability of global positioning system and semiautomated video-based performance data during elite soccer match play. *Journal of Strength and Conditioning Research*, **25**(8), pp. 2334–2336.

Portas, M.D., Rush, C., Barnes, C. and Batterham, A., 2007, Method comparison of linear distance and velocity measurements with global positioning satellite (GPS) and the timing gate technique. *Journal of Sports Science and Medicine*, **10**, pp. 001–009.

Portas, M.D., Harley, J.A., Barnes, C.A. and Rush, C.J., 2010, The validity and reliability of 1-Hz and 5-Hz global positioning systems for linear, multidirectional, and soccer specific activities. *International Journal of Sports Physiology and Performance*, **5**, pp. 448–458.

Post, S., Hollander, A.P. and Reilly, T., 2010, Measurement error and global positioning systems for analysing work-rate. In *International Research in Science and Soccer: The Proceedings of the First World Conference on Science and Soccer*, edited by Drust, B., Reilly, T. and Williams, A.M. (London: Routledge), pp. 77–84.

Randers, M.B., Mujika, I., Hewitt, A., Santisteban, J., Bischoff, R., Solano, R., Zubillaga, A., Peltola, E., Krustrup, P. and Mohr, M., 2010, Application of four different football match analysis systems: A comparative study, *Journal of Sports Sciences*, **28**(2), pp. 171–182.

Part 8

Movement Analysis

CHAPTER 38

An exploratory evaluation of measures of space creation and restriction in soccer

Martin Lames, Malte Siegle and Peter O'Donoghue

38.1 INTRODUCTION

Soccer matches involve two teams interacting as they contest the match. When in possession of the ball teams try to create space (Bangsbo and Peitersen, 2004) while the defending team tries to deny space (Bangsbo and Peitersen, 2002). Therefore, many performance variables reflect both one team's attacking play and the other team's defensive play. Player locations on playing surfaces can now be tracked automatically or semi-automatically using a range of technologies with varying degrees of reliability (Carling *et al.*, 2008). These systems can provide information on player movement such as distances covered in different speed ranges as well as the locations of any sprints and accelerations. Some systems also include outputs where player locations can be animated allowing qualitative assessment of sub-units within teams such as the defenders (Dijk, 2011). The player trajectory data that is available to clubs may also be used to provide quantitative information on tactical aspects of movement (Lemmink and Frencken, 2011; Lames and Siegle, 2011). Spatial aspects of performance such as depth and width (Daniel, 2003), concentration of players and delay (Worthington, 1980) and balance of defence (Olsen, 1981) have been discussed in soccer coaching literature which predates player tracking technology. Some simple research has been done on team centroids (Lames *et al.*, 2011; Duarte *et al.*, 2011; Lemmink and Frencken, 2011) and more advanced algorithms have been produced to determine sectors of coverage (Grehaigne *et al.*, 1997), balance of the defence (O'Donoghue, 2011) and other spatial variables relating to tactics (Robles *et al.*, 2011; Duarte *et al.*, 2012). There is, however, still a great need to define variables to represent the concepts of space creation and restriction described by Bangsbo and Peitersen (2002, 2004), Daniel (2003), Olsen (1981) and Worthington (1980) as well as to develop algorithms to measure these variables using player tracking data.

The aim of the current research was to evaluate space creation and restriction by elite soccer teams. This immediately leads to the question of what is meant by space. Is it mean distance from the nearest opponent or nearest goal-side opponent? Are we concerned with space for all players or a subset of the team? Is it better to use the mean space for players of interest or is the minimum or maximum space of any player more important? Are we concerned with space throughout a possession, or at the beginning of the possession, or at the end of the possession, or some temporal pattern of change in space available during a possession? Given the limited understanding of what precise spatial variables are the most important, the current research was an exploratory study to determine which variable(s) most distinguish between possessions of different outcomes. The effectiveness of possessions can be characterized by their outcomes. Tenga *et al.* (2009) classified possessions as ending in the defensive, middle and attacking thirds of the pitch as well as by whether they lead to scoring opportunities or not. Given the exploratory nature of the current study and the small sample involved, it was decided to classify outcome into three broad types; possessions failing to reach the attacking third, possessions reaching the attacking third but not generating a scoring opportunity and possessions leading to a scoring opportunity. The purpose of the study was to measure multiple spatial variables relating to possessions and compare these between possessions resulting in different outcomes.

38.2 METHODS

An exploratory case study was used to explore spatial variables in different types of performances. Two types of data from the first half of a Bundesliga match were used in the current investigation; player position data generated by an automatic player tracking system (Amisco system, Amisco, Nice, France) and manual notation data for possession details. The manual notation recorded the start time, end time, team in possession and outcome of each possession. The first half of the match contained 107 possessions; there were 16 possessions that lead to a scoring opportunity (2 goals, 11 shots on target and 3 shots off target), 25 positions where the team in possession entered the attacking third without creating a scoring opportunity and 66 possessions where they did not enter the attacking third.

An intra- and inter-operator agreement test was carried out on the manual possession analysis method. During the intra-operator reliability test, there were two possessions identified in one observation of the half that were not identified in the other. For the possessions identified on both occasions, there was total agreement for the team in possession and the outcome of the possession. The 95 per cent limits of agreement were 0.12 ± 1.92 s for the duration of possessions. During the inter-operator reliability study, there was one possession that one observer identified that was not identified by the other observer. For the possessions identified by both observers, there was total agreement for the team in possession and the outcome of possession. However, the 95 per cent limits of agreement were -0.52 ± 3.50 s meaning that there is limited objectivity for the first and last 3 s to 5 s of possessions.

The median duration of a possession was 12s with the lower and upper quartiles being 5s and 19.5s respectively. With possessions lasting a range of durations, it was necessary to determine a period of time to analyse at the beginning or end of each possession. Carling *et al.* (2005, p. 118–119) showed that the majority of goals scored in the 1998 and 2002 Federation of International Football Associations (FIFA) World Cup tournaments were from possessions of four passes or less. The possessions that lead to goals in the 1997–98 English Premier League were even shorter; over 55 per cent of goals were scored from possessions of less than 5s (Carling *et al.*, 2005, p. 118–119). It was, therefore, decided to examine the first and final 3s to 5s of possessions, comparing these between possessions of different outcomes.

An algorithm was developed in Matlab version 7.1.0.246 (The Matworks Inc., Natick, MA) to determine mean distance variables from nearest goal-side opponents for the team in possession. This used Pythagoras theory to calculate distances based on pitch coordinates of players. This was done for the forward-most 1 to 10 players in the team for the first and last 3s, 4s and 5s of possessions as well as the difference in mean distance to the nearest goal-side opponent between the first and last 3s, 4s and 5s of possessions. This gave a total of 90 ($10 \times 3 \times 3$) mean distance variables (10 forward-most players $\times$ 3 durations (3s, 4s and 5s) $\times$ 3 times within possessions (beginning, end and difference between beginning and end)). Requiring possession of at least 3s, 4s or 5s duration reduced the number of possessions that could be included in each analysis as shown in Table 38.1.

Table 38.1 Number of possessions of different durations

Duration	Outcome			
	Scoring opportunity	Attacking third but no scoring opportunity	Not in attacking third	All
3s+	12	20	45	77
4s+	10	20	37	67
5s+	9	20	30	59

The 90 mean distance variables were compared between possessions of the three outcome types using a series of Kruskal Wallis H tests with p values of less than 0.05 being deemed as significant. Where the Kruskal Wallis H test revealed a significant difference, Bonferroni adjusted Mann-Whitney U tests were used to compare different pairs of possession types based on the three broad outcomes. Any p values of less than 0.017 produced by the Mann-Whitney U tests were deemed as significant. Cohen's d was also reported between pairs of possessions of different outcomes.

38.3 RESULTS

There were no significant differences between possessions of different outcomes for any of the 30 mean distance variables for the first 3 s to 5 s of possessions (p > 0.05). There were also no significant differences between possessions of different outcomes for the 30 variables measuring the difference in mean distance between the first and last 3 s to 5 s of possessions (p > 0.05). However, 8 of the 30 variables for the 1 to 10 forward-most players and time (3s to 5s) at the end of possession (10×3) were significantly different between possessions of different outcomes as shown in Table 38.2 (p < 0.05). These significant differences also had moderate to large effect sizes ($0.59 \leq d \leq 1.34$) according to Cohen's (1988) criteria. The most significant variable was the mean distance to the nearest goal-side opponent for all 10 outfield players during the final 5s of the possession (p = 0.007).

Table 38.2 Mean distance to nearest goal-side opponent (m) for forward-most players of team in possession (mean ± SD)

Forward-most players	Time period at end of possession (s)	Scoring opportunity ($9 \leq n \leq 12$)	Attacking third, but no scoring opportunity (n = 20)	Not in attacking third ($30 \leq n \leq 45$)	p (KWH)	Effect size A	Effect size B
1	3	4.2 ± 2.2	3.2 ± 2.3	4.5 ± 2.5	0.085	0.45	0.09
	4	4.5 ± 2.4	3.1 ± 2.2	4.4 ± 2.3&	0.048	0.62	0.04
	5	4.6 ± 2.5	3.1 ± 2.2	4.4 ± 2.4	0.056	0.65	0.08
2	3	4.2 ± 1.6	3.6 ± 2.4	4.2 ± 2.0	0.154	0.31	0.00
	4	4.4 ± 1.6	3.5 ± 2.2	4.2 ± 2.0	0.069	0.48	0.09
	5	4.7 ± 1.5	3.5 ± 2.2	4.2 ± 2.1	0.066	0.66	0.29
3	3	4.2 ± 1.3	4.1 ± 1.9	4.5 ± 1.8	0.518	0.04	0.17
	4	4.3 ± 1.2	4.0 ± 1.7	4.6 ± 1.8	0.428	0.19	0.16
	5	4.5 ± 1.1	4.1 ± 1.7	4.5 ± 1.9	0.386	0.32	0.00
4	3	4.4 ± 1.1	4.2 ± 1.3	4.8 ± 1.5	0.352	0.18	0.25
	4	4.5 ± 1.0	4.2 ± 1.2	4.9 ± 1.5	0.198	0.24	0.35
	5	4.6 ± 0.8	4.2 ± 1.2	4.8 ± 1.5	0.413	0.34	0.17
5	3	5.0 ± 0.7	5.1 ± 1.9	5.2 ± 1.6	0.870	0.04	0.12
	4	5.0 ± 0.6	5.0 ± 1.8	5.3 ± 1.5	0.765	0.05	0.29
	5	5.0 ± 0.6	5.0 ± 1.7	5.1 ± 1.4	0.808	0.02	0.12
6	3	5.8 ± 1.2	5.6 ± 2.0	6.1 ± 2.1	0.611	0.1	0.17
	4	6.0 ± 1.4	5.6 ± 1.9	6.4 ± 2.0	0.324	0.22	0.22
	5	5.7 ± 1.0	5.6 ± 1.7	6.3 ± 2.1	0.618	0.09	0.34
7	3	6.4 ± 1.0	6.3 ± 1.7	7.2 ± 2.1	0.115	0.10	0.44
	4	6.6 ± 1.1	6.3 ± 1.5	7.4 ± 1.9	0.052	0.19	0.57
	5	6.3 ± 0.9	6.3 ± 1.4	7.4 ± 1.8	0.064	0.00	0.75
8	3	7.0 ± 0.9	7.4 ± 1.2	7.6 ± 1.9	0.131	0.37	0.44
	4	6.9 ± 0.9	7.4 ± 1.2	7.9 ± 1.5^	0.044	0.43	0.79
	5	6.7 ± 0.7	7.4 ± 1.2	7.8 ± 1.4^	0.037	0.67	0.97
9	3	6.8 ± 1.1	7.6 ± 1.1	7.7 ± 1.5	0.053	0.65	0.69
	4	6.8 ± 1.1	7.5 ± 1.1	8.0 ± 1.2^	0.021	0.65	0.99
	5	6.6 ± 1.0	7.5 ± 1.1^	7.9 ± 1.1^	0.009	0.87	1.20
10	3	6.8 ± 0.9	7.6 ± 1.1^	7.8 ± 1.4^	0.014	0.86	0.89
	4	6.7 ± 1.0	7.6 ± 1.0^	8.0 ± 1.1^	0.011	0.86	1.21
	5	6.6 ± 0.9	7.6 ± 1.1^	7.9 ± 1.1^	0.007	1.11	1.34

^ Mann-Whitney U test revealed significant difference to possessions where there was a scoring opportunity (p < 0.017).
& Mann-Whitney U test revealed significant difference to possessions where the team entered the attacking third without creating a scoring opportunity (p < 0.017, d = 0.59).
Effect size A: Cohen's d for the difference between scoring opportunities and entering the attacking third without creating a scoring opportunity.
Effect size B: Cohen's d for the difference between scoring opportunities and possessions failing to enter the attacking third.

The mean distance to the nearest goal-side opponent for the 10 outfield players was 6.6 ± 0.9 m during the last 5s of the 9 possessions of at least 5 s that resulted in a scoring opportunity. This was significantly closer than the 7.9 ± 1.1 m ($p < 0.017$, $d = 1.34$) and 7.5 ± 1.1m ($p < 0.017$, $d = 1.11$) for the last 5 s of the 30 possessions of at least 5 s that did not enter the attacking third and the 20 possessions that entered the attacking third without a scoring opportunity respectively.

38.4 DISCUSSION

The outcome of possession was used as a means of testing validity of space variables within the current investigation. The research question was ultimately whether any mean distance variables showed differences between possessions of different outcomes. There are a number of observations that can be made from the analysis of possessions.

The first observation is that a team as a whole (represented by 10 outfield players) has less space in possession when they create a scoring opportunity than when they fail to; the 0.8 m to 1.3 m differences were meaningful given the normal variability between possessions of the same outcome ($0.86 \leq d \leq 1.34$). This may seem to contradict coaching literature that states that teams should create space when in possession of the ball to create scoring opportunities (Bangsbo and Pietersen, 2004). However, a player with the ball may create space for a team mate by dribbling the ball towards an opponent, committing the opponent to challenge the ball carrier and creating space for a team mate who can then be passed to (Bangsbo and Pietersen, 2004). Therefore, spatial variables may need to consider ball carrying players differently to other players. A limitation of the current study is that specific players in possession of the ball during possessions were not notated.

Although the results focused on the most significant variable (mean distance to the nearest goal-side opponent for the 10 outfield players of the team in possession during the last 5s of a possession), there were 7 other significant variables with moderate to large effects that should be considered. In particular, the distance from the forward-most player to his nearest goal-side opponent during the last 4s of a possession has the greatest contrast to the other 7 significant variables. The forward-most player was 3.1 ± 2.2 m from the nearest goal-side defender during the last 4s of a possession when his team entered the attacking third but failed to create a scoring opportunity. This was a significantly lower distance than the 4.4 ± 2.3 m when the team failed to enter the attacking third ($p < 0.017$, $d = 0.59$) but not significantly less than the 4.5 ± 2.5 m when a scoring opportunity was created ($p > 0.017$, $d = 0.62$). Both of these differences have moderate effect sizes (Cohen, 1988). The forward-most player often provides the greatest threat to the opposition, especially when the team takes the ball into the attacking third. This result agrees with coaching literature that defending teams can prevent scoring opportunities by denying space to their opponents (Bangsbo and Pietersen, 2002).

There are other limitations to the current investigation in addition to those already mentioned. First, this exploratory study used one half of one match. Further data are needed to confirm the patterns observed in the current investigation. Another limitation is that distance from the nearest goal-side defender was used as an indication of space. Space is an area concept rather than a distance concept. Spatial variables based on polygons formed by three or more players have been analysed (Duarte *et al.*, 2012) and could be compared between possessions of differing outcomes.

The technology exists to track players during competition. However, it was still necessary to integrate player coordinate data with notated data about possessions. If the technology can be developed to also track the ball, then algorithms can be written to automatically identify which team and player is in possession of the ball or whether the ball is between players. This would give greater possibilities for the development of algorithms to consider spatial-temporal aspects of possessions in soccer.

38.5 ACKNOWLEDGEMENT

The authors wish to thank Oskar Kretzinger who was one of the observers for the inter-observer agreement study.

38.6 REFERENCES

Bangsbo, J. and Peitersen, B., 2002, *Defensive Soccer Tactics: How to Stop Players and Teams from Scoring*, (Champaign, IL: Human Kinetics).
Bangsbo, J. and Peitersen, B., 2004, *Offensive Soccer Tactics: How to Control Possession and Score More Goals*, (Champaign, IL: Human Kinetics).
Carling, C., Bloomfield, J., Nelson, L. and Reilly, T., 2008, The role of motion analysis in elite soccer: Contemporary performance measurement techniques and work rate data. *Sports Medicine*, **38**, pp. 839–862.
Carling, C., Williams, A.M. and Reilly, T., 2005, *The Handbook of Soccer Match Analysis*, London: Routledge.
Cohen, J., 1988, *Statistical Power Analysis for the Behavioural Sciences, 2nd edn*, (Hillside, NJ: Lawrence Erlbaum Associates).
Daniel, J., 2003, *The Complete Guide to Soccer Systems and Tactics*, (Spring City, PA: Reedswain Publishing).
Dijk, J. 2011, Training and performance management in the top. *World Congress of Science and Football VII, Book of Abstracts*, p. 32.
Duarte, R., Araújo, D., Davids, K., Folgado, H., Marques, P. and Ferreira, A., 2011, In search of dynamic patterns of team tactical behaviours during competitive football performance, *World Congress of Science and Football VII, Book of Abstracts*, (Nagoya, Japan), p. 114.
Duarte, R., Travassos, B., Araújo, D., Marques, P. and Taki, T., 2012, Identifying individual tactical profiles according to playing position in association football,

World Congress of Performance Analysis of Sport IX, Book of Abstracts, (Worcester, UK), p. 26.

Gréhaigne, J.F., Bouthier, D. and David, B., 1997, A method to analyse attacking moves in soccer, *Sciences and Football III*, edited by Reilly, T., Bangsbo, J. and Hughes, M., London: E & FN Spon, pp. 258–264).

Lames, M. and Siegle, M., 2011, Positional data in game sports: Validation and practical impact, Keynote address, *8th International Symposium of Computer Science in Sport*, (Shanghai, China).

Lemmink, K.A.P.M. and Frencken, W., 2011, Tactical match analysis in soccer: New perspectives?, *World Congress of Science and Football VII, Book of Abstracts*, (Nagoya, Japan), p. 22.

O'Donoghue, P.G., 2011, Automatic recognition of balance and in soccer defences using player displacement data, Keynote address, *8th International Symposium of Computer Science in Sport*, (Shanghai, China).

Olsen, E., 1981, *Fotball taktikk*, (Oslo, Norway: Norwegian School of Sport Sciences).

Robles, F., Castellano, J., Perea, A., Martinez-Santos, R. and Casamichana, D., 2011, Spatial strategy used by the World Champion in South Africa'10, *World Congress of Science and Football VII, Book of Abstracts*, (Nagoya, Japan), p. 75.

Tenga, A., Kanstad, D., Ronglan, L.T. and Bahr, R., 2009, Developing a new method for team match performance analysis in professional soccer and testing its reliability. *International Journal of Performance Analysis in Sport*, **9**, pp. 8–25.

Worthington, E., 1980, *Teaching Soccer Skills*, (London: Henry Kimpton Publishers Ltd).

CHAPTER 39

Analysis of team and player performance using recorded trajectory data

Robert Timmermann and Michael Dellnitz

39.1 INTRODUCTION

Beginning in the early 1990s, a number of tracking systems for team sports have been developed (Santiago *et al.*, 2010). To record the player trajectories, these systems usually rely on either video footage from the games, which is processed using software tools, or on sensors which are attached to the players. The collected data need to be post-processed to be usable by players, coaches, or others interested in team or player performance. In this article we will use data recorded by the Sports Performance Analyzer's (SPA) tracking system (Wilhelm *et al.*, 2010) and illustrate its methods for performance analysis, varying from low level statistical trajectory analysis to higher level play recognition and matching.

In Section 39.2.1 we briefly introduce the Sports Performance Analyzer, explain a method to segment a sports game into action and break sequences, and present a framework for the extraction of plays and matching of similar plays in sports games. The results of our work are presented in Section 39.3; an outlook on future work follows in Section 39.4.

39.2 METHODOLOGY

39.2.1 Sports Performance Analyzer

The SPA uses two high definition video cameras to record a sports game. These cameras are mounted below the ceiling of a sports hall, offering a bird's eye view of the action. These videos are tracked using either particle-filter or template matching based algorithms (Perš and Kovačič, 2000). Both algorithms are fast and reliable and need only little supervision by an operator. The players' trajectories are stored in (x,y)-coordinates and can be used for further analysis. Figure 39.1 illustrates the setup of the system and the steps of the tracking process.

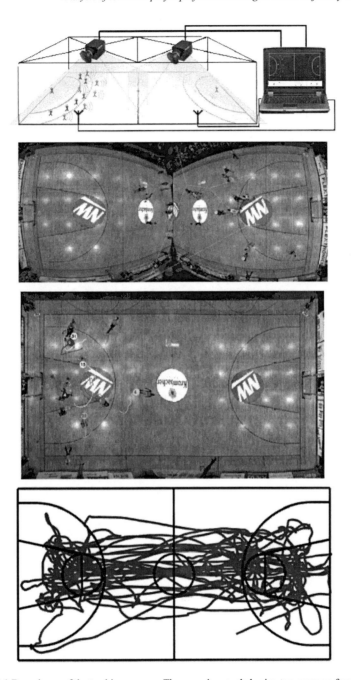

Figure 39.1 Four phases of the tracking process: The game is recorded using two cameras from a bird's eye view (top). The fisheye-images are used to track the players on the field (second). The two video feeds are combined and transformed into one rectangular video with player markers (third). The trajectories in (x,y)-coordinates are available for further analysis (bottom)

39.2.2 Net time segmentation

In order to generate reliable and meaningful game statistics and to conduct higher level analysis, such as the detection of single plays, we separate the course of the game into action and break sequences. By action we mean the time when the game was actually running and by break we mean all sequences when the game was interrupted by the referee. This includes e.g. fouls, timeouts, free throws and other situations.

Machine learning algorithms (see e.g. Bishop, 2006, for an introduction) are utilized to make assumptions about the state of the game (action or break) based on the current game situation only. Let $t_1,...,t_N \in \mathbb{R}$ be the discrete time-steps at which the players' trajectories were recorded (in seconds). Then the trajectories $P_j = (x_j y_j) \in \mathbb{R}^{N \times 2}$, $j = 1,..., p$, where p is the number of players, can be used to calculate the average player position

$$\bar{P} = (\bar{x} \ \bar{y}) = \frac{1}{p}\sum_{k=1}^{P} P_k = \frac{1}{p}\sum_{k=1}^{P}(x_k \ y_k). \tag{39.1}$$

Additionally we compute velocity-like values $V = (v \ \varphi) \in \mathbb{R}^{N \times 2}$ to better describe the players' movements with

$$v_i = \frac{1}{p}\sum_{k=1}^{P}\left\| \begin{pmatrix} x_{i,k} \\ y_{i,k} \end{pmatrix} - \begin{pmatrix} x_{i-1,k} \\ y_{i-1,k} \end{pmatrix} \right\|_2, \tag{39.2}$$

$$\varphi_i = \text{atan2}(\bar{x}_i - \bar{x}_{i-1}, \bar{y}_i - \bar{y}_{i-1}). \tag{39.3}$$

v_i is the average of the players' velocities at time t_i and φ_i the (angular) direction the average player position is moving. These two values are combined with (39.1) into a matrix $X = (\bar{x}, \bar{y}, v, \varphi) \in \mathbb{R}^{N \times 4}$.

In order to train a suitable machine learning model, we need a training set. These are points with known action/break state. This data is run through several machine learning procedures, an overview and results can be found in Table 39.1.

The results need to be post-processed in order to more closely resemble the real-world data. Initially the results contain unrealistically many switches between action and break which we filter out using a discrete zero phase filter. Afterwards, the results may still contain very short break sequences (<2 s), which we could not observe in the training data, and which we also delete from the action sets. The results of the action/break segmentation match our verification data very closely.

39.2.3 Play distance and matching

We use the player trajectories to compute the beginning and the end of a play. Without loss of generality, we say the observed team is in offense from right to left, in negative x-direction.

Definition 9.1 (Offensive Time Intervals) Let $N = [n_{0,k}, n_{f,k}] \subset \mathbb{N}$ a net interval, with $n_{0,k}, n_{f,k} \in \mathbb{N}$, then $\tau_0 \in N$ with $\tau_0 = j \Leftrightarrow \bar{x}_j < x_{off}$ and $\bar{x}_{j-1} \geq x_{off}$ marks the beginning of an offense and $\tau_f \in N$ with

$$\tau_f = j \Leftrightarrow x_{j+k,i} - x_{j+k-1,i} > 0 \, \forall i = 1, ..., p \text{ and } k = 0, ..., K.$$

An offense starts, when the average player position crosses the vertical line at x_{off} and it ends, once all players move backwards for a certain short time K. For each offensive time interval, we compute an offense $Off = \{P_1', ..., P_p'\}$ consisting of the short player trajectories

$$
P_i' = \begin{pmatrix} x_{\tau_0,i} & y_{\tau_0,i} \\ \cdot & \cdot \\ x_{\tau_f,i} & y_{\tau_f,i} \end{pmatrix}, i = 1, ..., p \tag{39.4}
$$

Finally we obtain the set $O = \{Off_1, ..., Off_n\}$ of all offenses.

Definition 9.2 (Weighted Average Distance) Let $P = \{P_1, ..., P_p\}$ and $Q = \{Q_1, ..., Q_p\}$ two offenses as defined above. Then the distance between these two offenses is defined as

$$
dist_{wavg} = \min_{s \in S_p} \sum_{k=1}^{p} d_{wavg}(P_k, Q_{S(k)}). \tag{39.5}
$$

Where S_p denotes the set of all permutations of p symbols, and d_{wavg} the distance between two single trajectories $P = (p_x, p_y) \in \mathbb{R}$ and $Q = (q_x, q_y^{My}) \in \mathbb{R}$ of lengths $M \in \mathbb{N}$ and $N \in \mathbb{N}$ is defined as follows

$$
d_{wavg}(P,Q) = \max \begin{pmatrix} \dfrac{1}{M} \sum_{i=1}^{M} v_i \min_{1 \leq j \leq N} \left\| \begin{pmatrix} p_{x,i} \\ p_{y,i} \end{pmatrix} - \begin{pmatrix} q_{x,j} \\ q_{y,j} \end{pmatrix} \right\|_2, \\ \dfrac{1}{N} \sum_{j=1}^{N} w_j \min_{1 \leq i \leq M} \left\| \begin{pmatrix} p_{x,i} \\ p_{y,i} \end{pmatrix} - \begin{pmatrix} q_{x,j} \\ q_{y,j} \end{pmatrix} \right\|_2 \end{pmatrix} \tag{39.6}
$$

with weights v and w.

We use (39.6) to compute the distance between two individual trajectories. The weights can be used to put an emphasis on the beginning of the trajectories. By, for example, choosing linearly descending weights from $w_1 = v_1 = 2$ to $w_N = v_M = 0$, we can take into account that the players follow the prescribed paths closely in the beginning and improvise freely in the end. Equation (39.5) computes the matching between $2*p$ trajectories, such that the combined distance is minimal.

In order to match similar plays, we train a self organizing map (SOM). Self organizing maps are a powerful tool for unsupervised data segmentation and have been used extensively in many different situations (Kohonen, 1998).

The procedure is straightforward: Let X the data space (in our case the set of plays) and $d_X : X \times X \rightarrow \mathbb{R}$ a metric on X (the distance d_{wavg}), $\mathcal{M} = \{x_i \mid x_i \in X; \ i = 1, ..., m\}$ the set of $m \in \mathbb{N}$ training elements, and $\mathcal{N} = \{(w_i, k_i) \mid w_i \in X, k_i \in \mathbb{R}^2, i = 1, ..., q\}, q \in \mathbb{N}$ e set of the SOM's nodes. The k_i form a two dimensional net and are usually chosen on a rectangular or hexagonal grid. An SOM is initialized with random w_i (the nodes are initialized with random plays) and trained using the following steps

(1) chose $x \in \mathcal{M}$ randomly
(2) find $(w, k) \in \mathcal{N}$ such that $d_X(w, x) = \min_{1 \le i \le q} d_X(w_i, x)$
(3) compute the set $\bar{\mathcal{N}} = \{(w_i, k_i) \in \mathcal{N} \mid \|k_i - k\|_2 < \delta_t\}$
(4) adjust all nodes in $\bar{\mathcal{N}}$ towards x: $w_i = w_i - \varepsilon_t (x - w_i) \forall (w_i, k_i) \in \mathcal{N}$

Iterating steps (1) to (4) and decreasing the learning radius δ_t and rate ε_t yields the trained self organizing map. This map contains cluster of nodes with low node to node distance. In our case, we are now able to classify offenses and assign them to one cluster by searching $n^* = (w^*, k^*) \in \mathcal{N}$ with $d_X(w^*, x) = \min_{1 \le i \le q} d_X(w_i, x)$.

39.3 RESULTS

39.3.1 Net time segmentation

In order to train a suitable machine learning model, we need a segmentation of our data into action and break situations: fortunately we have recordings of 70 basketball quarters from three seasons and various teams, in which the game clock is visible. Using a video processing algorithm, we observe the clock and decide whether the game was running or if it was interrupted. The resulting large data set contains about $1.43 \cdot 10^6$ action points and $1.24 \cdot 10^6$ break points. The results of the classification before and after post-processing can be seen in Table 39.1.

Table 39.1 Overview of the tested machine learning algorithms and their results

Algorithm	Correctly classified	Post processing
Gaussian mixture model	86.73%	91.78%
Bayesian networks	81.41%	86.35%
Bootstrap aggregation	86.15%	91.99%
Adaboost	85.56%	90.83%

This data can be used to calculate statistical information about running distance and time of the players, divided into net and gross time, to evaluate team and player performance in detail.

39.3.2 Grouping similar plays

We trained an example self organizing map with 36 × 36 nodes using plays from one basketball game. We extracted 49 offenses of the analyzed team, which were uninterrupted during their execution. The trained SOM is illustrated in Figure 39.2 (left). We presented a randomly chosen play from another game to the SOM and searched the best matching node (marked with a white circle). Comparison of the node's play with the random play reveals a high similarity (see Figure 39.2, right).

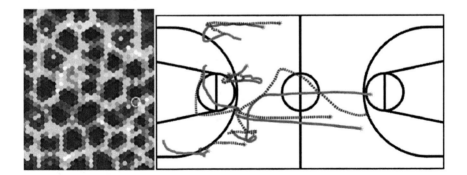

Figure 39.2 A self organizing map with 36 × 36 nodes and 10,001 training steps (left). This figure shows the two dimensional hexagonal grid of the SOM, colour coded with respect to the combined distance to the neighbouring nodes. Red (dark) indicates a large distance to the neighbours, blue (light colour) a low distance. On the right two similar plays are shown; the red one (solid lines) was picked randomly from another basketball game and the blue (dashed lines) one originates from the SOM (see white circle on the left) and is the one closest to the red play

39.4 DISCUSSION AND CONCLUSION

We presented a method for the segmentation of a sports game into action and break sequences which show a high accordance between the manually and automatically segmented (training) data. This data combined with the player's running distance and time can be very valuable for coaches and sports scientists. It enables them to specify the performance profile for a player or team and identify strengths and weaknesses. This method also lays the ground for the extraction of uninterrupted plays from a game. Using the proposed distance measure and an SOM, we are able to group the plays of a game and match other plays to the resulting clusters.

One application we bear in mind is the analysis of the opposing team: we aim to quickly recognize and understand its favourite plays and possible weaknesses, which might, for example, help in the preparation for an upcoming next playoff game.

Our future research will further evaluate the possibilities of self organizing maps. Larger examples have to be evaluated and the relationship between the clusters has to be fully understood. But nevertheless we think that self organizing maps offer a powerful tool for the analysis of sports games. In the future, we are going to combine the play information with the scored points, thus offering a way of evaluating the player and team performance.

39.6 REFERENCES

Bishop, C.M., 2006, *Pattern Recognition and Machine Learning*, (New York: Springer).
Kohonen, T., 1998, The self-organizing map. *Neurocomputing*, **21**, pp. 1–6.
Perš, J. and Kovačič, S., 2000, Computer vision system for tracking players in sports games. In *Proceedings of the 2nd International Symposium Image and Signal Processing and Analysis, ISPA*, pp. 177–182.
Santiago, C.B., Sousa, A., Estriga, M.L., Reis, L.P. and Lames, M., 2010, Survey on team tracking techniques applied to sports, *International Conference on Autonomous and Intelligent Systems*, Povoa de Varzim, Portugal.
Wilhelm, P., Thomas, P., Monier, E., Timmermann, R., Dellnitz, M., Werner, F. and Rückert, U., 2010, An integrated monitoring and analysis system for performance data of indoor sport activity. In *Proceedings of the 10th Australian Conference on Mathematics and Computer Sport*. Darwin.

CHAPTER 40

Running performance analysis in basketball using recorded trajectory data

Rasmus Jakobsmeyer, Reinhard Schnittker, Robert Timmermann,
Rene Zorn, Ulrich Rückert and Jochen Baumeister

40.1 INTRODUCTION

The evaluation of running performance in team sports, the estimation of specific requirement components and the application of this knowledge to obtain optimum training patterns and game strategies are very relevant to many disciplines of sports science. It is necessary to evaluate external characteristics of movement attributes (e.g. running intensity, running distance and running performance during a game) in an accurate way to understand the dependence on physiological parameters. In an optimal way both levels of performance (internal and external) are required to be recorded automatically and almost in real time. This study presents an application of the Sports Performance Analyzer (SPA), which is a system for performance analysis that gives its user the opportunity to combine internal physiological with external movement parameters (for a comprehensive introduction see Wilhelm *et al.*, 2010). The study presented focused on the external parameters, investigating player activity profile in basketball during competition, for the first time taking into account both teams at once and also comparing winner to loser. This study provides novel information with practical relevance for players, coaches and researchers in basketball.

There is an ambivalent judgement concerning the quality and quantity of video-based tracking systems available for use in sport performance analysis. While there exist an enormous number of high quality automatic tracking systems for football and other outdoor team sports, there are few systems appropriate for use with indoor team sports like basketball. The key to success lies in focusing on player detection as the principle of automatic tracking. Meaningful detection modes are based on algorithms concerning motion detection, template tracking or colour tracking (Perš and Kovačič, 2000). Challenges for indoor sports are the availability of cameras, the colours of jerseys and the fact that team sports are a dynamic system including confusing situations of attacks and ball possessions. Combined, these pose a significant challenge for automatic tracking systems for indoor team sports.

The activity profile in basketball is complex and its physical processes and parameters have been covered extensively in scientific literature. The discussion about the activity profile regarding external parameters like running distance and intensity reveals a heterogeneous prospect with the percentage of high intensity movements and its development in progression through the game appearing of greatest interest. While McInnes *et al.* (1995) found no changes in high intensity activities between quarters, Ben Abdelkrim *et al.* (2010) identified significant decreases from the first quarter to the second and the third to the fourth. The trend of decreases was not limited to level of play when comparing national level player to international level player (Ben Abdelkrim *et al.*, 2010). In contrast, Schmidt and von Benckendorff (2003) found a constant global distance compared the first to the second half and evaluated an increased distance for sprinting in the second half. This contradiction might be caused by different methods (manual vs. automatic tracking) or data (sample size, competition vs. practice) and motivates further research on running performance in basketball.

The aim of this study was to improve understanding of the physical requirements and demands placed on professional basketball players, especially during competition.

40.2 METHODOLOGY

The basis of the analysis was recorded trajectory data from the Sports Performance Analyzer (SPA). The data was recorded from two high resolution cameras mounted above the halves of the court at the ceiling of the sports hall. For the first time we used the system's particle-filter based tracking instead of template tracking.

The trajectory generation is divided into three parts. Verification of colour histograms is used to detect accurate body position. Position of the trunk is converted to calculate a foot position and then these positions are filtered to evaluate correct distances. The running intensity was subdivided into standing (<0.7 km.h^{-1}), walking (0.7–7.2 km.h^{-1}), jogging (7.2–14.4 km.h^{-1}), running (14.4–19.8 km.h^{-1}) and sprinting (>19.8 km.h^{-1}) (adapted from Rampinini *et al.*, 2007). Simultaneous recording of up to 30 people and monitoring both starting player and substitution player independently of their playing time makes tracking of a basketball game fast and easy to use. Net and gross times were calculated to illustrate and eliminate the influence of time-outs, for example. Net time, also known as live time, refers to the time when the ball was in play and the game clock was running (McInnes *et al.*, 1995).

The raw data were post-processed and controlled by an operator to avoid errors of measurement. The validation of the particle-filter tracking revealed a divergence of 5.09 per cent for distances and of 3.18 per cent for speeds in comparison to verified benchmark data. Therefore, we compared the SPA data with real data evaluated by measuring tapes and light barriers.

A sample of four games from the German Pro-A-League during the season 2010/2011 was evaluated and the running performance of eight teams (70 players; average age 25) was analysed. All players were tracked to generate an average activity profile composed of running distances and intensities with respect to net and gross time.

Ball possession as the main criteria of playing offence was derived from statistical BBL data. Another factor used in analysis was 'effectiveness' which is a calculated BBL qualitative parameter characterized by the difference between estimated positive, e.g. shots, rebounds, blocks and negative events, e.g. turnovers and shot success rate.

Data were processed descriptively in Microsoft Excel 2010 and statistically in SPSS 19 by significance of $p < .05$. Independent t-tests were used to determine group differences. If the data violated the assumptions of t-tests, Mann-Whitney U-tests were used. To evaluate practicable relevance, Cohen's d was calculated for significant group differences. Correlations were calculated according to Pearson (r).

40.3 RESULTS

Table 40.1 shows the results for the group mean of running performance averaged during the four games.

On average, a distance of 4364.64 m in net time and 6092.97 m in gross time was covered. Average speed of net time was 6.63 km.h^{-1} (1.84 m.s^{-1}) and 4.68 km.h^{-1} (1.3 m.s^{-1}) of gross time. Total net playing time was 2369.18 s and for gross time 4687.86 s. Divided into intensities in net time an average distance of 10.43 m was completed in the intensity standing (slow stepping), 1467.12 m in walking, 2008.72 m in jogging, 759.64 m in running and 118.73 m in sprinting (Table 40.2).

Table. 40.1 Group mean of running performance during the four games

Game	Team	Results	Distance (m) net	Distance (m) gross	Avg. Speed (km/h) net	Avg. Speed (km/h) gross	Time (s) net	Time (s) gross
1	A	80:94	4587.03	6379.44	6.81	4.81	2424.99	4778.70
	B		4376.58	6245.21	6.50	4.73	2425.69	4756.76
2	A	85:76	4366.61	6407.46	6.80	4.53	2311.73	5088.30
	B		4387.61	6329.36	6.84	4.49	2309.58	5069.87
3	A	81:91	4210.08	5736.67	6.40	4.72	2369.75	4374.43
	B		4263.30	5972.07	6.48	4.85	2369.10	4347.71
4	A	84:82	4347.72	5869.65	6.64	4.65	2358.65	4548.88
	B		4378.20	5803.93	6.61	4.60	2383.95	4538.27
Average of four games			4364.64	6092.97	6.63	4.68	2369.18	4687.86

Table 40.2 Overview of group average of running intensities

Intensity	Distance (m) net	Time (s) net	Distance (m) gross	Time (s) gross
Standing	10.43	89.18	60.31	606.43
Walking	1467.12	1391.60	2844.64	3084.91
Jogging	2008.72	701.63	2276.22	802.42
Running	759.64	167.01	789.91	173.85
Sprinting	118.73	19.76	121.90	20.25

The group mean for running intensities demonstrates that the longest net time was spent in walking (1391.6 s) and jogging (701.63 s), shortest duration was evaluated for sprinting (19.76 s). Distribution of percentage of net and gross time differed in intensities and distances. Walking distance dominated at gross time (46.69 per cent) whereas jogging distance dominated at net time (46.02 per cent). Time spent in walking dominated in gross (65.81 per cent) and net (58.74 per cent) time.

For net time we determined significant decreases between the two halves. Summarized distance decreased significantly from 5762.54 m in the first half to 5149.06 m in the second half ($t_{(30)} = 5.004$; $p \leq .001$; $d = 1.77$). Running distance decreased significantly from 1025.37 m to 873.74 m ($t_{(30)} = 2.960$; $p = .006$; $d = 1.05$) and sprinting distance from 181.91 m to 114.92 m ($t_{(30)} = 2.4$; $p = .023$; $d = 0.85$). An in-depth analysis of differences between the first and the second quarter revealed a significant decrease for summarized distance from 5942.9 m to 5582.19 m ($t_{(14)} = 3.209$; $p = .006$; $d = 1.6$). We also found significant decreases from the third to the fourth quarter in summarized distance (5436.07 m to 4862.05 m; $t_{(14)} = 4.171$; $p = .001$; $d = 2.08$) and running distance (983.15 m to 764.34 m; $t_{(14)} = 2.851$; $p \leq .001$; $d = 1.42$).

Comparison of running performance between winner and loser revealed marginal differences. No difference was of statistical significance.

Analysis of comparison between offence and defence was limited to global net distance as well as net running and sprinting distance. Global net distance did not differ significantly from offence (1268.96 m) to defence (1148.38 m), whereas net running distance differed significantly ($t_{(129.656)} = 3.56$; $p = .002$; $d = -0.60$) between offence (242.90 m) and defence (173.54 m). Net sprinting distance differed significantly ($t_{(138)} = 2.048$; $p = .042$; $d = -0.35$) from offence (38.39 m) to defence (28.16 m) as well.

Effectiveness of each player (n = 70; range −6 to 30) as an indicator for quality of play was correlated to running performance to investigate the relationship between running performance and overall game performance. The analysed parameters were normalized to effectiveness per second to eliminate individual time on court differences. Effectiveness per second correlated significantly with a player's average speed ($r = -.276$; $p = .21$). But we did not find significant correlations to the total running and sprinting distance. We further analysed group differences between high and low classified effectiveness per second (upper and lower 33.33 per cent from sample size) and did not find significant differences, either.

40.4 DISCUSSION AND CONCLUSION

This study provides recent information with practical relevance for players, coaches and researchers in basketball. We found decreases of running performance in the second half of a game and determined an average performance profile. Whereas the evaluated distances were similar to data from literature, the percentage of very high intensity movements was smaller than the proposed data. We have found a ratio of 0.8 per cent for sprinting and a ratio of 7.78 per cent when sprinting or running. McInnes *et al.* (1995) found a rate of about 15 per cent in high intensities and proposed that low intensities had a percentage of 60 per cent. Narazaki *et al.* (2009) detected 56.8 per cent for low intensities (walking), and Ziv and Lidor (2009) proposed a percentage of 65 per cent for intensities higher than walking. In summary, in contrast to presented literature, we calculated for net time a lower percentage in high and in low intensities (37.02 per cent for walking). One reason might be that, to our knowledge, this was the first analysis of real competition with an automatic tracking system. Second, the high intensity movements like shuffling and jumping are filtered in SPA. Furthermore, a unified classification of intensities does not exist in research.

Fatigue is an intensively discussed factor in research on team sports and it could be one reason for decreased running performance in the second half. Tactical order, the score and interruptions of the game could be reasons, too.

We found no significant difference between winner and loser in the four games, supporting the thesis that basketball is a complex system in which the running performance is just one part. Tactical order, technical aspects like the shot success rate and external stressors like the audience are other influencing, maybe crucial, factors.

Differences between offence and defence might be caused by different running directions (e.g. backwards running in defence). Effectiveness is not clearly related to running performance. It would be interesting to know whether there is a relationship between individual running performances and effectiveness over a large number of games in a longitudinal study.

We agree with Narazaki *et al.* (2009) and McInnes *et al.* (1995) and concluded that basketball produces high physiological exposure although the running speed is rather low. We analysed individual speed graphs and a permanent changing in speed with acceleration and deceleration supports this statement. Performance tests like the repeated-sprint-agility might be adequate to measure running performance in the context of competition (Carling *et al.*, 2009).

Recorded trajectory data is consistent and represents the progress in measuring running performance automatically. Especially, taking into account both teams on court during competition is important to note. The used tracking algorithm based on particle-filter is faster and more error-prone than template tracking. Thus it makes the Sports Performance Analyzer more reliable and easier to use.

For future research, it seems to be interesting to observe the ball, to perform long time studies on changes in running performance during a whole season and to value the tactical performance assessment with SPA.

40.5 REFERENCES

Ben Abdelkrim, N., Castagna, C., El Fazaa, S. and El Ati, J., 2010, The effect of players' standard and tactical strategy on game demands in men's basketball. *Journal of Strength and Conditioning Research*, **24** (10), pp. 2652–2662.

Carling, C., Reilly, T. and Williams, A.M., 2009. *Performance Assessment for Field Sports.* (New York: Routledge).

McInnes, S.E., Carlson J.S., Jones C.J. and McKenna M.J., 1995, The physiological load imposed on basketball players during competition. *Journal of Sport Sciences*, **13**, pp. 387–397.

Narazaki, K., Berg, K., Stergiou, N. and Chen, B., 2009, Physiological demands of competitive basketball. *Scandinavian Journal of Medicine & Science in Sports*, **19**(3), pp. 425–432.

Perš, J. and Kovačič, S., 2000, Computer vision system for tracking players in sports games. In *Proceedings of the 1st International Workshop on Image and Signal Processing and Analysis*, (Pula, Croatia), edited by Loncaric, S. (Zagreb: University Computing Center), pp. 177–182.

Rampinini, E., Coutts, A., Castagna, C., Sassi, R. and Impellizzeri, F., 2007, Variation in top level soccer match performance. *International Journal of Sports Medicine*, **28**(12), pp. 1018–1024.

Schmidt, G.J. and von Benckendorff, J., 2003, Zur Lauf- und Sprungbelastung im Basketball. *Leistungssport*, **1**, pp. 41–48.

Wilhelm, P., Thomas, P., Monier, E., Timmermann, R., Dellnitz, M., Werner, F. and Rückert, U., 2010, An integrated monitoring and analysis system for performance data of indoor sport activity. In *Proceedings of the 10th Australian Conference on Mathematics and Computer Sport*, edited by Bedford, A. (Darwin, Australia), pp. 137–144.

Ziv, G. and Lidor, R., 2009, Physical attributes, physiological characteristics, on-court performance and nutritional strategies of female and male basketball players. *Sports Medicine*, **39**(7), pp.547–568.

CHAPTER 41

Time-motion analysis of Pádel players in two matches of the 2011 Pro Tour

Jesus Ramón-Llin, Jose F. Guzmán, Rafa Martinez-Gallego,
Goran Vučković and Nic James

41.1 INTRODUCTION

Pádel is a relatively new sport sharing similar characteristics to tennis i.e. in relation to the playing surface and game characteristics. The main differences are that the court is smaller, 20 m × 10 m, walls around the perimeter are part of the game i.e. the ball can rebound off them; and a modified version of a racket, called a paddle, is used. Pádel is also only played in pairs (as for tennis doubles).

It was invented in Mexico in 1969 by Enrique Corcuera and has become very popular in Spain and South America (De Hoyo Lora *et al.*, 2008; Luna and Arazuri, 2008). The Pádel International Federation was established in Madrid in 1991 and the professional tournament circuit Pádel Pro Tour is almost entirely played in Spain. The popularity of Pádel has resulted in an exponential growth of facilities and explains why Pádel has become the top practiced sport in Spain (CSD, 2011).

Pádel has, until now, not been well researched, with the exceptions being the work of De Hoyo Lora *et al.* (2008) and Carrasco *et al.* (2010). They reported that players' heart rates averaged 148 beats/min, oxygen uptake was 24.06 ± 6.95 ml.kg^{-1}.min^{-1}, equating to 43.73 ± 11.04 per cent VO$_2$ max as assessed in a laboratory test and the main strokes used were volleys (forehand and backhand). However, these studies were undertaken on a sample of players aged under 17 years with very short duration of playing time.

The knowledge of the distance covered in a game allows coaches and players to plan training schedules more effectively and is the reason why this measure has been researched for so many sports, e.g. soccer (Bangsbo *et al.*, 1991; Barros *et al.* 2007), basketball (McInnes *et al.*, 1995), rugby (Deutsch *et al.*, 2007), field hockey (Johnston *et al.*, 2004), netball (Loughran and O'Donoghue, 1998), squash (Vučković *et al.*, 2002) and tennis (Fernandez *et al.*, 2007). In Pádel, Ramon-Llin *et al.* (2010) have presented the distance covered and speed of movements for three playing levels of Pádel (national, county and recreational). Results showed that players of county level covered more distance than the other groups and more distance was covered in balanced compared to unbalanced matches. However, these results only provided information for total match time whereas coaches also need to know activity profiles for the active periods of the match (ball in play time). Ramon-Llin and Guzmán (2012) have reported this information but that study was undertaken on only one match of national and recreational playing level.

In contrast, the purpose of this study was to analyze the distance covered and speed of movements in both active and passive periods of two matches involving the world number one pair, one of them closely contested and the other relatively easy.

It was hypothesized that Pádel Pro Tour (PPT) players would run faster compared to players of other playing levels, resulting in a greater distance covered for similar duration matches. With regard to match winners and losers two possible outcomes were thought possible based on previous literature. Hughes and Franks (1994) found that losers covered a greater distance than winners in squash whilst Vučković *et al.* (2004) found that winners covered more distance than losers. More recent studies have showed that players who use defensive tactics cover more distance than players with more attacking tactics (Martínez-Gallego *et al.*, 2012).

41.2 METHODS

41.2.1 Sample

Two matches (easy 1/8 final, closely contested final) of the Valencia 2011 Pádel Pro Tour (PPT) tournament, played on an indoor court, were recorded for analysis. The first match was between the PPT world ranked number 1 and 20 pairs and the second between the number 1 and 6 pairs.

41.2.2 Procedure and instruments

A video camera (Bosch Dinion IP 455, Germany) was placed above the court (12 m high) so that the whole area in which the players moved was in vision (Figure 41.1). The video format (MPEG-4) was converted in Bosch proprietary software to WMV format before converting to MPEG-2 format as the SAGIT software only accepted this format (Vučković *et al.*, 2009). The final distance and speed data were exported to and analyzed using Microsoft Excel software.

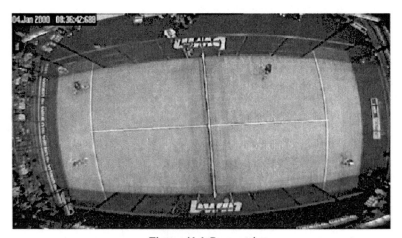

\Figure 41.1 Camera view

41.3 RESULTS

The mean distance covered for all players was 773.2 m ± 366.9 (Table 41.1) with great variability of players' workload evident between matches, but also between players in the same match and on occasion between partners.

Table 41.1 Distance covered, average speed of movement and duration of the game during the active part of a game (ball in play)

	Match 1				Match 2			
	Winner		Loser		Winner		Loser	
	1	2	1	2	1	2	1	2
1st game Distance (m)	401	450	521	401	1350	1470	1458	1446
2nd game Distance (m)	536	511	531	445	839	825	880	776
3rd game Distance (m)					633	707	599	684
1st game Speed (m.s^{-1})	1.07	1.20	1.39	1.07	1.13	1.23	1.22	1.21
2nd game Speed (m.s^{-1})	1.30	1.24	1.29	1.08	1.21	1.19	1.27	1.12
3rd game Speed (m.s^{-1})					1.11	1.24	1.05	1.20
1st game Duration (s)	375		375		1195		1195	
2nd game Duration (s)	412		412		693		693	
3rd game Duration (s)					570		570	

Wilcoxon Signed Ranks tests showed there was no difference ($z = 0.36$, $p = 0.72$) in mean distance covered between winning (772.2 m ± 367.7) and losing players (774.1 m ± 385.8). There was a high correlation between the distances covered by each pair ($r = 0.94$) with an average difference of 62.64 m ± 44.64.

During the active part of the game players' average speed of movement ranged between 1.07 and 1.39 m.s^{-1} with no difference between winning (1.19 m.s^{-1} ± 0.07) and losing (1.19 m.s^{-1} ± 0.11) couples (Table 41.1).

41.4 DISCUSSION

Elite players in this study moved slightly faster (mean = 1.19 m.s^{-1}) than previously found for other levels of player (recreational, 1.09 m.s^{-1}; national, 1.16 m.s^{-1}; Ramón-Llin and Guzmán 2012). Whilst this might be expected due to expert players being more likely to hit the ball harder and more accurately, hence making returning the ball more difficult and thus requiring faster speed to return the ball, these results were based on small sample sizes and so caution should be applied to the findings. This is exemplified by the fact that the distance covered by players was quite varied between games. Of course the distance covered is related to the length of time the match takes place over and this is determined by how closely contested the match is. The two matches analyzed in this study were quite different in terms of how closely contested they were and consequently the measured variables exhibited relatively large variation.

On the basis of these results it appears that the average speed of players is not related to the game duration. However, it may be hypothesized that in longer matches players may become fatigued resulting in some decrease in speed. This was not evident here but nevertheless may be a factor in Pádel. An alternative factor that may determine player speeds is the rally duration. Longer rallies are likely to be at least reasonably closely contested and therefore require all players to move relatively fast. Short rallies, on the other hand, may result in the partners of both the server and the returner of serve moving very little because they are not actively involved in the rally. This study did not differentiate between rallies and in future this may provide additional information regarding differences between playing standards and between winning and losing partners.

The analysis of distance covered by winning and losing players has produced conflicting findings, e.g. in squash it has been reported that losers run further than winners (Hughes and Franks, 1994; Vučković and James, 2010) whilst Vučković *et al.* (2004) found the opposite, winners covered more distance than losers. Recently, it has been suggested that the tactical style of players (offensive or defensive) may determine the distance covered more than who won the rally. For example Over and O'Donoghue (2010) reported that offensive tennis players do less physical work during the match than defensive players, as shown by Martinez-Gallego *et al.* (2012). In Pádel, teams tend to be attacking when they are at the net whilst the other team tries to move their opponents away from the net and are hence in a more defensive mode. It may be the case, therefore, that player movements in Pádel are determined by the amount of time spent at the net.

41.5 CONCLUSION

The analysis of player movements can provide useful information to coaches and players regarding training workloads but it seems that simply measuring whole matches without consideration of the game play may result in meaningless information. This study has showed that even when only measuring the best players in the world there can be relatively large differences in work rate data. This was thought to be due to how closely contested the matches were. However, previous studies have suggested that the playing characteristics, namely offensive and defensive strategies, could be more indicative of player work rates. In Pádel dominating the net is akin to being offensive and hence may be indicative of work rates. Using this logic it would seem that work rates are determined by the rally characteristics, e.g. short rallies, long rallies where only one team dominates the net etc., and to some extent tactics determines this. Future studies should therefore only consider work rate analysis with respect to the specific behaviors evident within the rally.

41.6 REFERENCES

Bangsbo, J., Nørregaard. L. and Thorsø, F., 1991, Activity profile of competition soccer. *Canadian Journal of Sport Sciences*, **16**, pp. 110–116.

Barros, R.M.L., Misuta, M.S., Menezes, R.P., Figueroa, P.J., Moura, F.M., Cunha, S.A., Anido, R. and Leite, N.J., 2007, Analysis of the distance covered by first division Brazilian soccer players obtained with an automatic tracking method. *Journal of Sport Science and Medicine,* **6**, pp. 233–242.

Carrasco, L., Romero, S., Sañudo, B. and de Hoyo, M., 2011, Game analysis and energy requirements of paddle tennis competition. *Science and Sports*, **26**(6), pp. 338–344.

CSD (2011). http://www.csd.gob.es/csd/estaticos/asoc-fed/Licencias-clubesfederados.pdf.

De Hoyo Lora, M., Corrales, B.S. and Páez, L.C., 2008, Demandas fisiológicas de la competición en pádel. [Physiological demands of paddle competition] *RICYDE*, **3**(8), pp. 53–58.

Deutsch, M.U., Kearney, G.A. and Rehrer, N.J., 2007, Time motion analysis of professional rugby union players during match-play. *Journal of Sports Sciences*, **25**, pp. 461–472.

Fernadez, J., Mendez, A., Pluim, B. and Terrados, N., 2007, Aspectos físicos y fisiológicos del tenis de competición II. *Archivos de medicina del deporte*, **25**(117), pp. 35–41.

Hughes, M. and Franks, I.M., 1994, Dynamic patterns of movement of squash players of different standards in winning and losing rallies. *Ergonomics*, **37**(1), pp. 23–29.

Johnston, T., Sproule. J., McMorris, T. and Maile, A., 2004, Time-motion analysis and heart rate response during elite male field hockey: Competition versus training. *Journal of Human Movement Studies*, **46**, pp. 189–203.

Loughran, B. and O'Donoghue, P., 1998, Time motion analysis of work rate in club netball. *Journal of Human Movement Studies*, **36**, pp. 37–50.

Luna, V.M. and Arazuri, E.S., 2008, Promoción del pádel de competición en las primeras etapas deportivas (6–12años). Un proyecto de intervención [Paddle promotion in first stages of sport initiation (6–12 years). An intervention project]. *Retos. Nuevas tendencias en Educación Física. Deporte y Recreación*, **13**, pp. 46–49.

Martínez-Gallego, R., Ramon-Llin, J., Guzmán, J.F. and Calpe-Gomez., V., 2012, Distancia recorrida por tenistas d eelite en función del resultado y del estilo de juego. In *Proceedings I Congreso Iberoamericano de la red europea de la actividad física y el deporte*, Murcia, España.

McInnes, S.E., Carlson, J.S., Jones, C.J. and McKenna, M.J., 1995, The physiological load imposed on basketball players during competition. *Journal of Sports Sciences*, **13**, pp. 387–397.

Over, S. and O'Donoghue, P., 2010, Analysis of strategy and tactics in tennis. *International Tennis Federation Coaching and Sport Science Review*, **50**(18), pp. 15–16.

Ramón-Llin, J., Guzmán, J.F., Vučković, G., Llana, S. and James, N., 2010, Players' covered distance according playing level and balance between teams: A preliminary analysis in pádel. In *Research in Sports Science 6*, edited by Hughes, M. (Szombathely, Hungary: West-Hungary University), pp. 188–193.

Ramón-Llin, J. and Guzmán, J.F., 2012, Distancia recorrida y velocidad de desplazamiento en pádel. en función de 2 niveles de juego. In *Proceedings I Congreso Iberoamericano de la red europea de la actividad física y el deporte.* (Murcia, España).

Vučković, G., Dezman, B., Erculj, F., Kovacic, S. and Pers, J., 2002, Computer tracking of players at squash matches. *Acta Kinesiol, 7*, pp. 216–220.

Vučković, G., Dezman, B., Erculj, F., Kovacic, S. and Pers, J., 2004, Differences between the winning and the losing players in a squash game in terms of distance covered. In *Science and Racket Sports III*, edited by Lees, A., Khan, J.F. and Maynard , I.W. (Oxon: Routledge), pp. 202–207.

Vučković, G., Perš, J., James, N. and Hughes, M., 2009, Tactical use of the T area in squash by players of differing standard. *Journal of Sports Sciences*, **27**(8), pp. 863–871.

Vučković, G. and James, N., 2010, The distance covered by winning and losing players in elite squash matches. *Kinesiologia Slovenica*, **16**(1–2), pp. 44–50.

Index